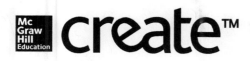

Annual Editions: Aging, 28/e

Elaina F. Osterbur

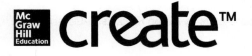

http://create.mheducation.com

ISBN-10: 1259359603   ISBN-13: 9781259359606

Contents

v

Preface

The global population of older adults is rising due in part to improved public health and economic conditions and is expected to reach 14% by the year 2040. According to the Population Reference Bureau, the average life expectancy at birth for women in Japan is 86 years, one of the highest in the world. Along with the observed increased life expectancy, the world total fertility rate is declining. The increase in longevity and the decrease in fertility rates have created this demographic shift whereby people 65 and over now account for a larger proportion of the world population.

What does this mean to an aging population? Historically, societies were plagued by infectious diseases that caused much of the morbidity and mortality of the times. Since then, aging societies have transitioned morbidity and mortality rates from infectious disease to noncommunicable chronic disease as the cause of disability and death. Living longer means greater planning on the part of both the older adult and his or her family. Thus older adults and families have reacted with the demand for increased medical technologies that will not only allow for longer life, but also allow older people to live at home longer with greater degree of independence. Increased longevity also means that financial planning from younger years may not spread far enough during the retirement years, and thereby older adults are requesting increased opportunities for work from employers. Greater options in health insurance coverage are demanded along with a variety of options for long-term care insurance. These advances in technologies are creating a peripheral legal marketplace that has reacted in ways that require advance directives, living wills, long-term care insurance options, and other lifespan planning devices. The culmination of opportunities, needs, and expectations of older adults brought forth through longevity has the popular press, researchers, and the media scrambling to provide pertinent information to the masses.

This volume represents the field of gerontology in that it is interdisciplinary in its approach, including articles from the biological sciences, medicine, nursing, psychology, sociology, and social work. The articles are taken from the popular press, government publications, and scientific journals. They represent a wide cross-section of author's perspectives and issues related to the aging process. They were chosen because they address the most relevant and current problems in the field of aging and present divergent views on the appropriate solutions to these problems. The topics covered include demographic trends; the aging process; the quality of later life; social attitudes toward old age; problems and potentials of aging; retirement; death; living environments in later life; and social policies, programs, and services for older Americans.

The articles are organized into an anthology issued for both the student and the teacher. Learning Outcomes outline the key concepts that students should focus on as they read the material. Critical Thinking questions allow students to test their understanding of the key concepts, and a list of recommended Internet References guides them to the best sources of additional information on a topic. The goal of *Annual Editions: Aging* is to choose articles that are pertinent, well written, and helpful to those concerned with the field of gerontology. Comments, suggestions, and constructive criticism are welcome to help improve future editions of this book.

Editor

Dr. Elaina F. Osterbur is an assistant professor at Saint Louis University in St. Louis, Missouri. After receiving a Master's Degree in Gerontology, Elaina received her PhD in Epidemiology at the University of Illinois Urbana-Champaign. Her research interests include gynecological cancer screening in older women and family caregiving.

Academic Advisory Board

Members of the Academic Advisory Board are instrumental in the final selection of articles for the *Annual Editions* series. Their review of the articles for content, level, and appropriateness provides critical direction to the editor(s) and staff. We think that you will find their careful consideration reflected in this book.

James Blackburn
Hunter College

Ric Ferraro
University of North Dakota

Stephen M. Golant
University of Florida

Lisa Hollis-Sawyer
Northeastern Illinois University

Unit 1

UNIT

Prepared by: Elaina Osterbur, *Saint Louis University*

The Phenomenon of Aging

The phenomenon of aging includes biological, psychological, sociological, and behavioral changes. Biologically, the body gradually loses the ability to renew itself. Various body functions begin to slow, and the vital senses become less acute. Psychologically, aging persons experience changing sensory processes; perception, motor skills, problem-solving ability, and drives and emotions are frequently altered. Sociologically, this group must cope with the changing roles and definitions of self that society imposes on individuals. For instance, the role expectations and the status of grandparents differ from those of parents, and the roles of retirees are quite different from those of employed persons. Being defined as "old" may be desirable or undesirable, depending on the particular culture and its values. Behaviorally, aging individuals may move more slowly and with less dexterity. Because they are assuming new roles and are viewed differently by others, their attitudes about themselves, their emotions, and, ultimately, their behavior can be expected to change.

Those studying the process of aging often use developmental theories of the lifecycle—a sequence of predictable phases that begins with birth and ends with death—to explain individuals' behavior at various stages of their lives. An individual's age, therefore, is important because it provides clues about his or her behavior at a particular phase of the lifecycle, be it childhood, adolescence, adulthood, middle age, or older age. There is, however, the greatest variation in terms of health and human development among older people than among any other age group. We find that by age 65, some people are in good health, employed, and performing important work tasks. Others of this cohort are retired but in good health or are retired and in poor health. Still others have died prior to the age of 65.

Another important phenomenon includes demographic changes in an aging world. Every day, 10,000 people all over the world turn 65. This trend will continue for the next 20 years. In the United States alone, waves of the 78 million baby boomers have begun to turn 65 years. This generation will have great expectations regarding healthcare, long-term care, housing, finances, technology, work, and even the return to college. The articles in this section attempt to explain the phenomenon of aging and the resulting choices in lifestyle as well as the wider, cultural implications of an older population.

Article

5, 7, 12, 20, 22, 31

Prepared by: Elaina F. Osterbur, *Saint Louis University*

Healthy Aging in the 22nd Century

MARTA M. KEANE

Learning Outcomes

After reading this article, you will be able to:

- Identify the four major components of health.
- Discuss the future technologies and how they affect the four components of health.
- Understand how societal views on aging will evolve in the future.

What will the term *elder* mean in the future? And at what age will someone be considered an elder in 2100?

To be born in 2012 and only be 88 years old in 2100 will probably mean middle age rather than elderhood. Elders will be those who have lived triple-digit years and have been through several careers and cycles of education, career, and leisure. These elders will have exponentially more knowledge and experience, and they will continue to be contributing to society. Technology will be a key element allowing individuals to age with more independence and more choice.

Here, we examine each component of health (as defined by the World Health Organization) and how each will be manifested in 2100.

- **Physical health.** People's physical health will be monitored daily in their homes. The smart home will be outfitted with readers to take vital signs and send them directly to a medical professional to review, and provide feedback on any medications or supplements that need to be altered that day. Rather than prescriptions as we have known them, medications will all be personalized to individuals' DNA, keeping all healthier for longer.

Elders will be able to live in their own homes longer. With driverless cars, limitations on transportation will be a thing of the past. And the smart home will adapt to people's changing needs so that they will not need to move from their current home to maintain a safe environment.

- **Social-emotional health.** As elders continue to work longer and cycle through more periods of leisure during their lifetimes, they will have more friends and engage in more activities that will allow them to stay involved. Twenty-second-century elders will see their generation continue to be involved in social-action projects, coming together for the specific project and meeting new people, and continuing some relationships and letting others end with the project.

As with work, there will be cycles with marriage and family dynamics. It will be unlikely that there will be marriages that will last 100 years, so there will be multiple groupings of families that will have a fresh approach to embracing each addition to the family and expanding the definition of the extended family.

- **Spiritual health.** Views of a "divine power" will be transformed by advances in science and technological power. As scientific breakthroughs increase longevity, the fear of mortality and what follows will disappear. Spiritual practices and beliefs will become more individualized; many elders, for instance, will continue to be concerned for the environment, and in so doing, get back in touch with nature and the earth.
- **Intellectual health.** Elders will be honored for their knowledge and experience. The many cycles of work and relationships will enrich their lives and be an inspiration to others. The ability to live longer will focus importance on lifelong learning and continuing to experience the world through all the senses.

The year 2100 will be an exciting time to be "old." Technology and societal views will encourage a new attitude about aging. Elderhood will be viewed as the period in one's life with the most opportunity for independence and quality choices about one's own life.

Critical Thinking

1. This article discusses the evolution of societal thoughts on aging. Describe this evolution.

2. Envision the types of resources needed in communities and in institutions to provide the technology that the article describes.

Create Central

www.mhhe.com/createcentral

Internet References

CDC Healthy Aging
    www.cdc.gov/aging
Medline Plus: Healthy Aging
    www.nlm.nih.gov/medlineplus/healthyaging.html

Keane, Marta M. Originally published in *The Futurist*, September/October 2012, pp. 40, 42–43. Copyright © 2012 by World Future Society, Bethesda, MD. Used with permission. www.wfs.org

Article   Prepared by: Elaina F. Osterbur, *Saint Louis University*

Demography Is Not Destiny: The Challenges and Opportunities of Global Population Aging

The world's population is aging: eventually there will be more older people than younger. Population patterns in three countries offer a projected, diverse view of the possibilities that await.

PETER UHLENBERG

Learning Outcomes

After reading this article, you will be able to:

- Identify the challenges of an aging population.
- Identify the reasons for an aging world.
- Discuss the social changes necessary to appreciate an aging population.

The world is undergoing a major demographic restructuring of its population: in nearly every country around the globe, the proportion of children is declining and the proportion of old people is increasing.

Population aging began in Sweden and France in the nineteenth century as a consequence of their declining fertility rates, and was pervasive across all developed countries by 1950. Nevertheless, as recently as 1950, only 5 percent of the world's population was older than age 65, and 34 percent were children under age 15. (Unless otherwise noted, all population statistics are taken from the United Nations Department of Economic and Social Affairs, 2011).

Population projections suggest that by 2060, the proportion of people older than age 65 will almost equal the proportion younger than age 15 (18 percent versus 20 percent). And in the more developed regions of the world in 2060, there will be 156 people older than age 65 for every 100 children younger than age 15.

Demographers thoroughly understand the reasons for global population aging and the patterns of population aging across countries. The more interesting and complex questions concern the social, political, and economic implications of this phenomenon. This article offers a brief explanation of why populations

around the world are growing older, compares patterns of population aging in three countries to illustrate the diversity that exists, and provides a foundation for thinking about a future where older people are more numerous than children.

Why Populations Age

The age composition of a population is determined by its past patterns of fertility, mortality, and international migration. Of these three variables, fertility decline is by far the most important factor leading to population aging. As women have fewer children, the proportion of children in the population declines and the proportion of older people increases. The reason developed countries have older populations than do developing countries is because fertility decline occurred far earlier in developed countries than it did in developing countries. In Western Europe, where low fertility rates persisted over most of the twentieth century, 20 percent of the population will be older than age 65 in 2015. In Eastern Africa, where fertility rates remained high until recently, only 3 percent of the population will be older than age 65 in 2015. Looking ahead, fertility rates are falling in Eastern Africa, and projections indicate that by 2060, the proportion of older adults in the population will increase to 7 percent. But because very low fertility is expected to persist in Western Europe, that region of the world is expected to have more than 27 percent elders by 2060. In Japan, where there is extremely low fertility, 35 percent of the population is projected to be older than age 65 in 2060.

The effect of declining mortality on population aging is more complex than declining fertility. Declining mortality among infants and children actually works to make populations younger. On the other hand, decreasing death rates at older ages increases the proportion of older adults in a population. Historically, declining mortality among the young caused gains in life expectancy as countries moved from high to moderate levels of mortality. But as most people survive to old age, declining death rates in later life become the primary reason for increased levels of life expectancy; future improvements in life expectancy in low-mortality countries will contribute to further aging of their populations. But the impact of declining mortality on population age composition is small compared with that of fertility change.

The effect of declining mortality on population aging is more complex than declining fertility.

Contrary to some popular thinking, international migration has only a small effect on population aging. Net positive immigration of young adults has an immediate effect of making a population younger, but in the long run, these immigrants age. A steady flow of in-migrants will lead to a slightly younger population over time, but demographers agree that immigration at any reasonable level will not significantly affect population aging in countries with low fertility (Keely, 2009). The relatively small effect of even large-scale immigration on population aging can be illustrated by comparing two projections of what percent of the U.S. populace will be older than age 65 in 2050. Assuming a steady stream of 820,000 immigrants annually produces a projection of 20 percent of the populace being older than age 65; assuming zero immigration yields a projection of 22 percent (United States Census Bureau, 1996). Without immigration, the population would be older, but only slightly.

Variability of Global Population Aging

In discussing global population aging, it is important to recognize the large demographic and social variability across regions and countries. The demographic contrast between Western Europe and Eastern Africa was mentioned above. Equally important are the large differences that exist across societies regarding the role of the state versus the family in caring for dependent elders. Because of this, population aging may have different implications for different societies. A comparison of population aging in three countries (Sweden, China, and the United States) illustrates the importance of examining aging within a social and historical context.

Sweden

Sweden was one of the first countries to experience population aging—8 percent of its population was older than age 65 in 1900. Across the twentieth century, the percentage of elders in Sweden more than doubled (to 17 percent in 2000), and this trend will continue in the coming decades, reaching a level of 26 percent of the populace older than age 65 in 2060. Although

Sweden no longer has the oldest population (Japan tops the list), what is occurring there is of interest because of Sweden's long history of population aging, combined with its generous welfare state. One goal of the Swedish welfare state has been to allow elders to maintain a high standard of living and to keep their independence in old age by providing them with state pensions, healthcare, housing, and access to social services. Providing these benefits requires a high tax rate on the working population. How viable this welfare-state model is—as the older population expands significantly relative to the working population-is a major question being asked in more developed countries at this time.

Population aging may have different implications for different societies.

While future adjustments to the welfare state in Sweden are uncertain, the choices made thus far suggest that changes can be made without abandoning popular welfare policies. The pension system was redesigned in the late 1990s to provide strong incentives for delaying retirement age and continuing to work past age 60, and average age at exit from the labor force increased by two years between 2001 and 2010. Greater restrictions on public financing of homecare and institutional care have increased the importance of family care for older people needing assistance. Survey evidence shows that only 5 percent of older Swedes in need of assistance with activities of daily living depend exclusively on in-home help if they are married and have a child, while 80 percent depend exclusively on family help (Sundstrom, 2009).

The tax base supporting the welfare state is being expanded by policies that increase the percentage of the population in the workforce and increase the hours worked by those who are employed. Sweden provides an example of a country that, in the face of aging, has made adjustments to welfare polices while continuing to provide a high level of support for its older population (and its younger populations).

Critics of a generous welfare state model have argued that as the state assumes more responsibility for the welfare of its population, the role of the family in providing care is undermined. However, a growing body of evidence suggests this has not been the case in Sweden. Not only does the family continue to be responsive to its older members, but elders continue to be involved in caring for their grandchildren. Given the high level of welfare support for children and working parents in Sweden, few Swedish grandparents co-reside with their grandchildren or provide regular childcare. But most Swedish grandparents care for grandchildren on an occasional basis, and they overwhelmingly agree that grandparents should help their grandchildren when needed (Albertini, Kohli, and Vogel, 2007). All evidence suggests that intergenerational bonds remain strong in Sweden.

China

Population aging in China stands out—and merits special attention—because of its magnitude, the speed with which it will occur, and the timing of its occurrence relative to China's economic development. One-fifth of the older people in the world now live in China, and by 2060, the older population of China will exceed the total older population living in developed countries (357 million versus 343 million). While most discussions of population aging focus on aging in wealthy countries such as Japan and those in Europe and North America, a global perspective calls attention to the fact that two-thirds of all older people live in developing countries. That fraction will increase to four-fifths by 2060.

The proportion of China's population that is older than age 65 doubled (or soon will) between 1950 and 2015 (from 5 percent to 10 percent), but between 2015 and 2060, that proportion will triple again, to 30 percent. The rapidity of this aging is unprecedented in world history—to go from a 10 percent elderly population up to 28 percent is taking 100 years in Western Europe (from 1950 to 2050), but this phenomenon will occur in merely forty years in China (from 2015 to 2055). This accelerated pace is because of the dramatic decline in fertility that occurred after institutionalization of the one-child policy in 1979. Some authors have warned of the devastating economic and social consequences that China will face as it encounters this so-called old age tsunami, but alarmist prophecies about the future consequences of demographic change tend to miss the mark because they fail to appreciate how social institutions adapt to changing conditions.

There is no question that rapid population aging will present challenges to China over the next several decades. China will become old before becoming rich. In contrast to most developed countries, China's state pension system does not cover most of the workforce, and it is largely unfunded. The availability of working-age people to support the older population is now favorable in China, but that will change dramatically. In 2015, there will be 7.7 people of ages 15 to 64 for every person older than age 65; by 2060, there will be only 1.9. Traditionally older people in China have depended upon their children for support, but in the future, older adults will have relatively few children (Chen and Liu, 2009).

Another factor to consider is China's unbalanced sex ratio from selective abortion under the one-child policy; this means that daughters to provide care to elderly parents and other family members will be in short supply. Healthcare for the aging population also presents challenges because the cost of providing healthcare for the old greatly exceeds that of caring for the young. Despite these challenges, demography is not destiny. The failure of economists to foresee the economic growth that occurred in China in recent decades should be a caution for those who think that the challenges of population aging cannot be overcome.

The United States

Between 1900 and 2010 there was a gradual aging of the U.S. population as the percentage of those older than age 65 increased from 4 percent to 13 percent. However, a much more rapid aging of the population will occur between 2010 and 2030 as the baby boomer cohort enters old age. By 2030, 20 percent of the population will be older than age 65. After 2030,

population aging will again be gradual, with those older than 65 reaching 22 percent by 2060. The aging of baby boomers in the United States has stimulated a great deal of discussion about the challenges of population aging. Most attention has been directed at issues facing Social Security, Medicare, and Medicaid—although both experts and average citizens disagree about what changes should be made to these programs. Equally important, but less discussed, is a question about how population aging might impact the supply of informal care for older people by spouses, children, and siblings. Data from the 2004 National Long-Term Care Survey shows that 79 percent of the care received by older people with disabilities who lived in the community was provided by family members (Houser, Gibson, and Redfoot, 2010). But the declining fertility that leads to population aging also leads to a decrease in the number of adult children and siblings available to provide informal care. How serious are these concerns? The following four observations provide some perspective.

Compared to other developed countries, the United States is exceptional in having a low level of population aging. Projections show 26 percent of the population in the more developed regions of the world, and 33 percent in Spain, will be older than age 65 in 2050, compared to only 21 percent in the United States. Why? Because fertility in the United States remains relatively high.

Other countries already have populations as old as the United States' population will be in 2030, after the baby boomer cohort passes age 65. But reaching this level of population aging has not inevitably resulted in significant social and economic upheaval. For example, Sweden now has an age composition similar to that expected in the United States in 2030. While no one knows how the United States will respond to population aging over the next several decades, other countries can provide insight into what is possible.

Alarmist writing on implications of population aging tends to exclude considerations of elders as resources. If reaching age 65 meant dependency and an end to productive activity, one might have cause for deep concern. But viewing old age as a long stage of life marked by dependency and unproductivity is a negative stereotype unsupported by empirical evidence. Along with growing labor force participation among those older than age 65, findings show high levels of volunteer work and engagement in family caregiving. Furthermore, aging is malleable and there is potential for greatly increasing the productivity of older people through greater opportunities and incentives, such as reducing age discrimination toward older workers, increasing recruitment of older volunteers, and providing them with more support and training and recognition.

Concerns have also been raised about the effects of population aging on the well-being of children (Uhlenberg, 2009). As the proportion of the populace that is older than age 65 increases from 15 percent to 21 percent between 2015 and 2050, the proportion that is younger than age 15 declines only from 20 percent to 19 percent. In other words, the demands on the working population to support children will not decrease as the demands of supporting the older population increase. The potential tension between supporting the old and supporting the young, sometimes referred to as the intergenerational equity issue, could be further complicated by the changing racial-ethnic composition of age groups. In 2050, it is expected that a majority of elders (66 percent) will be non-Hispanic whites, but only 43 percent of children will be in this category (United States Census Bureau, 1996). While conflict across generational lines has not yet been revealed in survey data on attitudes toward old-age entitlements, attention should be given to possible growing competition for scarce resources.

Thinking Clearly about Population Aging

In response to population aging, all societies face a number of common issues. The following points may provide a starting place for future discussions of global population aging.

There is no viable demographic way to avoid population aging. Countries with very low fertility might try to slow aging by encouraging women to have more babies, but efforts to implement pronatalist policies have not succeeded. No country is likely to adopt a policy of increasing death rates for the older population. And the level of immigration required to make a significant difference is politically infeasible. In a world with low fertility, low mortality, and restricted immigration, countries must deal with the reality of having 20 percent or 30 percent of their populations older than age 65.

As a country experiences the transition from high to low birth rates, shifts in its age composition are dynamic. In the early phase, which lasts at least three or four decades, the proportion of children in the population drops, while the proportion of elders hardly changes. Consequently, the ratio of the working-age population to the dependent age groups (children and older adults) grows substantially. This growth in the support ratio (number in the working ages divided by number in dependent ages) is referred to as the "demographic dividend," because it provides an opportunity for less spending on dependents and more savings to foster economic growth (Lee and Mason, 2006).

China provides a clear example of how the support ratio changes with a decline in fertility. Between 1950 and 2015, the ratio of the population ages 15 to 64 to the population younger than age 15 and older than age 65 increased from 1.6 to 2.7. But moving forward, this demographic dividend will disappear as the proportion of elders grows at the expense of the working-age population. By 2060, the support ratio will be only 1.3. All countries can expect this pattern of growth, followed by a decline of the support ratio, during the demographic transition, although the speed of change is variable and depends on how rapidly the fertility decline occurs.

The hope is that countries will take advantage of the demographic dividend to make investments that accelerate economic growth and establish an infrastructure that will provide long-term economic benefits. In the long run, countries must be prepared for much older populations and lower support ratios.

Business will need to adapt to the new demographic reality of older populations. Up to now, ageism in the business sector has presented an obstacle to constructive response to aging populations. Such ageism has led both to discrimination against older workers and to the neglect of older adults as a market. But change in the business sector is happening and will likely accelerate in coming decades.

The challenge for the global community is to champion social change that capitalizes on the worth of an increasing older population.

Business must re-evaluate the potential for older workers to make productive contributions. Empirical research challenges the stereotype that older workers are unhealthy, unable to learn, and too expensive (Biggs, Carstensen, and Hogan, 2012; Seiko, Biggs, and Sargent, 2012). In developed countries, cohorts reaching age 65 are increasingly composed of individuals who are well-educated and healthy, and who expect to live for another twenty to thirty years. To take advantage of older workers' potential, several straightforward responses by business are needed. The workplace can be made friendlier to older workers by increasing flexibility—offering gradual retirement, part-time work, and flexible hours. Employers can help workers avoid becoming obsolete by providing lifelong education and physical fitness programs. The linear career plan can be replaced with one that allows the transfer of older workers into less demanding jobs at lower salaries. Such adaptation by organizations can both improve the quality of life for older people and reduce the economic burden of population aging.

Recognition of the older population as a major market for business is beginning, as evidenced by an increasing number of articles about the "silver market." Because a great deal of wealth is held by the older population and the number of elders is increasing relative to other age groups, it makes sense for business to design products appealing to the older market, and to direct advertising to them. Consumption by the older population can stimulate the economy. The economic power of older adults also can act as a force to change the ageist stereotypes often perpetuated by advertising.

Finally, the way in which people age and the cultural meaning of old age can change. As sociologists put it, aging is to a large extent socially constructed. Social institutions can (and do) change over time, so the implications of a large portion of the population cresting age 65 are not static. As noted above, the way work is organized can change to take advantage of older workers' potential. Education can change to foster lifelong learning. Healthcare can move toward an emphasis on preserving good health and promoting healthy lifestyles that reduce disabilities and dependency in later life. New technology can be developed that enables people in later life to experience fewer limitations. Public policy can change to provide incentives for volunteering in later life. Religious organizations can move beyond seeing older people merely as a group in need of help to seeing them as a resource for ministry.

Little good comes from viewing population aging as the "gray peril." Large-scale population aging will inevitably occur in all countries around the world, and the challenge for the global community is to champion social change that capitalizes on the worth of an increasing older population. There is vast potential for improving and enhancing opportunity and incentive structures for people in later life. If we do this, we can help forge a future that includes a more balanced view of aging—one in which we collectively view older people more as a valuable resource than as a burden.

References

Albertini, M., Kohli, M., and Vogel, C. 2007. "Intergenerational Transfers of Time and Money in European Families: Common Patterns—Different Regimes?" *Journal of European Social Policy* 17(4): 319–34.

Biggs, S., Carstensen, L., and Hogan, P. 2012. "Social Capital, Lifelong Learning and Social Innovation." In Beard, J. R., et al., eds. *Global Population Ageing: Peril or Promise?* (pp. 39–41). Geneva, Switzerland: World Economic Forum. www3.weforum .org/docs/WEF_GAC_GlobalPopulationAgeing_Report_2012. pdf. Retrieved January 8, 2013.

Chen, F., and Liu, G. 2009. "Population Aging in China." In Uhlenberg, P., ed. *International Handbook of Population Aging* (pp. 157–72). Dordrecht, the Netherlands: Springer.

Houser, A., Gibson, M. J., and Redfoot, D. L. 2010. *Trends in Family Caregiving and Paid Home Care for Older People with Disabilities in the Community: Data from the National Long-Term Care Survey.* AARP Public Policy Institute Research Report 2010-09. Washington, DC: AARP Public Policy Institute.

Keely, C. B. 2009. "Replacement Migration." In Uhlenberg, P., ed. *International Handbook of Population Aging* (pp. 395–405). Dordrecht, the Netherlands: Springer.

Lee, R., and Mason, A. 2006. "What Is the Demographic Dividend?" *Finance and Development* 43(3). www.imf.org/external/pubs/ft/ fandd/2006/09/basics.htm#author. Retrieved September 12, 2012.

Seiko, A., Biggs, S., and Sargent, L. 2012. "Organizational, Adaptation and Human Resource Needs for an Aging Population." In Beard, J. R., et al., eds. *Global Population Ageing: Peril or Promise* (pp. 46–50). Geneva, Switzerland: World Economic Forum. www3.weforum.org/docs/WEF_GAC_ GlobalPopulationAgeing_Report_2012.pdf.

Sundstrom, G. 2009. "Demography of Aging in the Nordic Countries." In Uhlenberg, P., ed. *International Handbook of Population Aging* (pp. 91–111). Dordrecht, the Netherlands: Springer.

Uhlenberg, P. 2009. "Children in an Aging Society." *The Journals of Gerontology: Social Sciences* 64B (4): 489–96.

United Nations Department of Economic and Social Affairs (UN DESA), Population Division. 2011. *World Population Prospects: The 2010 Revision, Volume I: Comprehensive Tables.* ST/ESA/ SER.A/313.esa.un.org/unpd/wpp/unpp/panel_indicators.htm. Retrieved September 12, 2012.

United States Census Bureau. 1996. *Population Projections of the United States by Age, Sex, Race, and Hispanic Origin: 1995 to 2050.* Current Population Reports P25–1130. census.gov/prod/1/ pop/p25-1130.pdf. Retrieved September 12, 2012.

Critical Thinking

1. What are the global effects of an aging population?
2. How does an aging population affect healthcare resources globally?

Create Central

www.mhhe.com/createcentral

Internet References

National Council on Aging
www.ncoa.org

World Health Organization: Aging and Life Course
www.who.int/ageing/en

PETER UHLENBERG, PH.D., is professor of sociology and a Fellow of the Carolina Population Center at the University of North Carolina at Chapel Hill, North Carolina.

Uhlenberg, Peter. From *Generations,* Spring 2013, pp. 12–18. Copyright © 2013 by American Society on Aging. Reprinted by permission.

Article   Prepared by: Elaina Osterbur, *Saint Louis University*

The Booming Dynamics of Aging
Meeting the Challenges of the Emerging Senior Majority

The U.S. population is aging rapidly, led by baby boomers who will hit fifty this year. By 2056, for the first time in history, the United States' population sixty-five and older will outnumber those eighteen and under. The ramifications will be significant.

DORCAS R. HARDY

Learning Outcomes

After reading this article, you will be able to:

- Identify the major impact areas of global population growth among older adults.

- Discuss the solutions offered to prepare individuals, businesses, and communities.

- Understand how the "emerging senior majority" will affect the delivery of federal programs in the United States.

Very soon seventy-eight million baby boomers will become the new "Senior Majority." This demographic phenomenon presents significant challenges for our nation. It also represents tremendous opportunities for Certified Senior Advisors (CSAs).

A Global and National Phenomenon

Each day, ten thousand people turn sixty-five. These celebrations will continue daily for the next twenty years. By 2056, for the first time in history, the United States' population sixty-five and older will outnumber those eighteen and under.

Our older population is aging. The oldest-old (eighty years and older) is the fastest growing segment of our population. The eighty-five years and older population is expected to increase to 14.1 million in 2040, and by 2050, nineteen million.

Is our country ready for this? In a word, *no*, and we are not alone.

This demographic phenomenon is not happening only in the United States. By mid-century, approximately 25 percent of the world's population will be sixty and older. By 2050, nearly 17 percent of the global population will be sixty-five and older, twice what we have today.

Boomers: The Emerging Senior Majority

Born between 1946 and 1964, the first wave of American boomers began turning sixty-five in 2011. The youngest of this group will start turning fifty this year. By 2030, all of the boomers will have moved into the ranks of the older population. By 2060, the youngest baby boomers will be ninety-six years old.

Just as they have throughout their lives, boomers have a range of expectations that are having a dramatic effect on every aspect of life in America—from health care to long-term care to housing, finances, employment, business development, technology, communications, retirement and relaxation, and more.

What Does All This Mean for CSAs?

CSAs are in the right place at the right time to help the new senior majority." With some strategic planning, CSAs can, and should, become the "go-to" experts in their communities for people looking for help and advice as they plan for their own or their loved ones' later years.

The role of CSAs is broad and includes:

- an understanding of future challenges created by a demographic shift never before experienced;
- consideration of thoughtful, creative, and cost-effective solutions at the individual and business levels;
- uniquely defining and marketing skills to understand and best serve clients and community.

The issues that concern today and tomorrow's older adults and their families are numerous and multifaceted. The challenges are not going to disappear. They will multiply and become more complex as boomers age. The work that CSAs do is vital and critical to the well-being of older adults. The boomer cohort and all the challenges that accompany them are opportunities for CSAs to use their skills. The services CSAs provide are extremely important, especially now.

How Do We Address Future Challenges?

It has been nearly ten years since the White House Conference on Aging (WHCoA) of 2005. At that decennial event, policymakers and delegates addressed key issues on which our nation needed to focus for the next ten years, in order to be better prepared for a dynamic, new aging population. A key message from the WHCoA, "Don't get caught off guard," still applies today. For better or worse, many of the issues that were discussed then continue to be with us, some becoming more critical and time sensitive.

The challenges our country faces require tough decision making and innovative solutions. Take, for example, the convergence of aging baby boomers with the state of our economy: They have begun to draw on their savings, their pensions, their Social Security, and Medicare. Many have also continued to remain in the workforce. Entitlement programs will continue to be under great pressure. Our country is not ready for this.

Who will pay for our major federal entitlement programs? Medicare and Medicaid, long-term care, and Social Security will expand exponentially in the future.

By 2025, Medicare is projected to include more than seventy-three million beneficiaries (50 percent greater than today). Medicare's unfunded liabilities are more than $38 trillion over the next seventy-five years. That translates to an amount over $325,000 owed by every household in the United States. Some believe that is a low estimate.

The 2013 Medicare Trustees report acknowledged that slower growth in health care cost has improved Medicare's financial outlook, extending the trust fund to last until 2026, two years later than forecast in 2012. But the long-range projections do not support a positive outlook for seniors and taxpayers.

Today, more than sixty-one million people receive some form of Social Security benefits. By 2035, that number is projected to soar to ninety million, with an accompanying shortfall of $134 trillion over the next seventy-five years. If no changes are made in the Social Security retirement program, benefits will be about 30 percent less in 2033.

Federal entitlement programs were never meant to be the sole sources of financial security in retirement. Boomers have been called the largest, healthiest, and most affluent generation of all time. More than three-fourths of the nation's wealth is currently owned by people fifty and older. Yet, they are not saving enough for their longer lives. For example:

- twenty-five percent of boomers have no retirement savings;
- half of American workers have less than $10,000 for retirement;
- total savings and investments for 60 percent of American workers are less than $25,000.

Long-Term Care

Most of us are unprepared for long-term care. At any given moment, any one of us—or a family member, friend, or neighbor—could need long-term care. The demand is expected to increase almost two-fold by 2020.

Medicaid is a means-tested Federal/State program, and the primary provider of long-term care services for older adults. Costs continue to rise, and States are reviewing their programs to determine the best approaches for the future.

Many boomers are shocked to learn that the *median* cost of a private room in a nursing home in 2012 was $81,030, according to the 2012 Genworth Financial Cost of Care Survey. The median monthly cost of assisted living in 2012 was $3,300. These are staggering figures to many, especially those who have not planned ahead or saved enough to finance their own long-term care needs as they age.

Our present delivery system is fragmented and frustrating. If we were to take inventory of all the federal programs that are currently being used for any form of long-term care, whether institutional, homebased or community care, our list would look like a maze.

How do we get boomers to buy into the reality that they need to be more focused on their long-term care needs in the future? How do we ensure they are not caught off guard?

Aging in Place

Eighty percent of boomers say they want to remain in their homes and communities for as long as possible as they age.

Helpful Suggestions for CSAs

- Look for new opportunities. CSAs have the expertise and credentials. It is what sets them apart.
- Be straightforward. Boomers and seniors do not want an aggressive sales pitch. They want current information, honest advice, and direct guidance.
- Encourage your clients to "have the conversation" with their loved ones. Families need to talk about these hard topics. Knowing what people want makes it easier to be helped.
- Be a "Life Course Planner." See the big picture. Be the person who can help identify, navigate, understand, negotiate, and select from an array of options.
- Network, network, network. Get out there; be where seniors and boomers are.

We must develop a well-coordinated system to ensure that people who want and are able to age in place can do so successfully. If you develop a chronic health condition, like diabetes, arthritis, or Alzheimer's disease, aging in place means more than just staying put. You need a place to live that fits your needs and abilities. If driving becomes more difficult, you may need to access a range of paid services, including caregivers, or use extra funds for home modifications that can extend the time you can live at home.

Americans of all ages value their ability to live independently. But without a plan for aging in place, it can be hard to stay in control of your life. Knowing your health risks and financial options can make a big difference in your ability to stay in a familiar place.

Caregiving

For most of our history, the family has been the major provider of care. In many cases, this support has allowed seniors to remain at home longer. One in four families (13 percent of the population) is involved in caregiving of family, neighbor, or friend, with some boomers caring for both children and parents. Most become caregivers because of a crisis, and the great majority of those caregivers are not prepared for what that entails.

About forty-two million Americans were unpaid caregivers who provided $450 billion worth of care to adult relatives and friends in 2009. This is care for which we as a nation would otherwise have had to pay.

Caregivers need our support. At any point in time, anyone could become a caregiver. Would you be ready for this? Would you be able to advise your client about caregiving?

CSAs Leading the Way

CSAs should be considering how best to develop solutions and incorporate additional knowledge into their own business plans. CSAs should be ready for the senior majority to help them to not get caught off guard for challenges that may lie ahead. The questions CSAs should ask themselves are:

- How can you become that go-to person in your community?
- How do you earn—and keep—your clients' faith and trust?
- What sets you apart from other individuals who advise older adults?

How will seniors access information about services? Who will coordinate the needs of future "seasoned citizens"? CSAs might consider thinking of their business as a "hub" working with all the spokes. Consider your business becoming the go-to place, a fully integrated service that presents information and potential solutions for your clients and your communities.

Our challenges as a nation and as individuals need to be addressed sooner rather than later. All of us hope to remain active members of our families and communities as we age. With the proper tools and knowledge, CSAs can help build a positive future as leaders of the emerging "Senior Majority."

Don't get caught off guard! After all, the future is us. •CSA

References

A Place for Mom. "Elder Care Costs Comparison." http://www. aplaceformom.com/senior-care-resource. Accessed March 14, 2014.

Genworth Financial. Genworth 2012 Cost of Care Survey. 2012. Genworth Financial, Inc., Richmond, VA. Available from www. genworth.com.

Moeller, Phillip. 2013. "Long-Term Care Costs Favor Home-Based Treatment." *U.S. News and World Report.* April 9, 2013, http://money.usnews.com/money/blogs/the-best-life/2013/04/09/long-term-care-costs-favor-home-based-treatment. Accessed March 2014.

National Alliance for Caregiving (NAC). Selected Caregiver Statistics. Updated November 2012. http://www.caregiver.org/selected-caregiver-statistics. Accessed March 2014.

The Scan Foundation. June 27, 2010. "Brookings/ICF Long-Term Care Financing Model: Model Assumptions." http://thescanfoundation.org/brookingsicf-long-term-care-financing-model-model-assumptions.

The Scan Foundation. "Growing Demand for Long-Term Care in the United States." Updated June 2012. www.TheSCANFoundation. org/growing-demand-long-term-care. Accessed March 2014.

U.S. Census. 2010. Table 1. Projections and Distribution of the Population Aged 85 and Over by Race for the United States: 2010, 2030, and 2050. www.census.gov/prod/2010pubs/p25-1138.pdf.

—. 2012. "Projections Show a Slower Growing, Older, More Diverse Nation a Half Century from Now." Press Release, Dec, 12, 2012. http://www.census.gov/newsroom/releases/archives/population/cb12-243.html.

United Nations. 2009. World Population Prospects: The 2008 Revision. www.un.org/esa/population/publications/wpp2008/wpp2008_highlights.pdf. Accessed March 2014.

U.S. Department of Health and Human Services. Centers for Medicare and Medicaid Services. 2013 Annual Report of the Boards of Trustees of the Federal Hospital Insurance and Federal Supplementary Medical Insurance Trust Funds. May 31, 2013. http://www.cms.gov/Research-Statistics-Data-and-Systems/Statistics-Trends-and-Reports/ReportsTrustFunds/index.html?redirect=/reportstrustfunds.

—. 2006. 2005 White House Conference on Aging Final Report. "The Booming Dynamics of Aging; From Awareness to Action." http://permanent.access.gpo.gov/lps74930/05_Report_1.pdf.

Critical Thinking

1. What is the impact of global population growth among older adults in the areas of entitlement programs and Social Security in the United States?

2. What are some of the key areas that will be impacted by the population growth among older adults?

Internet References

Administration on Aging
   http://www.aoa.gov

United Nations Population Fund (UNFPA)
   http://www.unfpa.org

World Health Organization
   http://www.who.int/en/

DORCAS R. HARDY, former Commissioner of Social Security, is the Principal of DRHardy & Associates, a government relations and public policy firm serving a diverse portfolio of clients in the health services, disability insurance, financial and association industries. She serves on the board of the new Home Care Standards Bureau and chairs the National Advisory Board of Early Bird Alert, Inc., a healthcare communications technology firm. She also serves on the Board of Trustees of Wright Investors Service Mutual Funds and is appointed by the Speaker of the U.S. House of Representatives to the Social Security Advisory Board and by the Governor of Virginia to the Board of Visitors of the University of Mary Washington.

Article Prepared by: Elaina Osterbur, *Saint Louis University*

Headed for the Future
A Boomer's Guide to Returning to College

KAREN GORBACK

Learning Outcomes

After reading this article, you will be able to:

- Identify the benefits and challenges of returning to college.
- Discuss the reasons that baby boomers offer for wanting to return to school.
- Understand policies that inspire degree-seeking older adults.

At seventy-eight million strong, baby boomers continue to change the world, obliterating the notion that age is a meaningful variable in the decision about going back to college. According to Hunt (2012), "Adults returning to college today make up almost 20 percent of enrollments, which is double what it used to be when they were the young eighteen-year-old demographic."

Older adults engage in higher education for many reasons. Some go back to fulfill "dreams deferred" and transition into encore careers. Others, who may have lost retirement savings during the recession, go back to update existing skills and maintain employability; and some return to class for mental stimulation, to remain socially engaged, and indulge a love of learning. Regardless of motivation, it is useful for advisors and their clients to discuss both the benefits and challenges of *going back* in order for this new cohort of college students to fulfill their personal and professional goals.

Hollywood and Beyond

With the motto, *Curiosity Never Retires,* the Osher Lifelong Learning Institute (OLLI) conducts scholarly courses for individuals ages fifty and older at 117 colleges and universities across the country, with 113,000 members paying annual dues from two to six hundred dollars a year (Hasson 2013). Osher offers a wide variety of classes with topics tasty enough to satisfy any intellectual appetite, from "The Hollywood Novel," "Current Research Topics in Astronomy," and "American Environmental History."

Online examples of lifelong learning opportunities without tuition include those provided by the Emeritus Program through Continuing Education at the San Diego Community College District and by the State of Ohio, where "under Ohio law, residents sixty and older can audit classes for free at thirteen public universities and twenty-three community colleges, space permitting, with the professor's approval" (Brown 2011).

While the benefits of lifelong learning have been well documented, a recent study suggests that the well-being of entire communities is based, in part, on the extent to which their older citizens participate in formal and informal learning activities (Merriam and Kee 2014). Further, and with a wider perspective, higher education among older adults impacts the economy and welfare of the national and global community as well, as explained in a Lumina Foundation report (Pusser et al. 2007), "Returning to Learning: Adults' Success in College is Key to America's Future." The study notes that fifty-four million adults lack a college degree and thirty-four million have no college experience at all, suggesting insufficient preparation among the nation's adults to compete in a dynamic global economy.

The New Currency

The urgency for adults to pursue higher education has also been addressed by President Obama, as reported by U.S. Secretary of Education Arne Duncan in the *Adult College Completion Tool Kit* (Tolbert 2012) who notes, "Shortly after taking office, President Obama set a bold goal: By 2020, the U.S. will once again have the most highly educated, best-prepared workforce in the world. In order to meet this goal, the President challenged every adult to complete at least one year of postsecondary education. In today's knowledge economy, education is the new currency. Put simply, we must dramatically increase overall rates of educational attainment to ensure the success of individuals in the workplace and safeguard our country's prosperity in the global economy. To do this, adult learners across America must enter and succeed in postsecondary education in ever greater numbers."

Researchers Kelly and Strawn (2011) add that the country needs to graduate 10.1 million students between the ages of twenty-five and sixty-four with Associate and Bachelor degrees by 2020 in order to match the best performing countries throughout the world in college attainment.

A major, nationwide program addressing this issue is the *Plus 50 Initiative.* In 2008, the project started with ten community colleges across the country to encourage creative curricula designed to address the needs of baby boomers to remain "active, healthy and engaged in careers and projects that matter to them" (AACC 2014). Examples of projects from early grants include retraining experienced nurses to mentor new nursing students, training individuals to become seasonal guides at national parks, and providing business education through online classes in tax preparation and medical transcription.

But this was just the beginning. In 2010, the *Plus 50 Completion Initiative* was launched for eighteen community colleges throughout the nation to focus on degree and certificate completion for adults over age fifty. The three-year evaluation report released in August 2013 demonstrates the success of the program and the desire of boomers to participate in workforce education. With a goal of serving nine thousand students, instead it enrolled 16,507 participants earning 7,192 professional credentials in the fields of accounting, agriculture, business, health, human services, culinary arts, early childhood education, and many others (Learning for Action 2013).

The most recent iteration of *Plus 50* began in 2012 as the *Plus 50 Encore Completion Program.* This initiative is designed to help ten thousand baby boomers complete degrees or certificates in the high demand fields of education, health care, and social services (AACC 2014). Training in these areas is intended to provide pathways to employment as well as a means for boomers to give back to their communities and to the world.

When Life and Learning Collide

But nobody said it would be easy. At age fifty, Erik Amerikaner had held executive positions at companies across the country. But when asked to relocate in China, the vice-president and former CEO opted instead to pursue a teaching credential at Chapman University in San Luis Obispo, California. Today at age sixty-two, he has been teaching information technology for twelve years and has been honored as a Certified Educator by the National Board for Professional Teaching Standards. Although he loved going back to college, he notes, "The hardest part was working full time during the day while going to school at night."

Although Americaner had the tenacity to push through to completion, most do not. Data from the National Center for Educational Statistics show that just slightly more than a quarter (28 percent) of fulltime, and a mere 5 percent of part-time older students go on to finish their college studies (Schepp 2013). In discussing the explanation behind their poor completion rate, Schepp reports findings from the Apollo Research Institute indicating several reasons why adults drop out. Examples include anxiety over college-related expenses, guilt about spending too little time with loved ones, and concern over their ability to succeed.

While the cost of higher education is an understandable stressor, new online tools can help potential students select an educational program that best fits their finances. They include the United States Department of Education College Affordability and Transparency Center (2014), and the College Navigator (2014) produced by the Institute of Educational Sciences of the National Center for Educational Statistics. In addition, potential students need to apply for federal financial aid, as well as the myriad of scholarships available each year. A comprehensive resource addressing the cost of education is *501 Ways for Adults Students to Pay for College,* by Tanabe and Tanabe (2013), underscores the value of spending serious time seeking out scholarships that support adults.

In addressing the guilt stemming from spending less time with family and friends, advisors can help clients learn to clearly communicate their needs by using "I messages." An example is for the student to replace angry, accusatory statements such as "Don't make me feel guilty all the time" with "I care about you and I'm sorry that I can't go to the family picnic on Sunday. But at this time in my life, I'm choosing to attend college and I need to study. This is important to me, and I hope you'll understand."

Finally, potential students need to consider whether colleges that run by semesters, quarters, or rapid-fire, month-long terms will best fit into their lives. Online education with classes that are generally asynchronous and can be accessed any time of the day or night, continue to grow in popularity. Although some believe that online education is less demanding than traditional classes, this is false. Online offerings are obligated to demonstrate the same rigor as their classroom counterparts. However, for online students to be successful, they must be comfortable with technology, exceptionally motivated, and have enough self-discipline to persevere without the commitment of classroom attendance. In her book, *The Adult Student: An Insider's Guide to Going Back to School,* Dani Babb, Ph.D. (2012) discusses online learning, including considerations about attending public versus private programs, and an explanation of the issues regarding a college's accreditation and the potential impact on a student's career choices.

While college degrees and professional certificates generally result in lower unemployment and better paying jobs, job hunting is rarely easy at any age. However, a wide variety of resources are available to assist older adults in their job search. "New Trends in Retirement Jobs" is a CSA online article providing job seekers and advisors with extensive, practical suggestions for a successful outcome. Lastly, they should visit the websites of their local state employment offices, to inquire about workshops designed specifically for those seeking encore jobs or careers.

Mindfulness

When baby boomer Tamara Sprigel started college, her youngest of four children was twelve. She was going through a divorce and anxious to complete a degree in psychology. "At one point I carried twenty-three units. The toughest part was keeping the family going while I was in school, but I loved college." She now has a Ph.D. in clinical psychology and is a licensed marriage and family therapist. Gail Smith also went back to college after her children were grown. She earned a bachelor's degree in behavioral psychology, but not for specific career aspirations. Her goal was to feed something deeper—a validation of her ability to succeed. "As a result, I now have an 'I can' attitude rather than 'maybe not me.'"

To prove it's never too late, this year, at age sixty-four, Susan Miedzianowski proudly earned her Ph.D. in Human Services and Gerontology. After obtaining a master's degree on her fortieth birthday, she returned to school to reach the ultimate academic milestone. Now an adjunct professor at multiple universities, she hopes her perseverance will inspire other older adults to pursue their lifelong dreams.

It is not uncommon among adult learners to express a sense of pleasure about their college experience. Professors enjoy having older adults in class and often observe that they're among the most engaged. Mary Lange, Supervisor of Programs for Older Adults at Mt. San Antonio College in Walnut, California, and Chair of the California Community of College Educators of Older Adults adds, "As an educator, embracing the fact that older adult learners bring to the classroom a rich background of real-world experiences that add to the academic setting is very empowering for both students and faculty. Therefore, uniting

faculty and students to foster knowledge that encourages student participation, mentoring, and personal education goals is a synergistic approach that is beneficial to all generations."

Accordingly, with support from policy makers and leaders like Lange, along with colleges and universities across the country, the new "senior class" is changing the paradigm of higher education as an institution for young adults. Kanter (2006) recommends the term *even higher* education to describe the college experience for older adults. She explains, "This isn't going back to school. It's using school to move forward."

Thus, as boomers use college to move forward, they exemplify the concept of "mindfulness," described by researcher Ellen Langer (2014) as "the process of actively noticing new things. It is the essence of engagement." CSAs and other professionals who work with older adults can support their clients' mindful engagement in higher education by:

1. Helping clients define their goals and then locating appropriate educational programs to fulfill those goals.
2. Exploring all avenues for financial aid.
3. Researching a wide variety of instructional delivery options.
4. Facilitating clients' use of effective communication skills.
5. Teaching clients simple methods for time management, memorization, note taking and expository writing.
6. Encouraging clients to utilize college and university tutoring services, as well as study groups to solidify academic skills.

With support from advisors, family, and friends, older adults will continue going back to school for both lifelong learning and professional development fully engaged, and headed for the future. •**CSA**

References

American Association of Community Colleges. 2008. "New Plus 50 Initiative by Community Colleges Reaches Out to Baby Boomers." http://plus50.aacc.nche.edu/Documeiits/PressReleases/AP%20Finai%20Plus%2050%20release4-28-08.pdf. Accessed March 5, 2014.

—. 2013. "Plus Fifty Students: Tapping into a Growing Market." http://plus50.aacc.nche.edu/documents/Plus_50_Students_Tapping_Into_a_Growing_Market.pdf. Accessed March 5,2014.

Babb, Dani, Ph.D. *The Adult Student: An Insider's Guide to Going Back to School.* 2012. Weston, CT: Mandevilla Press.

Brown, Gayle. "Lifelong Learning with No Tuition." 2011. AARP Bulletin, http://www.aarp.org/personal-growth/life-long-learning/info-12-2011/lifelong-learning-with-no-tuition-oh. Accessed March 5, 2014.

Cummings, Betsy. *How to Find a Job After 50.* 2005. New York: Warner Business Books.

Freedman. Marc. *Encore. Finding Work That Matters in the Second Half of Life.* 2007. New York: Public Affairs.

Hannon, Kerry, *Great Jobs for Everyone 50+: Finding Work That Keeps You Happy, Healthy and Pays the Bills,* 2012. Hoboken, NJ: John Wiley & Sons.

Hasson, Judi. 2013. "Retirees Return to College Just for the Fun of It." Kiplinger's Retirement Report, http://www.kiplinger.com/article/retirement/T037-C000-S004-retirees-return-to-college-just-for-the-fun-of-it.html. Accessed March 13, 2014.

Hunt, Lauren. 2010. "Statistics on Adults Returning to College." EzineArticles. http://ezinearticies.com/?Statistics-on-Adults-Returning-to-College&id=3639820. Accessed February 24, 2014.

Kanter, Rosabeth Moss. 2006. "Back to College at Midlife." *AARP the Magazine,* http://www.aarp.org/personal-growth/life-long-learning/info-2006/back_to_college_at_midlife.html. Accessed February 24, 2014.

Kelly, Patrick, and Julie Strawn. 2011. "Not Just Kid Stuff Anymore: The Economic imperative for More Adults to Complete College." Center for Law and Social Policy (CLASP) and the National Center for Higher Education Management Systems (NCHEMS).

http://www.clasp.org/resources-and-publications/publication-l/NotKidStuffAnymoreAdultStudentProfile-1.pdf. Accessed March 13, 2014.

Langer, Ellen. "Mindfulness in the Age of Complexity." 2014. Harvard Business Review. 92: 68–73.

Learning for Action. 2013. "Plus 50 Completion Strategy: Year Three Evaluation Results." Report prepared for the American Association of Community Colleges and the Lumina Foundation. San Francisco: Learning for Action, http://plus50.aacc.nche.edu/Documents/Plus%2050%20Completion%20Strategy_Year%20Three%20Report_FINAL.pdf.

Pusser, Brian, David W. Breneman, Bruce M. Gansneder, Kay J. Kohl, John S. Levin, John H. Milam and Sarah E. Turner. 2007. "Returning to Learning: Adults' Success in College is Key to American's Future." Indianapolis, IN: Lumina Foundation, http://www.luminafoundation.org/publications/ReturntolearningApril2007.pdf.

Schepp, David. 2013. "Top 6 Reasons Adult College Students Drop Out." WestlakePATCH. November 27, 2013. http://westlake.patch.com/groups/jobs/p/top-6-reasons-adult-college-students-drop-out_l. Accessed March 4, 2014.

Tolbert, Michelle. 2012. "Adult College Completion Tool Kit." U.S. Department of Education, http://www2.ed.gov/about/offices/list/ovae/resource/adult-college-completion-tool-kit.pdf. Accessed March 6, 2014.

Tanabe, Gen, and Keliy Tanabe. 2013. *501 Ways for Adult Students to Pay for College.* Belmont, CA: Super College LLC, 4th ed.

Internet Resources

American Association of Community Colleges (AACC). 2014. "About Plus 50 Initiative." http://plus50.aacc.nche.edu. Accessed March 5, 2014.

California State University, Channel Islands. 2014. "Extended University and International Programs." Osher Lifelong Learning Institute. http://ext.csuci.edu/community-ed/osher. Accessed March 5, 2014.

College Navigator. Institute of Educational Sciences of the National Center for Educational Statistics. http://nces.ed.gov/collegenavigator. Accesed March 8, 2014.

Khan Academy. https://www.khanacademy.org. Accessed February 24, 2014.

Merriam, Sharan B. and Yougwha Kee. 2014. "Promoting Community Wellbeing: The Case for Lifelong Learning for Older Adults." http://aeq.sagepub.com/content/early/2014/01/03/0741713613513633.abstract. Accessed February 27, 2014.

San Diego Community College District Continuing Education. www.sdce.edu/classes/emeritus. Accessed March 1, 2014.

Society of Certified Senior Advisors. "New Trends in Retirement Jobs." www.csa.us/freeresources/socialinterestlibrary/jobtrends/. Accessed March 6, 2014.

United States Department of Education College Affordability and Transparency Center http://collegecost.ed.gov/catc. Accessed March 8, 2014.

www.workforce50.com. Accessed February 24, 2014.

Critical Thinking

1. What was the goal set forth by the Obama Administration that has led to adult learners entering college?
2. What are some of the barriers that older adults face when contemplating the return to college?

Internet References

Administration on Aging
http://www.aoa.gov
American Association of Community Colleges
http://www.aacc.nche.edu
Bureau of Labor Statistics
http://www.bls.gov

KAREN GORBACK earned a Ph.D. in education from the University of California, Santa Barbara. She is currently a commissioner on the Council on Aging for the City of Thousand Oaks, California. She recently published her debut novel titled *Freshman Mom,* a contemporary story about a divorced mother who goes back to college.

Article   Prepared by: Elaina F. Osterbur, *Saint Louis University*

Long Live . . . Us

In never-say-die America, life expectancy is longer than ever.

MARK BENNETT

Learning Outcomes

After reading this article, you will be able to:

- Identify the life expectancy in the United States for all persons, regardless of sex, in 2009.
- Identify the life expectancy of men and women in the United States in 2009.

Six members of the Class of '74 sit around a restaurant table.

They sip red wine and munch on a trail-mix-style bowl filled with fish oil, flaxseed oil and DHEA gel tabs. A joke about a classmate's spring break photo with her great-grandson's frat brothers on Facebook sparks hysterical laughter. As the chuckles subside, they check their iPhone clocks, realize the abs-crunch marathon fundraiser for the Macrobiotic Diet Consortium starts in an hour, and get busy planning their 85th reunion.

A retro "Dancing with the Stars" theme wins unanimous approval. One guy tweets his mother-in-law about next week's library tax protest, the class president picks up the tab, and they scatter out the door.

Sure, the ages of the folks in that futuristic dinner party would be around 103, but in never-say-die America, life expectancy is longer than ever, according to a report issued this month by the U.S. Centers for Disease Control and Prevention.

A baby born in 2009 will live an average of 78 years and two months. If that kid is a girl, she will likely linger on Earth for 80.6 years, compared to 75.7 for a boy. Back in 1930, a man's life expectancy was 58 and a woman's 62.

The CDC won't say why Americans live longer until the second half of its life expectancy report is released later this year, but the agency has a pretty good guess. Improved medical treatment, vaccinations and anti-smoking campaigns have helped drop the death rate to a record low as deaths from strokes, Alzheimer's, diabetes, heart disease and cancer decreased during the past 12 months.

Plus, our ancestors had no idea that red wine contained antioxidants and resveratol that protect blood vessels and reduce "bad" cholesterol. Or that DHEA supposedly repairs damage to cells in our bodies. Or that fish oil and flaxseed oil fight free radicals, which are cell-damaging molecules, not 1960s fugitives.

So, with almonds stashed in our shirt pockets instead of Marlboros, we've nearly tacked an extra decade onto our lives since 1970, when life expectancy in the U.S. was 70.8 years.

"It does go up every year, little by little," CDC statistician Ken Kochanek said by telephone from Washington, D.C., last week.

Seemingly, this age-defying trend could extend and create bizarre cultural dynamics, not unlike the aforementioned class reunion committee meeting. In Britain, for example, government researchers estimate that by 2014—just a little more than two years from now—the number of Brits ages 65 and older will surpass that of the under-16 population. Think of the implications—there are more people sitting around the UK who look like Keith Richards than fresh-faced kids. Actually, the Stones guitarist (now 67) would be considered a mere pup, if a BBC report is true. That story quoted a *Science* magazine analysis that concluded there is no natural limit to human life. The greeting card companies may be printing a new "Happy 200th" line someday.

Mel Brooks' 2,000-year-old man comes to mind. When asked if he knew Joan of Arc, Mel's character responded, "Know her? I went with her, dummy."

Reality continues to apply, though. Humans are managing to live longer, but not indefinitely. Though 36,000 fewer Americans died in 2009 than the year before, a total of 2.4 million still passed on in '09. The leading causes were, in order, heart disease, malignant neoplasms, chronic lower respiratory diseases, cerebrovascular diseases, accidents, Alzheimer's, diabetes, flu and pneumonia and nephritis. "In general, you have the same problems that have existed for a long time," said Kochanek.

Men show up in those statistics sooner than women, apparently because we do dumb stuff more often, such as smoking and exceeding the speed limit. "Men take more risks, and that affects life expectancy," Kochanek said. Both genders eat less wisely, too, even if we're popping those Omega-3 pills. Americans in the sixtysomething age range are, on average, 10 pounds heavier than folks of a similar vintage a decade earlier, according to FDA statistics cited by *U.S. News & World Report*.

The impact of poor choices in our lifetimes can be tabulated. For those dying to know how much time they've got, Northwestern Mutual Life Insurance Co. provides an online calculator. Just punch in your age, height, weight, then answer 11 other questions about your lifestyle, family history and habits and—voilà!—your final number appears. If you want something handy enough to stick onto the front of the fridge, the U.S. Census Bureau offers a less detailed chart subtitled "Average Number of Years of Life Remaining."

Of course, those are national figures. Averages. They vary by location. According to a nationwide study by the Robert Wood Johnson Foundation of the University of Wisconsin Population Health Institute, Vigo County's mortality rate ranks 69th out of 92 counties in Indiana, which isn't good. The mortality rate is a measure of premature death—the years of potential life lost prior to age 75.

Why do Vigo Countians die so young?

Well, in terms of health behaviors (smoking, binge drinking, car crashes, diet and exercise, STDs and teen birth rates), Vigo County rates an abysmal 80th out of 92 counties. (Apparently, very few of the wine-drinking, fish-oil-eating, fitness-crazed baby boomers described earlier call Vigo County home.) When calculating mortality rates, health behaviors account for nearly one-third of the influencing factors, along with clinical care, socioeconomics and physical environment, the Population Health Institute study said.

Given those real numbers, the secret of long life may not be such a secret after all. Author and psychologist Howard Friedman's new book, *The Longevity Project*, explores the topic. In a *Time* magazine interview this month, he explained that "conscientiousness" was a primary enhancer of life expectancy.

"The most intriguing reason why conscientious people live longer is that having a conscientious personality leads you into healthier situations and relationships," Friedman told *Time*. "In other words, conscientious people find their way to happier marriages, better friendships and healthier work situations. They help create healthy, long-life pathways for themselves. This is a new way of thinking about health."

That should give Keith Richards something to consider every time the Stones play "Time Is On My Side."

Critical Thinking

1. Why is the life expectancy of men lower than the life expectancy of women?

2. What were the leading causes of death in the United States in 2009?

3. How has the weight of persons over 60 changed in the last ten years?

4. Why does Howard Friedman believe that conscientious people live longer?

Create Central

www.mhhe.com/createcentral

Internet References

The Aging Research Centre
www.arclab.org
National Center for Health Statistics
www.cdc.gov/mchs/agingact.htm

Article   Prepared by: Elaina F. Osterbur, *Saint Louis University*

How to Live to 100

The latest research suggests the key to longevity lies in changing daily habits.

KIMBERLY PALMER

Learning Outcomes

After reading this article, you will be able to:

- Identify the elements of longevity.
- Discuss the positive behaviors associated with long life.
- Discuss the behaviors that do not contribute to longevity.

Why do some people live long, healthy, and happy lives, while others struggle with dementia, heart disease, and depression? Are there steps we can take to protect ourselves from those outcomes, or is it all a matter of luck (and good genes)? What do the latest scientific advancements say about helping us get the most out of our lifespans, and how can we afford our longer lives?

Those are the questions *U.S. News* sought to answer with this project, *How to Live to 100*. Promises of magic elixirs abound: in television ads for skin-care products, in doctor's offices, and even at the grocery store. Every day, new research seems to suggest something new: Drink red wine, skip red meat, take vitamin C, drink coffee. We sought to find out the truth about steps we can all take to increase our chances of staying healthy, happy, and affording it.

The financial side of longevity is playing an increasingly visible role as people begin to routinely live 10, 20, and even 30 years after retirement. "People have many more years to worry about and take care of, and we're living at a time when a lot of their resources have been diminished. The drop in the value of homes has probably wiped out an average of two-thirds of home equity for American homeowners. And your job might not be there as long as you had hoped," says Mort Zuckerman, editor-in-chief of *U.S. News*.

In addition to interviewing the country's top researchers on health, longevity, happiness, and finances, we sought out people who seem to have discovered the answer to successful aging. They often echoed each other's thoughts about consciously choosing healthier diets, opting to spend more time with family over work, and finding meaning by giving back to communities and connecting with others long past retirement. As actress

Betty White, perhaps the nation's most famous nonagenarian, recently put it to CNN's Piers Morgan, "Old age is all up here," gesturing to her head.

That's certainly the case for 77-year-old marathoner Ruth Heidrich, a breast cancer survivor who changed her diet and exercise habits after her diagnosis in 1982. "That's what started me on this whole road," she says, referring to her all-raw diet and extreme exercise habits, including triathlons and Iron Man competitions.

Heidrich, who lives in Honolulu, eats a large bowl of leafy greens for breakfast, mixed with a banana, a mango, and raw steel-cut oats. She sprinkles cinnamon and ginger on top, and drinks green tea mixed with a tablespoon of pure unsweetened cocoa, along with some Stevia to sweeten the drink. A typical dinner includes more leafy greens and fruit along with broccoli and salsa. For dessert and snacks, she munches on blueberries, walnuts, prunes, apples, and popcorn. "I started eating at least a cup of blueberries a day after I read that blueberries are good for the brain," she says. She doesn't drink coffee or alcohol.

Today, she no longer competes in Iron Man competitions but continues to work out for three hours daily, typically running, biking, or swimming before breakfast, and plans to continue doing so, albeit at a slower pace. "I will keep exercising forever," she says. "My energy levels are through the roof and I'm having fun. I feel like I've got to tell everybody, 'You've got to eat right and exercise right . . . Walking is not exercise. You've gotta sweat, you've gotta breathe hard.'"

Robert Kuhns, 69, found fulfillment in retirement through a second career: The retired IBM executive works as a forest ranger in Virginia's Shenandoah National Park during part of the year, leading hikes, giving talks on animal habits, and taking photographs for park brochures. From the end of March through the end of November, he works 40 hours a week, which includes plenty of exercise, hiking up and down trails as he shares information about native species of insects and trees with visitors. "It's one of the most rewarding things I've done in my life," he says. He plans to continue for as long as he can, perhaps another 10 years.

Kuhns earns extra cash from the gig, too. "[My wife and I] have more available funds when I'm working than during the months when I'm not," he says, and this year he got promoted to a higher pay grade.

Doreen Orion, 52, and her husband, Tim Justice, 54, decided to scale back work and hit the road in their 340 square-foot RV, so they could focus on adventure, each other, and reducing their dependence on material goods. She documented their trip in her 2008 memoir, *Queen of the Road.* As psychiatrists who work for insurance companies, they can do much of their work remotely. "We had a really good marriage before, but being thrust into new situations all the time and having to problem-solve, it can't help but bring you closer together," she says. Orion and her husband recently decided to put their Colorado home on the market and live in their RV full-time.

While still in her twenties, Nicole Mladic, a communications director in Chicago, realized she was never going to save enough for retirement if she continued on her current trajectory of little or no savings each month. So she started slowly by saving 2 percent of her salary each month. A few months later, she raised it to 3 percent, then 4 percent, and eventually reached her goal of 10 percent. Today, Mladic is in her early thirties and her net worth is over $100,000. "The thought of saving 10 percent of my salary for retirement each month seemed impossible when I first started working," says Mladic. "But by starting small, it was easy to get to 10 percent, and far less of a shock to my budget."

George Vaillant, a professor of psychiatry at Harvard Medical School, has overseen the longest-running longitudinal study of health and happiness. His study has tracked the lives of more than 500 Harvard students and men from inner-city Boston since the 1930s, and has drawn some intriguing conclusions, including that stable relationships are one key to a long and happy life. Divorce, he says, "is very bad for your health."

Vaillant says what makes him happiest now, at age 77, are his grandchildren. His advice is sometimes at odds with what one usually hears: He urges people to take money out of their retirement accounts to go on vacation, because learning how to relax and spend time with loved ones is essential to one's happiness later in life. "Just remember, if you get nothing else out of talking to me, to put some of your IRA money into vacations," he says.

As for what brings happiness to that retirement, he says it almost always comes down to relationships. "There were three things that correlated with a fun retirement: 1) whether your marriage was good, 2) whether you took fun vacations before you retired, and 3) whether you have always liked doing things for other people. So it's being more interested in others than yourself that leads to a happy retirement, and having somebody you enjoy being with. And it's having learned before you retire how to play." That's why he suggests investing in vacations long before retirement—to practice.

Love of grandchildren, he found, can trump even disease. "People in poor health with 13 grandchildren are happy . . . I'm 77, and what I enjoy most are my grandchildren."

There are seemingly endless findings about what you can do now to increase your odds of being a healthy and happy

77-year-old, 90-year-old, and beyond. Getting your heart rate up by exercising at least 150 minutes a week, for example, can cut your chances of heart disease and cancer. Eating a Mediterranean diet, which is heavy on olive oil and fish, capping red meat at 18 ounces per week, flossing daily, sleeping at least six hours a night, and having no more than two drinks a day for men and one for women also appear to promote good health.

To boost your chances of happiness, build a long and loving marriage, cultivate gratitude and optimism, and commit to constant self-improvement. To afford your long life, start a vigorous savings plan as early as your twenties, make frugal lifestyle choices, such as living in a smaller home and cooking more meals at home, and work as long as possible, well past age 65.

Changing ingrained habits, of course, isn't easy. Sometimes it takes a major life event, such as a cancer diagnosis, as it did for Ruth Heidrich. But habits can also be changed with conscious effort. *New York Times* reporter Charles Duhigg, author of *The Power of Habit,* found that changing a habit requires first identifying a cue, such as putting your running shoes on before breakfast, that your brain connects to going for a run. Then, he suggests rewarding yourself after the run, with a piece of chocolate or a long shower.

"There has to be some sort of reward at the end of the routine to make it a habit," he says. Exercise does contain its own reward, because people feel good after running, but he says it can take a few weeks for the brain to pick up on those internal rewards, which is why he suggests supplementing with a more obvious, external reward. "That's how the neurology learns to encode that behavior," he adds.

One worthy new habit might be earning supplemental income, even before retirement, to help fund those decades. Says Zuckerman: "Understand that there is no point in your life when you have to stop learning. Continue to read, try and learn and understand what is going in the world, and hopefully train yourself for other work."

Critical Thinking

1. How will increased longevity impact the U.S. healthcare system?

2. Why do positive health behaviors contribute to long life and quality of life?

Create Central

www.mhhe.com/createcentral

Internet References

The Aging Research Centre
  www.arclab.org
Harvard Health Publications
  www.wifle.org/pdf/Living_to_100.pd

Article

Prepared by: Elaina Osterbur, *Saint Louis University*

7 Career Mistakes You Don't Even Know You're Making

ANN BRENOFF

Learning Outcomes

After reading this article, you will be able to:

- Identify the seven career mistakes that older adults make.
- Discuss the strategies to avoid career mistakes.

Older workers have a harder time finding jobs and remain the demographic that once unemployed, stays out of work the longest. So hanging on to their jobs is of paramount importance. Yet here are 7 mistakes older workers unwittingly make:

1. They don't think they need to pick up new skills while they are still employed.

Jobs are not static anymore. The workplace is constantly evolving and they need to evolve along with it. If an employer offers training classes, some older workers wrongly believe the classes are intended for new company hires and don't go. Instead, they should be taking as many of those earn-as-you-learn classes as possible.

Should they lose that job, training is hard to come by. Government training programs are geared toward those who are receiving public assistance. The goal is to get those folks off the public dole and into tax-generating jobs.

Retraining programs for college-educated professionals kind of don't exist. That, or they do a terrific job of hiding themselves from the public. In fact, a "60 Minutes" segment featured a Connecticut program in 2012 for just one reason: It was such a rarity. In that program, college-educated professionals, who had lost their jobs when they were in their 40s or 50s and who had been out of work for a full 99 weeks, were given a crack at some internships that could lead to permanent jobs. These former six-figure earners were grateful for the foot in the door for one big reason: Most of their peers don't even get that.

Take-away: If you have a chance to broaden your skills, jump at it.

2. They think community colleges are just for kids.

The community college system has borne the brunt of retraining the displaced older workforce. There's a program that launched in 2010 called the Plus 50 Completion Strategy which basically helps post-50 students complete their post secondary degrees, and aims to give older workers the skills they need to get jobs in fields that are actually hiring—like health care. So far, the Plus 50 initiative has served about 24,000 students, which—not to diminish this rare drop in the bucket—is about how many out-of-work journalists I hear from in any given week.

Even if you are working, it still makes sense to keep an eye on what lies around the corner for you professionally. Many of these classes can be taken online. If you are in one of those careers that is contracting, use the "hospice time" to prepare for what you will be doing next. And a community college is a great place to start.

3. They don't sufficiently value reverse mentoring.

Older employees have some amazing teachers right under their noses, says Robert L. Dilenschneider, an author and business leader who lectures older workers around the country about staying relevant. "Younger employees are fluent not just in the new technologies but in the best ways to deliver business messages and marketing in such technologies," he said, and older workers should seek them out. When workers can learn from each other, the workplace is strengthened.

Mentoring is a two-way street and the older workers who embrace that—instead of thinking that their age and experience alone make them the only teachers in the room—improve their value to the company.

4. **They wrongly assume that working beyond 66 will be their choice.**

This is a silly assumption, especially with companies eager to reduce costs and an economy that can provide many eager-to-work millennials who can be paid less than an older, more-experienced worker. The reality is that there is a guillotine lurking in every future and no job is secure for a lifetime anymore. It's another argument for making yourself as invaluable as possible to the company by being willing and able to do multiple tasks.

Most boomers have gotten over the notion that they will be able to retire as young as their parents did. Now the goal is to hang on to the jobs they have for as long as possible.

5. **They inflict self-damage when they joke about being tech-illiterate.**

Stereotypes are bad things. And one of the popular stereotypes is that older people resist technology. It hurts them in the workplace and can be the death knell if they are job-hunting. And never mind that it isn't a universal truth.

It's important not to fuel the myth. Telling your younger boss that you need your teenager to program your new phone isn't a funny joke; it's a check mark in your "not capable" column.

6. **They don't make time to socialize with the younger people in the office.**

While you may not think you have oodles in common with your decades-younger coworkers, it's important to secure your place in the office universe.

Go out to lunch when they invite you, make time for the occasional drink after work, be interested in their weekend plans. Aside from the fact that having office friends will actually make coming to work more fun, it's also easier to lay off the people who nobody knows.

7. **They don't actually have an exit strategy or a retirement plan.**

A Fidelity study reported that 48 percent of boomers won't be able to afford basic expenses in retirement. It begs the question: What are you doing about it?

The simplest answer is to try and save more and look for ways you are wasting money now. Another thing to think about is your housing costs, which are pretty much everyone's big ticket item. While you are still working is the perfect time to look into more affordable places to live or how you can adapt your home expenses to be more aligned with your reduced retirement income.

Critical Thinking

1. What are the reasons that older adults make career mistakes?
2. What are some strategies that younger pre retirement adults can use while they are still employed that will spare them the mistakes during their older years?

Internet References

AARP
   http://www.aarp.org
Administration on Aging
   http://www.aoa.gov
Bureau of Labor Statistics
   http://www.bls.gov

Ann Brenoff, "7 Career Mistakes You Don't Even Know You're Making," *Huffington Post,* July 3, 2014.

Unit 2

UNIT

Prepared by: Elaina Osterbur, *Saint Louis University*

The Quality of Later Life

Although it is true that one ages from the moment of conception to the moment of death, children are usually considered to be "growing and developing," but adults are often thought of as "aging." Having accepted this assumption, most biologists concerned with the problems of aging focus their attention on what happens to individuals after they reach maturity. Moreover, most of the biological and medical research dealing with the aging process focuses on the later part of the mature adult's life cycle. A commonly used definition of *senescence* is "the changes that occur generally in the postreproductive period and that result in decreased survival capacity on the part of the individual organism" (B.L. Shrehler, *Time, Cells and Aging,* New York: Academic Press, 1977).

As a person ages, physiological changes take place. The skin loses it elasticity, becomes more pigmented, and bruises more easily. Joints stiffen, and the bone structure becomes less firm. Muscles lose their strength. The respiratory system becomes less efficient. The individual's metabolism changes, resulting in different dietary demands. Bowel and bladder movements are more difficult to regulate. Visual acuity diminishes, hearing declines, and the entire system is less able to resist environmental stresses and strains.

Increased medical technologies will probably increase the life expectancy for the 65-and-over population, resulting in longer life for the next generation. Although people 65 years of age today are living only slightly longer than 65-year-olds did in 1900, the quality of their later years has greatly improved. Economically, Social Security and a multitude of private retirement programs have given most older persons a more secure retirement. Physically, many people remain active, mobile, and independent throughout their retirement years. Socially, most older persons are married, involved in community activities, and leading productive lives. Many older adults are able to live independently, live their own homes, direct their own lives, and involve themselves in activities they enjoy.

Although more people survive to age 65 today, many will live with at least one disabling chronic disease such as diabetes, arthritis, heart disease, effects of stroke, and cancer. These are the most common, costly, and preventable of all health problems according to the Centers for Disease Control and Prevention. The articles in this section attempt to explain how the older adults can improve the quality of their lives with or without chronic disease through nutrition, exercise, creativity, social relationships, and other activities that bring happiness and purpose to the lives of older adults.

Article   Prepared by: Elaina F. Osterbur, *Saint Louis University*

Age-Proof Your Brain

10 Easy Ways to Stay Sharp Forever

BETH HOWARD

Learning Outcomes

After reading this article, you will be able to:

- Name the foods a person can eat that would reduce the risk of developing Alzheimer's disease.
- Identify the chronic health problems that are often associated with dementia.

Alzheimer's isn't inevitable. Many experts now believe you can prevent or at least delay dementia—even if you have a genetic predisposition. Reducing Alzheimer's risk factors like obesity, diabetes, smoking and low physical activity by just 25 percent could prevent up to half a million cases of the disease in the United States, according to a recent analysis from the University of California, San Francisco.

"The goal is to stave it off long enough so that you can live life without ever suffering from symptoms," says Gary Small, M.D., director of the UCLA Longevity Center and coauthor of *The Alzheimer's Prevention Program: Keep Your Brain Healthy for the Rest of Your Life.* Read on for new ways to boost your brain.

1 Get Moving

"If you do only one thing to keep your brain young, exercise," says Art Kramer, Ph.D., professor of psychology and neuroscience at the University of Illinois. Higher exercise levels can reduce dementia risk by 30 to 40 percent compared with low activity levels, and physically active people tend to maintain better cognition and memory than inactive people. "They also have substantially lower rates of different forms of dementia, including Alzheimer's disease," Kramer says.

Working out helps your hippocampus, the region of the brain involved in memory formation. As you age, your hippocampus shrinks, leading to memory loss. Exercise can reverse this process, research suggests. Physical activity can also trigger the growth of new nerve cells and promote nerve growth.

How you work up a sweat is up to you, but most experts recommend 150 minutes a week of moderate activity. Even a little bit can help: "In our research as little as 15 minutes of regular exercise three times per week helped maintain the brain," says Eric B. Larson, M.D., executive director of Group Health Research Institute in Seattle.

2 Pump Some Iron

Older women who participated in a yearlong weight-training program at the University of British Columbia at Vancouver did 13 percent better on tests of cognitive function than a group of women who did balance and toning exercises. "Resistance training may increase the levels of growth factors in the brain such as IGF1, which nourish and protect nerve cells," says Teresa Liu-Ambrose, Ph.D., head of the university's Aging, Mobility, and Cognitive Neuroscience Laboratory.

3 Seek Out New Skills

Learning is like Rogaine for your brain: It spurs the growth of new brain cells. "When you challenge the brain, you increase the number of brain cells and the number of connections between those cells," says Keith L. Black, M.D., chair of neurosurgery at Cedars-Sinai Medical Center in Los Angeles. "But it's not enough to do the things you routinely do—like the daily crossword. You have to learn new things, like sudoku or a new form of bridge."

UCLA researchers using MRI scans found that middle-aged and older adults with little Internet experience could trigger brain centers that control decision-making and complex reasoning after a week of surfing the net. "Engaging the mind can help older brains maintain healthy functioning," says Cynthia R. Green, Ph.D., author of *30 Days to Total Brain Health.*

4 Say *"Omm"*

Chronic stress floods your brain with cortisol, which leads to impaired memory. To better understand if easing tension changes your brain, Harvard researchers studied men and women trained in a technique called mindfulness-based stress reduction (MBSR). This form of meditation—which involves focusing one's attention on sensations, feelings and state of mind—has been shown to reduce harmful stress hormones. After eight weeks, researchers took MRI scans of participants' brains. The density of gray matter in the hippocampus increased significantly in the MBSR group, compared with a control group.

5 Eat Like a Greek

A heart-friendly Mediterranean diet—fish, vegetables, fruit, nuts and beans—reduced Alzheimer's risk by 34 to 48 percent in studies conducted by Columbia University.

"We know that omega-3 fatty acids in fish are very important for maintaining heart health," says Keith Black of Cedars-Sinai. "We suspect these fats may be equally important for maintaining a healthy brain." Data from several large studies suggest that seniors who eat the most fruits and vegetables, especially the leafy-green variety, may experience a slower rate of cognitive decline and a lower risk for dementia than meat lovers.

And it may not matter if you get your produce from a bottle instead of a bin. A study from Vanderbilt University found that people who downed three or more servings of fruit or vegetable juice a week had a 76 percent lower risk for developing Alzheimer's disease than those who drank less than a serving weekly.

6 Spice It Up

Your brain enjoys spices as much as your taste buds do. Herbs and spices like black pepper, cinnamon, oregano, basil, parsley, ginger and vanilla are high in antioxidants, which may help build brainpower. Scientists are particularly intrigued by curcumin, the active ingredient in turmeric, common in Indian curries. "Indians have lower incidence of Alzheimer's, and one theory is it's the curcumin," says Black. "It bonds to amyloid plaques that accumulate in the brains of people with the disease." Animal research shows curcumin reduces amyloid plaques and lowers inflammation levels. A study in humans also found those who ate curried foods frequently had higher scores on standard cognition tests.

7 Find Your Purpose

Discovering your mission in life can help you stay sharp, according to a Rush University Medical Center study of more than 950 older adults. Participants who approached life with clear intentions and goals at the start of the study were less likely to develop Alzheimer's disease over the following seven years, researchers found.

8 Get a (Social) Life

Who needs friends? You do! Having multiple social networks helps lower dementia risk, a 15-year study of older people from Sweden's Karolinska Institute shows. A rich social life may protect against dementia by providing emotional and mental stimulation, says Laura Fratiglioni, M.D., Ph.D., director of the institute's Aging Research Center. Other studies yield similar conclusions: Subjects in a University of Michigan study did better on tests of short-term memory after just 10 minutes of conversation with another person.

9 Reduce Your Risks

Chronic health conditions like diabetes, obesity and hypertension are often associated with dementia. Diabetes, for example, roughly doubles the risk for Alzheimer's and other forms of dementia. Controlling these risk factors can slow the tide.

"We've estimated that in people with mild cognitive impairment—an intermediate state between normal cognitive aging and dementia—good control of diabetes can delay the onset of dementia by several years," says Fratiglioni. That means following doctor's orders regarding diet and exercise and taking prescribed medications on schedule.

10 Check Vitamin Deficiencies

Older adults don't always get all the nutrients they need from foods, due to declines in digestive acids or because their medications interfere with absorption. That vitamin deficit—particularly vitamin B_{12}—can also affect brain vitality, research from Rush University Medical Center shows. Older adults at risk of vitamin B_{12} deficiencies had smaller brains and scored lowest on tests measuring thinking, reasoning and memory, researchers found.

Critical Thinking

1. What food that a person consumes seems to reduce the risk of Alzheimer's disease?
2. What is the advantage of an active social life for reducing the person's chances of developing dementia?
3. How does learning new skills reduce the risk of dementia?

Create Central

www.mhhe.com/createcentral

Internet References

Aging with Dignity
  www.aging with dignity.org
The National Council on Aging
  www.ncoa.org

Reprinted from *AARP The Magazine*, February/March 2012, pp. 53–54, 56. Copyright © 2012 by Beth Howard. Reprinted by permission of American Association for Retired Persons (AARP) and Beth Howard. www.aarpmagazine.org 1-888-687-2227.

Article   Prepared by: Elaina F. Osterbur, *Saint Louis University*

Poll: Obesity Hits More Boomers in U.S.

Learning Outcomes

After reading this article, you will be able to:

- Compare the percentage of the current baby-boomer population that is obese with that of people who are younger and older.

- Cite how much more Medicare pays for an obese senior than for one who is at a healthy weight.

Baby boomers say their biggest health fear is cancer. Given their waistlines, heart disease and diabetes should be atop that list, too.

Boomers are more obese than other generations, a new poll finds, setting them up for unhealthy senior years.

And for all the talk of "60 is the new 50" and active aging, even those who aren't obese need to do more to stay fit, according to the Associated Press-LifeGoesStrong.com poll.

Most baby boomers say they get some aerobic exercise, the kind that revs up your heart rate, at least once a week. But most adults are supposed to get 2½ hours a week of moderate-intensity aerobic activity—things like a brisk walk, a dance class, pushing a lawn mower. Only about a quarter of boomers polled report working up a sweat four or five times a week, what the average person needs to reach that goal.

Worse, 37 percent never do any of the strength training so crucial to fighting the muscle loss that comes with aging.

Walking is their most frequent form of exercise. The good news: Walk enough and the benefits add up.

"I have more energy, and my knees don't hurt anymore," says Maggie Sanders, 61, of Abbeville, S.C. She has lost 15 pounds by walking four miles, three times a week, over the past few months, and eating better.

More boomers need to heed that feel-good benefit. Based on calculation of body mass index from self-reported height and weight, roughly a third of the baby boomers polled are obese, compared with about a quarter of both older and younger responders. Only half of the obese boomers say they are regularly exercising.

An additional 36 percent of boomers are overweight, though not obese.

The nation has been bracing for a surge in Medicare costs as the 77 million baby boomers, the post-war generation born from

1946 to 1964, begin turning 65. Obesity—with its extra risk of heart disease, diabetes, high blood pressure and arthritis—will further fuel those bills.

"They're going to be expensive if they don't get their act together," says Jeff Levi of the nonprofit Trust for America's Health. He points to a study that found Medicare pays 34 percent more on an obese senior than one who's a healthy weight.

About 60 percent of boomers polled say they're dieting to lose weight, and slightly more are eating more fruits and vegetables or cutting cholesterol and salt.

But it takes physical activity, not just dieting, to shed pounds. That's especially important as people start to age and dieting alone could cost them precious muscle in addition to fat, says Jack Rejeski of Wake Forest University, a specialist in exercise and aging.

Whether you're overweight or just the right size, physical activity can help stave off the mobility problems that too often sneak up on the sedentary as they age. Muscles gradually become flabbier until people can find themselves on the verge of disability and loss of independence, like a canoe that floats peacefully until it gets too near a waterfall to pull back, Rejeski says.

He led a study that found a modest weight loss plus walking 2½ hours a week helped people 60 and older significantly improve their mobility. Even those who didn't walk that much got some benefit. Try walking 10 minutes at a time two or three times a day, he suggests, and don't wait to start.

"I don't think there's any question the earlier you get started, the better," says Rejeski, who at 63 has given up running in favor of walking, and gets in 30 miles a week. "If you allow your mobility to decline, you pay for it in terms of the quality of your own life."

When it comes to diseases, nearly half of boomers polled worry most about cancer. The second-leading killer, cancer does become more common with aging.

"It's the unknown nature, that it can come up without warning," says Harry Forsha, 64, of Clearwater, Fla., and Mill Spring, N.C.

Heart disease is the nation's No. 1 killer, but it's third in line on the boomers' worry list. Memory loss is a bigger concern.

In fact, more than half of boomers polled say they regularly do mental exercises such as crossword puzzles.

After Harding retires, he plans to take classes to keep mentally active. For now, he's doing the physical exercise that's important for brain health, too. He also takes fish oil, a type of fatty acid that some studies suggest might help prevent mental decline.

Sanders, the South Carolina woman, says it was hard to make fitness a priority in her younger years.

"When you're younger, you just don't see how important it is," says Sanders, whose weight began creeping up when breast cancer in her 40s sapped her energy. Now, "I just know that my lifestyle had to change."

Critical Thinking

1. Why is dieting alone not the most efficient way to lose weight?

2. What is the most efficient way to stave off mobility problems in later life?

3. What is the biggest health problem on the worry list of the baby boomers?

Create Central

www.mhhe.com/createcentral

Internet References

Aging with Dignity
   www.agingwithdignity.org

The Gerontological Society of America
   www.geron.org

The National Council on the Aging
   www.ncoa.org

Article
Prepared by: Elaina Osterbur, *Saint Louis University*

Building the Foundation for Active Aging

Is your organization prepared to address the challenges and opportunities of population aging? This comprehensive and integrated model will guide you in creating a firm foundation for your active-aging efforts—whether it's a first foray into this arena or a longtime pursuit.

COLIN MILNER

Learning Outcomes

After reading this article, you will be able to:

- Identify and define the seven dimensions of wellness.
- Identify and define the nine principles of active aging.
- Discuss the ICAA Model.

Population aging is changing societies on a global level. Our current models have fallen short in addressing both challenges and opportunities presented by this demographic shift. Governments and organizations need new implementable models to address the accompanying wave of change. Globally, active aging is recognized as part of the solution.[1] Why?

Active aging promotes the vision of all individuals—regardless of age, socioeconomic status or health—fully engaging in life within all seven dimensions of wellness: emotional, environmental, intellectual/cognitive, physical, professional/vocational, social, and spiritual.[2]

Research shows that an active lifestyle can lessen the challenges and increase the opportunities associated with population aging.[3] Active aging provides environments, programs, and places that support individuals in living well and taking charge of their health and wellness.

The International Council on Active Aging® (ICAA) has created Nine Principles of Active Aging, a model to guide governments, product and service providers, employers, and the healthcare industry in how they respond to population aging. By implementing and operating by these guiding principles, organizations, and agencies will be able to build a foundation for their efforts and encourage active, engaged living for people of all ages.

It is also essential, when implementing the nine principles, to incorporate the seven dimensions of wellness into each principle. This integration is the "spine," or support structure, of the ICAA Model, and is crucial to meeting the needs, capabilities, expectations, dreams, and desires of the older consumer.

ICAA's Nine Principles of Active Aging

There were 810 million people over age 60 worldwide in 2012.[4] Every week *over one million people around the world turn age 65,* according to Harvard Professor David Bloom, PhD, a world-renowned demographer and economist.[5] Yet, addressing population aging is less about the numbers of older people and more about their diversity. That's why the first principle of active aging is Populations.

> 1. **Populations: The diverse population of older adults requires diverse solutions.**

A lifetime of diverse experiences, and the behaviors they have created, makes the 65-and-over age group an extremely unique segment of the population.[6] These experiences and behaviors impact everything, from where and how people live, to their health status and quality of life. Meeting this group's expectations and needs requires you to understand who they are. Consider, for example, their physical and cognitive abilities; health; age; work or marital status; sex; sexual orientation; race and culture, as well as whether or not they have children or grandchildren, access to transportation, and disposable income. This is why the older-adult market will challenge your creativity, strategic thinking, planning and implementation processes, and why one-size-fits-all solutions fail miserably with these individuals. To address this group, you will first need to establish this group's wants and needs. Once you do so, think about what kinds of products or services you will create and deliver to meet the expectations of this large, diverse market.

A thought to ponder: Is the lack of diversity in your offerings limiting your success?

2. Perceptions: Ageism and negative stereotypes of aging impede an inclusive society.

Aging used to be simple: People were born, moved through childhood into adolescence and adulthood, through midlife into old age (if they lived that long), and then died. They often established a home, a family and a vocation, before retiring to live out their "declining" years. Today, with 30-plus years added to the life span,[3] a new view of aging has emerged—one filled with anticipation and accomplishment. Standing in the way of optimal aging, however, is that familiar foe: ageism. Whether the older adult is viewed as a burden to family and society[7] or as a "superhero," unrealistic perceptions of aging can, and do, have a negative impact on the mental and physical health of this population.[8] The media and marketers use fear-based communications to sell "anti-aging" products and services, driving home the message that aging, a natural process in life, is negative and should be fought every step of the way.[6,9] The reality is we are all aging. And we all will experience old age, if we're lucky enough to live that long.[9]

While negative portrayals and messages of aging are common when marketers and the media address the older market, most of the time this population is practically invisible to them.[10] Only five percent of marketing dollars are spent on individuals over age 50.[10,11] Together with the lack of inclusive, appropriate products, this neglect can make older consumers feel irrelevant, even though they have money to spend.[10]

What the media and marketers miss in all the above is the reality. By addressing the real challenges that older adults face and fulfilling the opportunities they desire for lifelong experiences, you and your organization can significantly impact the self-perception of these consumers and their quality of life,[8] as well as the way others perceive them. To do so requires you and your staff, your organization, and your suppliers to become advocates for this consumer group. How? Promote the message and language of autonomy, while fostering a "can do" attitude among customers. You will see a return on this investment in many ways, from consumer loyalty, to increased business, to a positive position in the greater community.

Of course, to achieve the above, you may also need to address perceptions within your organization. The International Longevity Center in New York points out four categories of ageism: personal, institutional, intentional, and unintentional.[12] Living in an ageist society, we are often unaware of how stereotypes of aging shape our perceptions of older adults. Greater sensitivity begins with increased awareness.

Bottom line, perceptions become reality. The only way to change old perceptions is to create a new reality.

A thought to ponder: What is the societal cost of ageism and exclusion, versus self-empowerment and inclusion?

3. People: Trained and committed individuals are needed to meet the needs of older adults.

With fewer people entering the labor force, and the field of aging in particular,[13] where will your future staff come from? And, how can you ensure they have the expertise needed to meet your consumers' expectations? This challenge exists in large part because of principle number two, Perceptions. Until we change the negative perceptions associated with both aging and working with older adults, we will continue to see a shortage of expertise within our field and within society itself. So how do you implement this principle in your organization? The place to start is with a review of the competency levels of your staff. Keep in mind that people are one of the significant ongoing costs for most organizations. Poor people choices and poor training equal poor results.

Once you have established your staff's current level of expertise, set out to enhance it with additional training and knowledge gathering. Yes, this will cost you money. But incompetent staff will cost you much more over time in terms of lost business, a poor reputation and a disappointing return on investment.

Where should you look for training and knowledge enhancement? Seek out universities, colleges, or certification providers that offer courses geared to working with an older population. Then, make sure these courses focus on active aging and wellness as a way to support independence for older adults. (Training staff with outdated information will do nothing but continue poor results.) You can also partner with associations, governmental groups, and content providers to enhance staff development in areas ranging from communications to programming. In addition, consider seeking out student interns. This may help you build a solid base for future recruitment. No matter which avenues you use, it's vital for your organization to have the right people on staff and the right educational partner.

Still, time waits for no one. Although fewer people in the field of aging presents challenges for organizations that serve this group, it also creates opportunities for those open to exploring alternative solutions. This is highly evident in the field of robotics. From cutting lawns and cleaning pools to building cars and disarming bombs, robots are increasingly used today to perform tasks, even if we do not realize it. Honda's ASIMO, billed as "the world's most advanced humanoid robot," signals what robotics might offer our field.[14] Among its many capabilities, ASIMO can walk, carry things, ascend and descend stairs, and run at speeds of nearly four miles per hour. We can expect to see more of ASIMO in the future, as well as other robotic applications under development to address this shortage of workers. Dare we say it: The rise of the robots has begun.

A thought to ponder: How will this seismic demographic shift impact your organization's staffing, both now and in the future? Are you prepared?

4. Potential: Population aging is creating new economies.

Do you know what an "aged economy" is? According to the United Nations, an aged economy is one in which consumption by older people surpasses that of youth.[4] Thirty years ago, there were no "aged economies" in the world. In 2010, there were 23 such economies, and by 2040, there will be 89.[4]

Within the next four years, age 50-plus American consumers will control 70% of the disposable income in the United States,[11] dominating purchasing decisions for decades to come. For example, in 2010 alone, Boomers and their parents spent over US$3.4 trillion.[15] With this kind of spending power, this group expects you to meet its needs, wants, dreams and desires, if you intend to gain its business.

How can you and your organization benefit from population aging's surge? It comes back to focusing on providing a product or service that interests older adults. From housing to travel, career training to wellness programs and services, there is tremendous potential for organizations that become laser-focused on this market.

If you're wondering if you really need to adopt this focus, ask yourself the following questions:

- *What is the cost of **action?*** What changes will your organization need to make to maximize this opportunity? What will you need to invest in terms of time, energy and money to ensure your optimal return on investment?
- *What is the cost of **inaction?*** How much business might you lose if you take a wait-and-see approach? Will your competitor become the top-of-mind brand?

- *What is the cost of **reaction?*** What will it mean to your organization if you eventually have to make wholesale changes, instead of incremental ones, to address this group's needs?

The real question is: How will you respond to this opportunity?

A thought to ponder: An aged economy will be driven by the expectations that older adults have formed from a lifetime of experiences. This will create major opportunities for businesses that can meet these expectations, and significant challenges for those that can't.

5. Products: Products and services are needed that tailor to older-adult needs.

Many organizations today continue to focus their products and services toward youth, even though American adults ages 18–49 have US$3,000 in their bank accounts, on average.[16] Why? The following three reasons may shed some light:

- Research from the United Nations shows that this lack of interest in the older consumer stems from ageism and a limited understanding of the market.[4]
- Many companies are either unaware of the potential of the changing market and demand for products, or they have failed to respond and adapt.[17]
- A widespread lack of thought exists in this area, resulting in limited availability of goods, products, and services inclusive of, or appropriate for, people in older age groups.[18]

With your competition neglecting this market, where is the opportunity for you? Just look around. Not only is the older-adult population diverse, but so are the opportunities to provide needed solutions and offerings. Virtually every area of business can improve the way they design and deliver products for this market—from more functional furniture to cosmetics and supplements, to wellness (the fifth fastest-growing global segment in the packaged consumer goods industry[19]) and products to improve quality of life. One example: Once seen as a supplement for ailing and frail individuals, one rebranded nutritional drink now promises to help customers maintain bone and muscle. We're also seeing growth in the creation and recognition of Age-friendly Cities, an initiative that guides cities in shaping more accessible, inclusive urban environments for older citizens.[20]

Population aging is causing us to rethink the way we design and deliver products and services. How will you adjust your products or services to better meet the market's expectations?

A thought to ponder: What impact does the current lack of appropriate products and services have on the inclusion of older people in society? As we all grow old, how will this affect you and your family, plus future generations, if left unchanged?

6. Promotions: Older adults are a key market to attract.

Despite the immense purchasing power of adults ages 65-plus, most marketers have yet to take advantage of the opportunity afforded by population aging.[10,11] To gain the business of this group requires first the correct product, then a market effort that can effectively engage it. How can you accomplish this?

Effective promotions and marketing must be rooted in the realities of life for older adults. Messages about anti aging, the "super senior," or the frail, ill family matriarch fail to reflect the reality of today's older population.[9] As a result, older consumers are turned off by marketers' messages that target them, and they tune them out completely.[21]

Shifting today's marketing model to meet your consumer demand can sell product, while inspiring societal change. Here is a question to ask yourself: What do you need to create, or offer, to be a real (authentic), ageless and inclusive brand? And how do you need to communicate it? Your answers will dictate how your customers and community see you, as well as how your staff, partners and vendors view, and interact with, your organization.

A thought to ponder: It all starts with your story and those of your customers, so think about how you can tap into this extensive reservoir of life experience to tell it. Real people, real images and a real story, told in appropriate language, equal real results.

7. Places: Environments must be constructed to enable multiple functional abilities.

The environment(s) that we build or live in are vital to enhancing our quality of life and our life experiences. Environments can encourage, or discourage, people of all ages to lead an active, engaged life.[22,23,24] When it comes to creating compelling environments for your older consumer, think about how to design and build them so they are inclusive of all people and their abilities. Remember principle one: diversity of populations.

One place to start is with a visioning process. Bring together your staff, consumers, vendors, and key partners to share their thoughts on your current or proposed settings, and what they feel will make the environment more compelling. Many times it can be the little things that make a difference. From the colors you choose, to ease of use, and creativity to inclusiveness, how you incorporate details matters.

Another strategic approach is to hire a group of older adults to visit your current place of business and those of your competitors. Ask them to write down what they liked and what they did not. Did the lighting make it easy to see? How were the

bathrooms and locker rooms? Did the front desk, fitness areas, café, and so on enhance the experience or detract from it, and why? What would they change to make the environment more engaging? Once you have gained this market intelligence, create a large storyboard where recommendations, pictures and more can be placed in full view of your staff. (A meeting room or office area is the best location.) Start the process of improvement, and don't stop until you have addressed everything on the board. Then ask the same group to walk through your location again. What are their reactions now? This simple method can help you create a compelling, inclusive, and ageless environment for your business.

A thought to ponder: Environments provide experiences, good and bad, and good experiences create memories that bring consumers back. How will you make your environment(s) compelling?

8. Policies: The human rights of older adults should be protected.

In late 2001 and 2002 the United Nations, the World Health Organization and ICAA defined the concept of active aging.[25,26] Since then, there has been a solid stream of research, conferences, and initiatives that have driven policy change around the world pertaining to active aging. A recent example is the 65th World Health Assembly in Geneva, Switzerland, where a key resolution was passed. This resolution highlighted "strengthening" noncommunicable disease policies to promote active aging in the effort to ensure optimal health and well-being for older adults worldwide.[27]

In Europe, the European Commission and the United Nations Economic Commission for Europe (UNECE) launched the Active Ageing Index. This new statistical tool is designed to assist European Union member governments with assessing how their active-aging policies are working compared to other nations. By establishing this benchmark, countries can address where they fall short in meeting the needs of their older citizens. This Index is an example of how active aging is impacting all levels of government.[28]

In Sao Paolo, Brazil, active aging is at the center of an age-friendly state initiative.[29] Many other cities and regions around the world have embraced this kind of effort, joining the World Health Organization's Age-friendly Cities initiative.[20] In fact, countries are vying for the privilege of being the first age-friendly country in the world.

Bringing this principle back to you, what policies do you have in your organization to ensure inclusivity and respect for the rights of older adults? This includes policies for staff.

A thought to ponder: What policies can you influence within your organization, city, state or country to make a difference?

9. Programs: The seven dimensions of wellness anchor the principles.

Programming possibilities for older adults are limited only by our creativity and our biases—what we believe older adults can (or should) do or not do. The essential elements in programming include the following:

- all of the seven dimensions of wellness;
- adaptation for this group's diverse abilities and health issues, using functional levels;
- engagement that helps customers find and fulfill their purpose in life.

By implementing these three programming elements, you'll keep your customers coming back for more. Let's look at these areas in more detail.

Multidimensional wellness offers you a breadth of programming options to meet the diversity of needs, capabilities, and expectations in the older-adult market. ICAA endorses seven wellness dimensions, as outlined. An overview of each dimension also appears, giving you information to help you implement or augment wellness programing. Keep in mind, though, that wellness is not singular; it is like a good wool suit—best when woven tightly together.

With the seven dimensions of wellness, it's possible to offer a multitude of life-fulfilling opportunities. The benefits can be minimized, however, if your programing does not address consumers' diverse abilities, physical and cognitive, to ensure engagement.

Referring to **ICAA's functional levels** will help you adapt your programing to meet your target group's needs. A sidebar describes these functional levels, which are adapted from the work of Waneen Spirduso, EdD.[30] It summarizes the five levels of physical function, as well as the specific fitness abilities and immediate physical needs of older adults. You'll also find programming goals and areas of focus to help you engage customers.

Finally, **engagement** in life is emerging as a critical indicator of healthy aging. Providing a menu of diverse activities for older adults is an appropriate first step in encouraging an active lifestyle. To engage older adults requires knowing each person as an individual. An exploratory process can help your staff uncover each customer's hopes, past successes and personal goals.

In 2011, an ICAA work group wrote a white paper on engagement, providing the following definition:[31]

Engagement represents a dramatic business shift from traditional programming that is typically rooted in activity theory. Getting to know an individual's life story, desires and dreams requires more time and an additional skill set for staff. For example, an engagement approach positions program and activity directors as personal life coaches. Staff roles would shift from designing and delivering large group programs to the role of "engagement coach" with the purpose of helping each client to live the life that they chose to live. Providing programs and professionals who facilitate engagement is a more complex business model than simply offering older clients things to do.

A thought to ponder: Would it take you further than you are today if you addressed the diverse abilities of your older consumers, physical and cognitive, through an engagement strategy for the wellness experience? If so, what are you waiting for?

A Solid Foundation for Active Aging

We live in a world that is increasingly growing older and more diverse. To address this shift, we too need to become more diverse in the environments we provide, the programs and products we offer, and the way we position and promote these services. We also need to create the policies and hire the staff that will allow customers to feel comfortable in our organizations. By accomplishing this, we will help change perceptions of aging among older adults and within our organizations and communities, enabling us to benefit from the full potential of this market.

The comprehensive, integrated approach described in these pages will help you build a solid foundation for your active-aging efforts, whether it's a first foray into this arena or a long-time pursuit. The first step is always the hardest. But ICAA's Nine Principles of Active Aging are there to guide you along the way.

References

1. Beard, J. R., Biggs, S., Bloom, D. E., et al. (Eds.). (2011). *Global Population Ageing: Peril or Promise.* Geneva, Switzerland: World Economic Forum. Available at http://www.weforum.org/reports/global-population-ageing-peril-or-promise.
2. International Council on Active Aging. The ICAA Model. Retrieved on May 13, 2013, from http://www.icaa.cc/activeagingandwellness.htm.
3. Olshansky, S. J., Beard, J., & Börsch-Supan, A. (2011). The Longevity Dividend: Health as an Investment. Chapter 11 from "III. Pursuing Healthy Ageing: What Healthy Ageing Involves," in: Beard, J. R., Biggs, S., Bloom, D. E., et al. (Eds.). *Global Population Ageing: Peril or Promise.* Geneva, Switzerland: World Economic Forum. Available at www.weforum.org/reports/global-population-ageing-peril-or-promise.

4. United Nations Population Fund (UNFPA) and HelpAge International. (2012). Ageing in the Twenty-First Century: A Celebration and A Challenge. Chapter 1. Available at http://www.unfpa.org/public/home/publications/pid/11584.

5. Milner, C. (2013). Personal communication with David E. Bloom, PhD.

6. Larkin, M. (2011). Tackling Graywashing: What Drives It, How to Recognize and Avoid It. *Journal on Active Aging, 10*(4), 24–33; July/August.

7. Dahmen, N., & Cozma, R. (2009). Media Takes: On Aging. International Longevity Center—USA and Aging Services California. Available at http://www.mailman.columbia.edu/sites/default/files/Media_Takes_On_Aging.pdf.

8. Levy, B., Slade, M., Kunkel, S., & Kasl, S. (2002). Longevity Increased by Positive Self-Perceptions of Ageing. *Journal of Personality and Social Psychology, 83*(2), 261–270.

9. Milner, C., Van Norman, K., & Milner, J. (2011). The Media's Portrayal of Ageing. Chapter 4 from "I. The Backdrop. What We Must Contend with and Why We Must Act Now," in: Beard, J. R., Biggs, S., Bloom, D. E., et al. (Eds.). *Global Population Ageing: Peril or Promise.* Geneva, Switzerland: World Economic Forum. Available at http://www.weforum.org/reports/global-population-ageing-peril-or-promise.

10. Pickett, J. (2002). Marketing and Advertising to Older People. London, United Kingdom: Help the Aged.

11. Nielsen. (2012, August 6). Don't Ignore Boomers—The Most Valuable Consumer. Retrieved on May 13, 2013, from http://www.nielsen.com/us/en/newswire/2012/don%C3%A2%C2%80%C2%99t-ignore-boomers-%C3%A2%C2%80%C2%93-the-most-valuable-generation.html.

12. Anti-Ageism Taskforce at the International Longevity Center. (2006). Ageism in America. New York NY: International Longevity Center—USA. Available at www.mailman.columbia.edu/sites/default/files/Ageism_in_America.pdf.

13. Milner, C. (2012). A New Era: the BOOMing Opportunities of Population Aging. *Journal on Active Aging, 11*(1), 22–29; January/February.

14. Honda. ASIMO. Retrieved on May 13, 2013, from http://asimo.honda.com.

15. AARP. "Mapping the Longevity Economy," a presentation prepared for the 2012 What's Next Boomer Business Summit, March 28, 2012.

16. Fry, R. (2011, November 7). The Rising Age Gap in Economic Well-being. Pew Research Center. Retrieved on May 13, 2013, from http://www.pewsocialtrends.org/2011/11/07/the-rising-age-gap-in-economic-well-being.

17. Ageing Well Network. (2012, June). The New Agenda on Ageing: To Make Ireland the Best Country to Grow Old In. Available at http://www.atlanticphilanthropies.org/learning/report-new-agenda-ageingto-make-ireland-best-country-grow-old.

18. FUTURAGE. (2011). The FUTURAGE Road Map for European Ageing Research. Available at http://futurage.group.shef.ac.uk/road-map.html.

19. Euromonitor. 5 Key Trends for Health and Wellness. Retrieved on October 15, 2012, from http://blog.euromonitor.com/2012/10/5-key-trends-for-health-and-wellness.html.

20. World Health Organization. WHO Global Network of Age-friendly Cities and Communities. Retrieved on May 13, 2013, from http://www.who.int/ageing/age_friendly_cities_network/en.

21. Age Wave. (2006). TV Land's New Generation Gap Study. Available at http://www.agewave.com/research/landmark_tvlandGap.php.

22. White, M. P., Alcock, I., Wheeler, B. W., & Depledge, M. H. (2013). Would You Be Happier Living in a Greener Urban Area? A Fixed-Effects Analysis of Panel Data. *Psychological Science,* ePub ahead of print; doi:10.1177/0956797612464659.

23. National Seniors Productive Ageing Centre (2012, July). Neighbourhood Characteristics: Shaping the Wellbeing of Older Australians. Research Monograph 2. Available at http://www.productiveageing.com.au/userfiles/file/NeighbourhoodCharacteristics.pdf.

24. Inclusive Design for Getting Outdoors (I'DGO). (2012, April 26). Why Does the Outdoor Environment Matter? Available at http://www.idgo.ac.uk/pdf/Intro-leaflet-2012-FINAL-MC.pdf.

25. World Health Organization. (2002). Active Ageing: A Policy Framework. A contribution of the World Health Organization to the Second United Nations World Assembly on Ageing, Madrid, Spain, April 2002. Available at http://whqlibdoc.who.int/hq/2002/WHO_NMH_NPH_02.8.pdf.

26. International Council on Active Aging. History of ICAA. Retrieved on May 13, 2013, from http://www.icaa.cc/about_us/history.htm.

27. World Health Organization. (2012, May 26). News release: 65th World Health Assembly Closes with New Global Health Measures. Retrieved on May 13, 2013, from http://www.who.int/mediacentre/news/releases/2012/wha65_closes_20120526/en/index.html.

28. European Commission and the United Nations Economic Commission for Europe (UNECE). Active Ageing Index. Available at http://www1.unece.org/stat/platform/display/AAI/Active+Ageing+Index+Home.

29. Plouffe, L. A., & Kalache, A. (2011). Making Communities Age Friendly: State and Municipal Initiatives in Canada and Other Countries. *Gaceta Sanitaria, 25*(S), 131–137.

30. Spirduso, W. (2004). *Physical Dimensions of Aging* (second edition). Champaign IL: Human Kinetics.

31. Rogers, K., & Van Norman, K. (2011). The Case for Engagement: A Metric with Meaning for the Active-Aging Industry (ICAA Engagement Work Group discussion summary). International Council on Active Aging white paper. Available at www.icaa.cc/business/whitepapers/engagementstatement.pdf.

Critical Thinking

1. How do you create an age-friendly society?
2. What are some lessons for marketers about competing in the aging economy?

Internet References

Administration on Aging (AoA)
http://www.aoa.gov

International Council on Active Aging
http://www.icaa.cc

COLIN MILNER, founder and CEO of the International Council on Active Aging® (ICAA), is a leading authority on the health and well-being of the older adult. For the past five years, the World Economic Forum has invited Milner to serve on its Network of Global Agenda Councils, recognizing him as one of "the most innovative and influential minds" in the world on aging-related topics. An award-winning writer, he has authored more than 250 articles. Milner is a contributing blogger to the US Department of Health and Human Services' *Be Active Your Way Blog,* and has been published in journals such as *Global Policy.* He also contributed a chapter to the book *Global Population Ageing: Peril or Promise,* published by the Forum in 2011. Milner's speeches have stimulated thousands of business and governmental leaders, industry professionals and older adults worldwide, and inspired a broad spectrum of leading-edge publications to seek his insights. He hosts the *Age-friendly BC Community* video series released in spring 2012 by the British Columbia Ministry of Health.

Article Prepared by: Elaina Osterbur, *Saint Louis University*

The Arts and Health Project
Supporting Healthy Aging Through the Arts

"Community-engaged" arts programs promote health, well-being, and social inclusion for vulnerable older adults.

JENIFER MILNER

Learning Outcomes

After reading this article, you will be able to:

- Discuss how art and recreation affect health and well-being.
- Explain the difference between community-engaged and collaborative arts.
- Identify the benefits of group programs that allow participants to see the work of professionals.

I n the year 2000, as the world contemplated the potential of a new century, Gene D. Cohen, MD, PhD, contemplated the potential of aging. To this potential, as well as damaging myths of aging, Cohen drew the public's attention in his new book *The Creative Age: Awakening Human Potential in the Second Half of Life.*[1] He heralded "a new juncture" in the field of aging—one in which we move beyond studies of *what aging is* to *what is possible with aging.*

"Finally, we are ready to talk about what is possible, not despite aging, but *because* of it," Cohen observed. "There is no denying the problems that accompany aging. But, what has been universally denied is the potential. The ultimate expression of that potential," he wrote, "is creativity."

A geriatric psychiatrist who established the world's first federal research program on mental health and aging and a former acting director of the US National Institute on Aging, Cohen was director of George Washington University's Center on Aging, Health, and Humanities when *The Creative Age* was released. He also held positions at GWU as a professor of psychiatry and a professor of health care sciences. Through his research projects and life's work in the field, the eminent doctor had seen a capacity for creativity in older adults that he felt went unrecognized in society due to negative attitudes toward later life.[1]

To Cohen, creativity was more than simply artistic activity: It was the spark that illuminates the human spirit and ignites the desire to grow.[1] This quality is innate, he believed, adding that ". . . we can use our creativity to shape our lives and, especially as we age, unleash new potential for personal growth and expression."

"Arts and Health" Opens Up New Possibilities

In 2001, an opportunity arose to study the effects of creativity in older adults. As principal investigator for a multisite research project sponsored by the National Endowment for the Arts and others,[2] Cohen evaluated the impact of community-based, professionally led arts programs on health, well-being, and social functioning in older adults. The groundbreaking controlled research, unofficially called the Creativity and Aging Study, revealed a link between creativity and healthier aging.[2,3]

Compared to those in the study's control groups, arts program participants enjoyed better health (both physical and mental) plus increased overall activity when assessed over a two-year period. "These results point to powerful positive intervention effects of these community-based arts programs run by professional artists,"[2] Cohen and colleagues stated. They also concluded that the programs had "true health promotion and disease prevention effects."[2]

For organizations that support health and wellness in older adults, the Creativity and Aging Study suggested another way to make a difference. "The possibilities that opened up were exciting," says Claire Gram, a population health policy consultant at Vancouver Coastal Health (VCH), headquartered in Vancouver, British Columbia.

Since 2006, VCH has partnered with the City of Vancouver Board of Parks and Recreation, as well as community groups and artists, to provide "community-engaged" arts programs to vulnerable and marginalized older adults. A three-year pilot project—"Arts, Health and Seniors: Healthy Aging through the Arts" (AHS)—launched in 2006. Recognizing the project's merits, the partners expanded and extended the project a further three years in 2009, renaming it the "Arts and Health Project: Healthy Aging through the Arts."

According to Gram, VCH has an interest in finding and encouraging programs that support the older population's more vulnerable or marginalized members, which is one reason it initially became involved in the AHS project. As the regional health authority for a geographic area that includes the metropolis of Vancouver and neighboring cities, as well as a good number of Aboriginal and coastal mountain communities, VCH is responsible for delivering health services to more than one million Canadians. Most of these services are community or hospital based, Gram explains, "but we also have a role in public health." Part of this role includes addressing determinants of health—for example, income, racism, education, and sense of identity.

While VCH itself doesn't have a large capacity for older-adult health promotion, "we have a strong tradition of partnering with community health organizations to address things that affect public health and keep people well," Gram continues. "Care at the end of life is a very high percent of our healthcare budget, so the more we can keep people well, the better it is for the individual, for the community, and for the healthcare system."

What the health authority has discovered with its community partners, Gram adds, "is a fairly big gap between services offered for well older adults and those for frail seniors who come into care. Services provided through recreation, for example, are primarily for well individuals." So in 2005, when Gram discovered the Creativity and Aging Study and other developments in arts and health, she began looking into opportunities that might exist at VCH to pursue these programs.

"Fortunately, it was good timing for our SMART Fund," Gram says. As outlined in the Fund's strategic plan, this granting program "invests in innovative, community-based" initiatives that promote and improve health for people who live in the VCH service region.[4] Funded projects "respond to the health needs of vulnerable populations by supporting community capacity-building strategies that demonstrate results." The AHS project fit perfectly with those objectives.

Addressing the Needs of an Aging Population

At Vancouver Board of Parks and Recreation, as in many public sector offices in 2005, staff also were grappling with the needs of the fast-growing older-adult population. In Canada, not only is life expectancy at birth among the highest in the world, but the population is also aging more rapidly than in other developed nations due to the size of the post war Baby Boom.[5] By mid-century, statisticians expect that one in four Canadians will be 65 years of age or older.[6]

For the Park Board, demographics were "the single most significant consideration" in developing the AHS pilot project with VCH, says Margaret Naylor, who works in the Arts, Culture and Environmental Arts Department. Generally speaking, "programming is very limited for older adults," explains Naylor, coordinator of the Arts and Health Project: Healthy Aging through the Arts. "We need to provide a wide variety of programs for older adults, and we need to explore their needs and look for ways to address them."

Because health and well-being become increasingly important issues to people as they age, the initiative's potential to address those things was a major factor, Naylor notes. Also significant, "our definition of recreation is changing," she adds. "We now understand that recreation can be more expansive— for instance, we see the role of the arts in relation to health, and of arts and health in relation to recreation."

In March 2005, before Naylor was involved in the project, her colleague Jil P. Weaving encountered Claire Gram at the first Canadian Arts and Health Forum, held in Vancouver. Weaving, coordinator of arts, culture and environment for the Park Board, is a seasoned artist and cultural worker who has developed numerous community projects and partnerships involving the arts and artists. Unsurprisingly, she was enthusiastic when preliminary results from the Creativity and Aging Study were presented at the forum.

Recognizing this work's promise, Gram and Weaving agreed to explore the possibilities of a local project. "We knew people working in the field were supported by Cohen's study, so we didn't really see the need to do a pilot study just to see if the intervention would work," mentions Gram. "Rather, we wanted to turn it into more of a demonstration of how this approach works in a Canadian setting and in this area, as well as to build capacity to do more such programs."

Gram and Weaving decided that an initiative established by VCH and the Park Board would focus not only on measuring health outcomes, but also on implementing programs to offer older adults "real" hands-on workshop experiences with professional artists. Programs where older adults would engage with the artists as full creative participants in the work they created together—a practice known as community-engaged arts.

A Practice that Encourages Meaningful Participation

According to jil weaving, community-engaged arts programs "are hugely meaningful." "Some community-based arts programs are about individual skill building," she says, "while others are about participating in something that is really the creative work of the artist." While those are all useful projects, community-engaged arts offers a different kind of experience, weaving observes.

With a community-engaged arts practice, "you go into a project with the knowledge that everybody is creative, everybody has individual life knowledge, and these will be absolutely essential to what's created," explains weaving. "The work itself will have elements of this creativity and life knowledge integrated into its very fabric." Respect is a cornerstone of this approach, she stresses—respect for everyone involved and for the knowledge they offer the project.

Because community-engaged arts is not a practice where artists simply bring ideas for participants to realize, it's important that people understand from the start exactly what they're embarking on, weaving continues. "The artist, or the person who fulfills that role, needs to bring together everyone's creativity and life knowledge, so the collaborative work of the participants communicates beyond the group. That's a complex thing to do," she adds. "And that's why you need an artist whose heart is engaged in this kind of process."

Collaborative Approach Supports Participants and Programs

With the goal of establishing a community-engaged arts initiative in the Vancouver area, VCH and the Park Board consulted widely with local community associations, seniors groups, and other stakeholders for about a year, relates Margaret Naylor. This input helped in developing a plan to get the initiative underway in fall 2006.

According to a 2012 report,[7] partnerships were set up with several community organizations that serve older adults to deliver separate arts programs at four community centers in Vancouver and North Vancouver. Programs provided through these partnerships have aimed to strengthen the health, wellness and social inclusion of vulnerable older adults. While participant numbers have ebbed and flowed, 51 people took part in the AHS programs consistently over the initial three-year term. These participants ranged in age from 55 to 90 years, with women making up a large majority (80%). At three pilot sites, individuals "faced some form of barrier or marginalization beyond age, including language barriers, stigma related to sexual orientation, and/or economic challenges."[7]

Program participants are encouraged to work with each other and with professional artists on ideas that they consider important "and [represent] seniors in a fuller way to the community at large."[7] At the six program sites that currently exist, individuals have collaborated on writing (also digital photography, video, and theater); puppet theater, storytelling and dance; painting and drawing; mixed media arts; writing and digital video; and choral singing.

Each site's project team consists of a professional artist, an associate artist (in some cases, a co-lead artist), and a seniors'/community worker. The artists are responsible for developing programming and working with participants in weekly two-hour workshops that run from approximately September to June each year. The seniors' worker undertakes "organizational and administrative tasks," plus provides "social and cultural support."[7]

For example, at Strathcona Community Centre, Seniors' Worker Liza Tam was heavily involved at the program's start in recruiting participants among the area's Chinese-speaking elders. Previous attempts to offer arts programming in the area had largely failed due to insufficient interest from the community. When Tam approached people about the AHS arts program, they proved reluctant to participate, so she focused her pitch on health instead. In addition, she approached seniors programmers and other seniors programs to explain the benefits of participation. The health angle reframed the program in people's minds and a group of elders enrolled as participants. The program's overall success—and its ongoing popularity—can be traced to that initial recruiting result and the enthusiastic word-of-mouth by participants that followed.

Critical Components Enrich Overall Impact

Among other activities supported by the AHS pilot, now the Arts and Health Project, participants enjoy occasional arts experiences that allow them to see the work of professional artists in disciplines related to their group's work. In addition, the groups have public performances and exhibitions of their own work. An end-of-year showcase is the highlight. Members of all the groups gather together at the Park Board's Roundhouse Community Arts and Recreation Centre, where they show their work to peers, family and friends, and members of the community.

"We think it's essential that these works are performed or installed or exhibited," states jil weaving. "They are intended to extend beyond participants in a way that any artwork 'creates beyond its creator.' Public performances and exhibitions provide opportunities for others who haven't been involved in making these works to engage with them and the ideas they express. And that is why it's important for these programs to support creative, meaningful and communicative work that benefits the community."

Another critical project activity is the Arts and Health Community of Practice (CoP). Together with steering committee members, artists, seniors' workers and other staff from project sites participate in monthly meetings, where they discuss a wide range of topics. They also offer each other emotional and professional support. The original goal when the CoP formed was "to share newly acquired knowledge and to collectively and creatively address issues and situations that arose at the different project sites,"[7] the project report shows.

For VCH's Claire Gram, the CoP is at the heart of the arts and health initiative. "It builds knowledge and ability within the community—the competencies for successful implementation," she says. "From the start, we had this vision for a broader application."

Research Reveals and Reinforces Benefits

In addition to a capacity-building component, VCH, and the Park Board always intended the AHS project to include research. They turned to researchers from the University of British Columbia (UBC), also located in Vancouver, who agreed to partner with the project. "It was pretty clear that the group was inspired by Gene Cohen's study and envisioned a similar kind of evaluation," says Principal Investigator Alison Phinney, PhD, associate professor in the UBC School of Nursing. But the two projects differed in some significant ways, which the research would need to reflect.

"Cohen's research study was multisite, had a lot of funding, and evaluated three arts programs that had been ongoing," explains Phinney. In contrast, the Vancouver program was new, "and the evaluation structure could be integrated from the start." Health outcomes would be only one part of the project's evaluation as well. Other planned components included process evaluation, reports from participants, and the CoP.

The project's six months lead time and lack of research funding presented challenges, according to Phinney, who scrambled to pull together a research study that would not only measure health outcomes, but would also work quickly and inexpensively. According to the project report, quantitative tools were selected "with pre- and post questionnaires to measure aspects of physical well-being, emotional well-being, and social inclusion."[7] To "enrich the quantitative data," qualitative research would include focus groups and feedback.

In the end, the researchers were able to replicate Cohen's study (although on a small scale, Phinney points out), and illuminate the benefits of a real-world community-engaged

arts intervention. Study results showed that participants had "improved physical well-being, higher degrees of social inclusion, increased confidence and an enhanced sense of accomplishment."[7]

Phinney calls the quantitative results "compelling," particularly in the area of social inclusion. "The participants' sense of community and belonging was powerfully impacted," she says, a finding that she believes dovetails with the whole premise of community-engaged arts. Qualitative research supported these results. What was unexpected, and in-sightful, however, was how participants reacted to some of the questions on the survey. Many individuals objected to these questions, calling them "insulting," "hurtful" or senseless, according to the report.[7]

VCH's Claire Gram sheds some light: "The research we need to show for funding focuses on proving how vulnerable older adults are, but that undermines the nature of the programming itself. Participation is aimed at building people's confidence, self-esteem and self-efficacy," she says. "Quantitative research doesn't begin to explain the experience for them."

Participants had the chance to clarify what the AHS programs had brought into their lives in the focus group discussions. There, four common themes emerged, which the report summarizes as below:[7]

- "The program provided opportunities to develop social connections and foster a sense of belonging for the participants. This happened both within the AHS project and within the larger community."
- "The art projects provided seniors with an opportunity to engage in a challenging and valuable experience that led to a sense of confidence and a stronger sense of identity for participants."
- "The seniors experienced a level of discipline and focus that enabled them to engage in other activities that promote health."
- "The seniors involved in the program expressed the ability to find new ways to engage creatively and to gain a sense of accomplishment as artists."

The last finding seems to validate the personal promise of creativity and aging in community-engaged arts. Individuals in later life who don't believe they're creative, come to recognize this ability in themselves by participating in these programs, and they learn new ways to express themselves.

Project Focus Moves to Broader Dissemination

The Arts and Health Project is moving into a new phase in 2013, with the long-term goal of broader program dissemination. The existing six project sites "will graduate from financial funding at the end of 2012," notes the Park Board's Margaret Naylor. To prepare the organizers, "we've been working with them on developing grant-writing skills and exploring ways in which they can implement their programming in a sustainable way." While the financial relationship will end, sites will still participate in both the Arts and Health Community of Practice and the year-end showcase.

Moving forward, the plan is to choose two or more new sites every year (subject to funding) for a four-year mentorship. According to Naylor, "We'll work closely with organizational partners to build their capacity for community-engaged arts practice, work with seniors' workers and older adults, share lessons learned about programming, and finance these sites' programs for three years." As with the existing sites, the financial relationship will then end, but the professional relationship will continue.

In the past year, the British Columbia Recreation and Parks Association (BCRPA) has become the Arts and Health Project's fiscal agent, Naylor continues. BCRPA's broader geographical reach will allow project sites to be developed within the province, beyond the Vancouver area, she says. And with the association involved, the project's professional development capabilities will expand. Naylor mentions online learning tools, capacity-building workshops and a dedicated project website, expected to go live later next year.

What truly supports the Arts and Health Project, though, is the passionate conviction of all the people taking part in the project. "We all recognize that these community-engaged arts programs provide such positive experiences," states Naylor. "Older adults who take part have a new network of colleagues, which they value tremendously. Many feel healthier and better about themselves, and have become more active in their lives— something they usually attribute to the confidence they've gained from participating. People also feel like their relationships are stronger with their families and with the community at large."

Most significantly, Naylor adds, "participants believe that they are not only contributing to their culture by telling their stories, but they are also changing the way their culture understands older people and aging. And they feel that that's an important role for them to be playing in the community."

References

1. Cohen, G. D. (2000). *The Creative Age: Awakening Human Potential in the Second Half of Life.* New York: HarperCollins.
2. Center on Aging, Health and Humanities, George Washington University. (2006). Creativity and Aging Study: The Impact of Professionally Conducted Cultural Programs on Older Adults, April 2006 report (executive summary). Retrieved on October 15, 2012, from http://www.gwumc.edu/cahh/NEA_Study_Final_Report.pdf.
3. Cohen, G. D., Perlstein, S., Chapline, J., et al. (2006). The Impact of Professionally Conducted Cultural Programs on the Physical Health, Mental Health and Social Functioning of Older Adults. *The Gerontologist, 46*(6), 726–734. Retrieved on October 15, 2012, from http://www.gwumc.edu/cahh/TG-Creativity&Aging.pdf.
4. Vancouver Coastal Health. (2009, November). SMART Fund Strategic Plan 2009–2014. Retrieved on October 15, 2012, from http://www.smartfund.ca/docs/smart_strategic_plan.pdf.
5. Statistics Canada, Demography Division. (2008). Canadian Demographics at a Glance, p. 30. Catalogue no. 91-003-XWE. Retrieved on October 16, 2012, from http://www.statcan.gc.ca/pub/91-003-x/91-003-x2007001-eng.pdf.
6. Human Resources and Skills Development Canada. Canadians in Context—Aging Population. Retrieved on October 15, 2012, from http://www4.hrsdc.gc.ca/.3ndic.1t.4r@-eng.jsp?iid=33.
7. Phinney, P., Pickersgill, M., Naylor, M., et al. (2012). The Arts, Health and Seniors Project: A Three Year Exploration of the Relationship between Arts and Health.

Critical Thinking

1. What are some of the outcome goals of the AHS Project research?
2. What advice did the interviewees provide for organizations considering arts programs?

Internet References

City of Vancouver Board of Parks and Recreation: Arts and Health Project
http://vancouver.ca/parks-recreation-culture/arts-and-health-project.aspx

George Washington University's Center on Aging, Health and Humanities
www.gwumc.edu/cahh

National Endowment for the Arts: Arts in Aging
www.arts.gov/resources/accessibility/artsnAging_top.html

JENIFER MILNER is editor-in-chief of the *Journal on Active Aging.*® A former cultural worker, Milner has written numerous articles on the benefits of arts activities in various settings and for different populations.

Article   Prepared by: Elaina F. Osterbur, *Saint Louis University*

Age and Gender Effects on the Assessment of Spirituality and Religious Sentiments (ASPIRES) Scale: A Cross-Sectional Analysis

I. TUCKER BROWN ET AL.

Learning Outcomes

After reading this article, you will be able to:

- Discuss the Assessment of Spirituality and Religious Sentiments (ASPIRES) Scale.

- Identify the age and gender effects suggested by the ASPIRES Scale.

- Discuss the differing religious styles among younger and older generations.

A substantive and growing body of empirical research demonstrates the salience of spirituality and religiousness as stand-alone psychological constructs (Hill & Pargament, 2008; Hill et al., 2000; Kapuscinski & Masters, 2010; McCullough, Enders, Brion, & Jain, 2005; Piedmont, Ciarrocchi, Dy-Liacco, & Williams, 2009; Slater, Hall, & Edwards, 2001). In the early debate on the relevance and application of these numinous dimensions, some researchers posited that they were better accounted for by already existent, underlying psychological processes (Buss, 2002; Van Wicklin, 1990). In an effort to validate the empirical and practical significance, if not existence, of these constructs (e.g., that they are causal inputs as opposed to outcomes), research in the psychology of religion and spirituality has centered on their construct validity. For example, Piedmont (2004, 2005) has focused on establishing spirituality's unique predictive power over and above the Five-Factor Model of personality (FFM), as well as showing statistically significant correlations with a variety of psychosocial markers (Piedmont et al., 2009).

Studies of this sort, although necessary, are only as robust as the sound psychometric properties of the instruments used to measure the targeted spiritual and religious variables. There is clearly a need for more rigorously developed and conceptually anchored measures in the field (e.g., Kapuscinski & Masters, 2010). The Assessment of Spirituality and Religious Sentiments (ASPIRES; Piedmont, 2010) scale was developed to meet the need for an empirically sound instrument, based on a psychological model of personality, that articulates relevant and robust numinous qualities. Indeed, studies employing the ASPIRES—a 35-item scale measuring two independent though correlated psychological dimensions, Spiritual Transcendence and Religious Sentiments—showed that spirituality and religiousness: (a) function as motivational variables; (b) are both independent of established models of personality; (c) reflect different, yet interrelated, psychological systems; (d) exhibit potential causal influences on a variety of significant psychosocial outcomes; and (e) demonstrate conceptual and structural invariance across religious denominations and cultures (see Chen, 2011; Piedmont, 1999, 2004, 2005, 2007; Piedmont et al., 2009; Piedmont & Leach, 2002; Rican & Janosova, 2010).

Although interest in scale development garners much attention in the research literature (cf. Hill & Pargament, 2008; Hill et al., 2000; Kapuscinski & Masters, 2010), evaluation of how these numinous constructs evolve over the life span, and between genders, represent areas requiring further empirical investigation (Seifert, 2002). Though there are theoretical and empirical models based on the hypothesis that individuals experience systematic changes in levels of spirituality and religiousness over the course of their lives (e.g., Argue, Johnson, & White, 1999; Dalby, 2006; Dillon, Wink, & Fay, 2003; Ingersoll-Dayton, Krause, & Morgan, 2002; Koenig, McGue, & Iacono, 2008; Wink & Dillon, 2002, 2008), relatively few empirical studies have used standardized and cross-culturally validated measures, such as the ASPIRES.

Studies examining changes in spirituality and religiousness over time and between genders have been, for the most part, grounded in personality theory and research. This rigorous background of psychological inquiry has established a sound foundation upon which to advance emergent theory and social scientific investigation (cf. Piedmont, 2005). The vast majority of age and gender effects designs are based on data taken from single-item responses (e.g., "Are you spiritual" and "How often do you pray") and recoded interview segments contained within much broader sets of self-report measures primarily intended to assess other aspects of psychological functioning (e.g., Argue et al., 1999; Dillon et al., 2003; Good, Willoughby, & Busseri, 2011; McCullough et al., 2005; McCullough & Laurenceau, 2005; McCullough, Tsang, & Brion, 2003; Wink & Dillon, 2002, 2003).

Wink and Dillon (2002, 2008) collated longitudinal data evaluating the role of spirituality and religiousness across a life span of over 60 years. Drawing from a sample of more than 200 participants born in the 1920s, Wink and Dillon examined the development and expression of these numinous dimensions from young adulthood through old age. Their findings suggested that levels of spirituality increased significantly over the course of the life span, especially from middle to late adulthood, with women evidencing a higher level of spirituality than men. Men's spirituality, however, showed a more significant increase than women's from early to middle adulthood. For women, a high level of spirituality in late adulthood was related to the number of negative life events experienced in middle adulthood, most notably financial strain and spousal and parental conflicts.

Drawing from data collected in the Terman Longitudinal Study of high ability children, McCullough, Enders, Brion, and Jain (2005) identified three reliable models of religious experience, each with a unique arc or trajectory over time. There were individuals who scored low on religiousness in youth and remained low throughout their lives (i.e., homeostatic). A second group scored high on religiousness in youth and remained high longitudinally. Finally, there was a group that expressed a moderate level of religiousness in youth with an increase into middle adulthood and then a decrease in late life (i.e., nonlinear relationship).

These longitudinal studies were all limited in that they did not use standardized measures of spirituality and religiousness. Rather, they relied on an amalgam of available surveys and interview data. Without clear validity for scores on these indices, regardless of the sophistication of the statistical analyses used in the design, the meaning of the purported relationships across time and between genders cannot be reliably substantiated (cf. Brennan & Mroczek, 2003).

Despite these limitations, the longitudinal designs reviewed here suggest three plausible theoretical perspectives by which to approach potential age effects on spirituality and religiousness across the life span: (a) homeostasis, (b) increasing relevance, and (c) nonlinear relationship. According to the homeostatic model, levels of spirituality and religiousness stay the same from early to late life. In the increasing relevance approach, spirituality and religiousness rise steadily, in a linear fashion, throughout human development. From the perspective of a nonlinear relationship, it is hypothesized that levels of spirituality

and religiousness change by some combination of increase, decrease, and period of plateau, although the sequencing of these changes is not clearly identified. Taken as a whole, these longitudinal data demonstrate that levels of spirituality and religiousness may not be static across the life span.

Although the research literature suggests age- and gender-related effects for numinous constructs, little is known about the *content* that evolves in spirituality and religiousness over time and between genders. In other words, as people age and their experiences of their world evolve, does their understanding of what spirituality and religiousness mean also change? Is spirituality defined and understood differently for older and younger individuals? Answers to these questions have important implications for the assessment of numinous constructs. If peoples' understanding of the numinous changes, or if men and women experience the numinous differently, then there would be a need to develop instruments that capture these differences. It may be possible that scale scores that are valid for one age group, or one gender, may not be valid in another age group or for a different gender. Spirituality would need to be considered an evolving characteristic adaptation that works out of the changing life experiences of people. However, if it can be established that despite mean level changes in scores the underlying structure of the scale remains unchanged over time, then a strong case can be made for the numinous as a cohesive, common, dispositional aspect of human functioning.

The purpose of this study was twofold. First, the study intended to determine whether the observed gender and age effects noted in numerous longitudinal studies would be evidenced on the ASPIRES, a psychometrically sound, cross-culturally validated measure of spirituality and religiousness. As noted above, many longitudinal studies have relied on post hoc-developed indices of religiousness and spirituality that often differed across the assessment intervals. The lack of a single standardized measure suggests that the observed age effects may have been due to differences in instrumentation across the assessment intervals and not to real changes in the construct. Finding age and gender effects in the ASPIRES would add more confidence to the findings of the longitudinal studies. Second, this study sought to determine whether the underlying factor structure of the ASPIRES was consistent across both age and gender groups. Do people of different ages come to understand the numinous in significantly different ways? Or, is there an underlying understanding of the numinous that is constant across the life span? Thus, do mean level changes in scores reflect the varying salience of the numinous over time or fundamental changes in how the transcendent is understood and experienced?

This study offers a first step in evaluating the effects of age and gender on a *standardized* measure of spirituality and religiousness, in a cross-sectional sample. Furthermore, it allows for a first look at the structural nature (i.e., intrinsic meaning and factorial integrity) of the ASPIRES scales among age and gender groups. In so doing it sheds light on how spirituality and religiousness may operate in similar or different ways, both broadly and with respect to age and gender.

Method

Participants

Participants consisted of 1,539 women and 698 men, ranging in age from 17 to 94 ($M = 30$ years). Of these, 47% were Caucasian, 22% Asian, 6% Hispanic, 2% African American, 1% Middle Eastern, and 11% indicated other. Concerning faith tradition, 90% indicated a Christian tradition, 4% were Jewish, 2% were atheist/agnostic, 2% were Muslim, Buddhist, or Hindu, and 2% indicated "other." Concerning age, 1,603 individuals were between 17 and 29, 357 between 30 and 60, and 277 were between 61 and 94. These individuals represented a sample of convenience obtained from one of four locations: Maryland/Washington, DC area, Massachusetts/New Hampshire, Mississippi, and Illinois. All subjects volunteered. This sample consists of approximately 75% of the current normative sample (N = 2,999) for the ASPIRES. For more information about the normative sample see Piedmont (2010).

Measures

Assessment of Spirituality and Religious Sentiments (ASPIRES)

Developed by Piedmont (2010), this 35-item scale measures two major numinous dimensions: Spiritual Transcendence, the motivational capacity to create a broad sense of personal meaning for one's life; and Religious Sentiments, the extent to which an individual is involved in and committed to the precepts, teachings, and practices of a specific religious tradition. Spiritual Transcendence is measured by three correlated facet scales: Prayer Fulfillment (PF), the ability to create a personal space that enables one to feel a positive connection to some larger reality; Universality (UN), the belief in a larger meaning and purpose to life; and Connectedness (CN), feelings of belonging and responsibility to a larger human reality that cuts across generations and groups. Religious Sentiments consists of two correlated dimensions, Religious Involvement (RI), which reflects how actively involved a person is in performing various religious rituals and activities; and Religious Crisis (RC) which examines whether a person may be experiencing problems, difficulties, or conflicts with the God of their understanding.

Piedmont (2010) presented information on the reliability and validity of this scale. Alpha reliabilities for the self-report scales ranged from .60 (CN) to .95 (PF) with a mean alpha of .82. Structurally, the Spiritual Transcendence Scale (STS) consists of three correlated dimensions respectively defined by the items of the PF, UN, and CN subscales. The Religious Sentiments dimension was shown to have two subscales, which consisted of the items of the RI and RC scales. Scores on these scales were shown to predict significantly a range of psychosocial outcomes (e.g., well-being, self-esteem, prosocial behavior, social support, and sexual attitudes), even after the predictive effects of personality were removed. Support for the structural, predictive, and incremental validity of the ASPIRES has been demonstrated across religious faiths, cultures, and languages (Piedmont, 2007; Piedmont & Leach, 2002; Piedmont, Werdel, & Fernando, 2009; Rican & Janosova, 2010).

Procedure

The subjects in this study were the extant normative sample of the ASPIRES as of June, 2009. The ASPIRES manual contains all relevant descriptive information about this sample (Piedmont, 2010). Although overall gender and age effects have been conducted on the ASPIRES scales (and reflects why scores on the scale are normed on the basis of age and gender), no effort has been made to systematically study how scores change over time and whether the factor structures of the scales remain unchanged across these different demographic groups.

Results

A one-way MANOVA was conducted using gender as the independent variable and total STS, Religious Involvement, and Religious Crisis scores as the outcome criteria. A significant multivariate effect was found [Wilks $\Lambda = .975$, multivariate $F(3, 2225) = 19.30, p < .001$]. Univariate analyses indicated that women scored significantly higher ($M = 84.05$) than men ($M = 80.48$) on overall Spiritual Transcendence [$F(1, 2229) = 34.16, p < .001, \eta^2 = .02$], and men scored significantly higher ($M = 7.70$) than women ($M = 7.21$) on Religious Crisis [$F(1, 2229) = 13.13, p < .001, \eta^2 = .01$]. No difference was found for Religious Involvement scores.

Testing for Nonlinear Age Effects

A polynomial regression analysis was performed to examine the presence of nonlinear age effects on these three outcome variables. Three polynomial multiple regression analyses were conducted using each of the ASPIRES scale scores as the dependent variable. Using a hierarchical entry approach, age, its square, and cube were entered (which evaluate the presence of linear, quadratic, and cubic associations, respectively). Results indicated a significant quadratic effect for age on Total STS [$\Delta R^2 = .05, F(1, 2234) = 120.50, p < .001$, partial $\eta^2 = .13$], Religious Involvement [$\Delta R^2 = .04, F(1, 2234) = 93.62, p < .001$, partial $\eta^2 = .21$], and Religious Crisis [$\Delta R^2 = .01, F(1, 2233) = 22.22, p < .001$, partial $\eta^2 = .03$]. Based on theory drawn from life span and personality development, age was partitioned into three groupings (i.e., 17–29, 30–60, 61–94). Figure 1 presents how scores on the ASPIRES scales vary across these age groupings.[1]

To examine these mean level differences among the age groups, a one-way ANOVA was performed using age category as the independent variable and the ASPIRES scale scores as the outcomes. A significant age effect was noted on total STS scores [$F(2, 2234) = 148.87, p < .001, \eta^2 = .12$] and the LSD post hoc test indicated that STS scores were significantly higher in the middle adulthood group (i.e., 46–55) than in the early adulthood or old age cohorts. However, STS scores for the eldest group still were significantly higher than for the

---

[1] In examining the facet scales for the STS domain, significant quadratic effects were found for age on the Prayer Fulfillment [$\Delta R^2 = .04, F(1, 2234) = 91.94, p < .001$, partial $\eta^2 = .09$] and Universality [$\Delta R^2 = .06, F(1, 2234) = 164.85, p < .001$, partial $\eta^2 = .17$] facet scales. The patterns of effect mirrored that presented for the overall STS score. No age effects, linear or otherwise, were found for Connectedness.

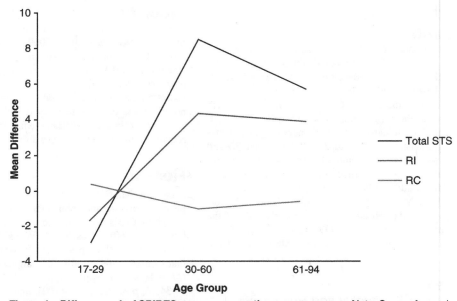

Figure 1   Differences in ASPIRES scores across three age groups.   Note: Scores for each scale are portrayed as each age group's difference from its respective overall group mean.

youngest group (see Figure 1). Concerning Religious Involvement scores, a significant age effect was also noted, $F(2, 2234) = 239.39$, $p < .001$, $\eta^2 = .18$. A post hoc analysis indicated that scores were significantly higher in the middle adulthood group and then stabilized in the old age cohort. Scores for the eldest group were not significantly different from the middle aged group, but they were significantly higher than the youngest group. A significant age effect was also found for Religious Crisis, $F(2, 2233) = 37.39$, $p < .001$, $\eta^2 = .03$. Scores were high in the early adulthood group and were significantly lower for the other two age cohorts, with the middle-aged and eldest groups being significantly lower than the youngest group, although these two groups did not differ between themselves.

To examine whether gender and age interact, a 2 (men vs. women) $\times$ 3 (age grouping) MANOVA was conducted using total STS, Religious Involvement, and Religious Crisis scores as the dependent variables. No significant interactions were found. Thus, age and gender operated as additive effects in influencing scores on the ASPIRES. The effects of gender and age were examined separately in this report.

Structural Invariance

A series of structural equation models (SEM) were conducted to determine the extent to which the putative factor structure of the STS and Religious Sentiments scales were recoverable across the different age and gender groups. LISREL 8.72 was used for these analyses. The STS scale was hypothesized to consist of three positively correlated facet scales, constituting the PF, UN, and CN dimensions. With regards to the Religious Sentiments domain, the RI and RC scales should represent two distinct, negatively correlated scales. These structures were examined within each age and gender group. The results of these analyses are presented in Table 1. As can be seen, the putative normative structure was clearly obtained in each instance. The weakest findings were obtained for the middle-aged and elderly groups on the Religious Sentiments domain. The overall structure of the scale remained consistent across age and gender groups.

In order to determine whether each dimension was similarly defined by its respective items, a series of confirmatory factor analyses (CFA) were conducted for each numinous domain across the gender and age groups. For the STS domain, three correlated factors were extracted and rotated, Although for the RS domain two correlated factors were extracted and rotated. The resulting pattern loadings from each analysis were then compared both to normative pattern loadings presented in Piedmont (2010) and among the various age and gender groups using congruence coefficients (CC). CCs determine the extent to which two sets of factor loadings on the same items across two groups are identical. Unlike a simple correlation coefficient which evaluates pattern similarity, CCs evaluate similarity in terms of both pattern and magnitude of loadings and are thus, the preferred method for examining profile similarity (see Gorsuch, 1983, pp. 284–288 for a fuller discussion of this index). The null distribution of CCs was determined by conducting a series of Monte Carlo studies that generated random loadings which were then compared with the normative values for both the STS and RS domains. A set of 10,000 iterations was conducted and the 95th, 99th, and 99.9th percentiles in each distribution of CCs were identified. An observed CC was determined to be significant if its value exceeded these cut-off values produced in the null distribution.

Age and Gender Effects on the Assessment of Spirituality and Religious Sentiments (ASPIRES) Scale by I. Tucker Brown et al.

49

Table 1 SEM Results Testing the Factor Structure of the ASPIRES Scales across the Age and Gender Groups

	χ^2	df	RMSEA	SRMR	NFI	CFI	GFI
Spiritual transcendence							
Age group							
Young[a]	184.21	104	.02	.04	.99	1.00	.99
Middle[b]	339.60	207	.04	.05	.96	.98	.92
Elder[c]	224.42	207	.02	.06	.94	.98	.89
Gender							
Men[d]	698.61	196	.06	.05	.96	.97	.92
Women[e]	1,161.86	185	.06	.04	.98	.98	.94
Religious sentiments							
Age group							
Young[a]	100.86	35	.03	.02	.99	1.00	.99
Middle[b]	94.05	41	.08	.06	.95	.97	.93
Elder[c]	165.64	45	.10	.09	.96	.97	.90
Gender							
Men[d]	76.68	39	.04	.02	.99	1.00	.98
Women[e]	115.90	36	.04	.02	.99	1.00	.99
Desired values			<.10	<.10	>.90	>.90	>.90

Note. RMSEA = Root Mean Square Error of Approximation; SRMR = Standardized Root Mean Residual; NFI = Normed Fit Index; CFI = Comparative Fit Index; GFI = Goodness of Fit Index.

[a] n = 1,608. [b] n = 359. [c] n = 270. [d] n = 1,534. [e] n = 697.

Table 2 presents the results of these analyses. Each age group was compared with the normative factor loadings as well as to each other. Similar analyses were done for gender. All resulting CCs were statistically significant indicating that the factor structure of the ASPIRES was identical across both age and gender groups. Table 3 presents the actual pattern loadings for each ASPIRES item on its respective factor across the identified age and gender groups. For comparison, normative values are also presented. As can be seen, each item on the ASPIRES loaded on its respective domain similarly across the age and gender groups. Although there are some anomalous loadings (e.g., the loading for item CN6 for the "young" group; the loadings for UN1, UN4, and UN5 for the "middle age" group), the values are quite consistent and compare very

Table 2 Congruence Coefficients for Age and Gender Comparisons for all ASPIRES Scales

	ASPIRES Scale				
Comparison	PF	UN	CN	RI	RC
Young[a]	.99	.95	.87	.99	.95
Middle[b]	.97	.76	.83	.99	.92
Elder[c]	.99	.85	.80	.97	.93
Female[d]	.99	.99	.99	.99	.95
Male[e]	.97	.97	.97	.99	.97
Gender	.95	.95	.95	1.00	1.00
Age 1	.97	.67	.59	.99	.98
Age 2	.98	.84	.78	.98	.99
Age 3	.97	.82	.65	.98	.97

Note. Each of these groups were compared with normative data (Piedmont, 2010); Gender = the congruence coefficients between men (n = 698) and women (n = 1,533); Age 1 = the congruence coefficients between young (n = 1,603) and middle age (n = 357) groups; Age 2 = congruence between young and elder (n = 277) groups; Age 3 = congruence between middle aged and elder groups. PF = Prayer Fulfillment; UN = Universality; CN = Connectedness; RI = Religious Involvement; RC = Religious Crisis. All coefficients are significant at p < .001.

[a] N = 1,608. [b] N = 359. [c] N = 270. [d] N = 1,534. [e] N = 697.

Table 3 Pattern Loadings for Each ASPIRES Item on its Respective Factor for Each Age and Gender Group

ASPIRES item	Young	Middle age	Elderly	Men	Women	Norms
PF1	.67	.75	.81	.63	.72	.73
PF2	.63	.74	.62	.64	.63	.61
PF3	.72	.57	.57	.78	.69	.78
PF4	.78	.73	.76	.77	.83	.81
PF5	.75	.77	.80	.73	.76	.76
PF6	.87	.77	.77	.83	.88	.86
PF7	.86	.72	.75	.86	.83	.86
PF8	.84	.84	.85	.82	.86	.81
PF8	.84	.64	.81	.80	.86	.83
PF10	.72	.70	.78	.76	.75	.73
UN1	.57	.26	.61	.54	.59	.66
UN2	.69	.76	.75	.45	.84	.75
UN3	.58	.61	.50	.30	.76	.59
UN4	.43	.28	.43	.66	.40	.69
UN5	.61	.27	.38	.50	.59	.66
UN6	.40	.56	.59	.25	.64	.57
UN7	.52	.60	.58	.40	.64	.62
CN1	−.12	.00	.01	−.15	−.06	.00
CN2	.79	.63	.61	.74	.82	.82
CN3	.78	.63	.67	.77	.82	.75
CN4	.49	.72	.32	.40	.59	.57
CN5	.26	.27	.63	.33	.24	.34
CN6	.01	.52	.57	.06	.22	.31
RC1	.80	.85	.81	.85	.83	.84
RC2	.70	.80	.76	.76	.78	.77
RC3	.77	.77	.84	.84	.77	.79
RC4	.80	.80	.83	.82	.84	.83
RC5	.83	.70	.86	.85	.83	.83
RC6	.83	.62	.76	.84	.80	.83
RC7	.75	.87	.80	.80	.78	.79
RC8	.43	.39	.55	.54	.46	.53
RS1	.85	.75	.93	.83	.84	.84
RS2	.85	.85	.90	.84	.87	.86
RS3	.81	.71	.71	.81	.80	.80
RS4	.55	.60	.33	.47	.54	.50

Note. PF = Prayer Fulfillment; UN = Universality; CN = Connectedness; RI = Religious Involvement; RC = Religious Crisis.

well to normative values. The items for the two Religious Sentiments and the Prayer Fulfillment scales evidenced the greatest levels of consistency. Despite significant mean level differences in scores across the different age cohorts and between genders, the underlying factor structure was invariant.

Discussion

These data clearly demonstrate that there are significant age and gender effects on the ASPIRES scales. Concerning gender, women scored significantly higher than men on all scales except Religious Crisis, where men scored higher. These observed differences parallel findings in the research literature, where women consistently score higher than men on measures of spirituality and religious involvement (e.g., Maselko & Kubzansky, 2006; Wink & Dillon, 2002). Fortunately, these gender differences do not impact the underlying factor structure of the scale; men and women appear to understand and experience spirituality in a similar manner (e.g., Gomez & Fisher, 2005).

Age effects were also found, which are consistent with longitudinal research that documents changes across the life span in spirituality and religiousness (e.g., Wink & Dillon, 2002). Levels of spirituality and religiousness appear to rise over the late adolescent and adult life course. Levels of Religious

Crisis begin high but decline over time. Again, Although mean levels may vary, the underlying factor structure of the scales remains unchanged. Thus, Although the outward expression of religious sentiments and spiritual motivations may change over time, and across genders, the nature of these constructs is constant. Spirituality and religiousness represent unitary qualities that are common to men and women, young and old. These data suggest that there are not different types of spiritualities and religious understandings (e.g., women's spirituality or an elderly spirituality; see Reich, 1997). Numinous qualities can be understood as cohesive, common dimensions that can be used to describe the human experience. These findings are also consistent with other measures of spirituality that have been found to be independent of the FFM, such as the Faith Maturity Scale (FMS; Benson, Donahue, & Erickson, 1993; Piedmont & Nelson, 2001). The FMS evidenced a common factor structure despite mean level differences between genders and across age groups and religious denominations.

However, the presence of mean-level differences underscores the need for users of spiritual/religious scales to control for age and gender effects in their work. Because most measures of spirituality and religiousness do not have normative data (the ASPIRES does have normative data that adjusts scores by age and gender), users will need to provide their own adjustments to obtained raw scores in order to control for these influences.

Interpreting the Age Effects
Cohort Interpretation

As a cross-sectional study the most direct, and simplest, interpretation of these findings would be to view them as cohort effects. The observed differences across the three age groups represent the unique developmental, cultural, and social experiences that shaped the values for each generation's world view. In the current study, on average, subjects in the three age groups were born in 1936 (the Silent Generation), 1960 (the Baby Boomers), and 1989 (the Millennial Generation), respectively; coming of age in the 1950s, 1980s, and now. The groupings and the related generational interpretations are based on data from the Pew Research Center (2010).

The Baby Boomers and Silent Generation share much in common in terms of religious involvements, both scoring high on this scale. Over 85% in each group are affiliated with religious denominations (Pew Research Center, 2010). Both groups came of age in times of social and political conservatism, periods in which group membership and conformity were more salient (Gitlin, 2011; Strauss & Howe, 1992). In the 1950s, society tried to settle into a uniform, comfortable reality as the chaos and social tumult of World War II began to recede (Strauss & Howe, 1992). The 1980s saw a similar increase in conventionality as the social and political upheavals of the late 1960s and early 1970s, along with the strong focus on the individual, began to fade away (Gitlin, 2011). However, the Baby Boomers seemed to develop a higher need for meaning and purpose along with their religious involvements. Perhaps this was a carry-over from the 1960s where there was an eschewal of material values and an emphasis on finding humanity's higher nature and purpose (Isserman & Kazin, 2011).

In the present study, the youngest group evidences a pattern quite different from the other two groups. The Millennial Generation is low on both spirituality and religious involvement. The Pew Research Center (2010) noted this group to exhibit lower levels of religious intensity than their elders today. The need for conformity and group membership in larger social/religious organizations is less than the other cohort groups. Fully 25% of those in this generational group are "unaffiliated" with any religious group and are more likely to define themselves as "atheist" or "agnostic." For those who do attend services, they do so at lower rates than the other two cohort groups did when they were the same age. With the arrival of the Internet and social media, the youngest generation may be finding their social needs gratified in connectivity through these electronic portals that provide a global community rather than in membership in static physical organizations (Jones, Cox, & Banchoff, 2012). The concomitant rise in both materialism and secularism during the past 20 years may explain the lower scores on spirituality, where the ethos focuses on consumption, acquisition, and upward financial mobility (Fischer, 2010; Pew Research Center, 2007).

Interestingly, though, the higher scores on Religious Crisis suggest that the Millennials are not just ignoring religion and spirituality, finding them irrelevant to their current world-view. Instead, there is a sense in this generation that they feel alienated, isolated, and punished by the God of their understanding. They may avoid religious and spiritual issues because that whole aspect of life is perceived as hostile and threatening. High scores on Religious Crisis have been linked to increased levels of Axis II pathology (Piedmont et al., 2007). Identifying the factors contributing to this process would be an important insight into the social mechanisms that give rise to spiritual isolation and its related psychological implications. Nonetheless, these data may be identifying important motivational and attitudinal shifts that are occurring in our society. Given that high scores on numinous constructs are related to higher levels of well-being, life satisfaction, emotional maturity, and prosocial attitudes, these shifts may carry with them important implications for how the American lifestyle may be evolving over the next half century.

Longitudinal Interpretation

Although the viewing of discontinuities in spiritual and religious styles between the younger and older generations may seem jarring, it may not be reasonable to expect that these mean level scores will remain constant over the life span of this younger group. As our initial review of the longitudinal literature indicated, spirituality and religiousness change in nonlinear ways over the life span. Thus, it may be more appropriate to view these intercohort scores as "snapshots" taken at discrete points in an ongoing, continuous developmental process. Although a cross-sectional study cannot speak to issues of process, it can be pointed out that the different patterns of scores are consistent with several longitudinal studies that have noted increasing levels of spirituality and religiousness over the life span (e.g., Wink & Dillon, 2002, 2008).

In fact, many theories of spiritual development expect individuals to increase in spiritual awareness, maturity, and commitment (e.g., Mattes, 2005). Piedmont (1999) explicitly stated that scores on spirituality should increase as one gets older. He argued that the increasing salience of mortality would be a powerful stimulator of spiritual motivations and religious involvements. When viewed through the lens of ongoing development, these findings offer another set of hypotheses for understanding spiritual and religious maturation that can be tested in future longitudinal work.

The lower scores on religiousness and spirituality for the Millennial cohort may be a consequence of several factors. Late adolescence is a time of great emotional exuberance, where young adults revel in feelings of infallibility, infertility, and immortality. The processes of self-exploration and self-understanding focus on the immediate sense of personhood and may overwhelm any concerns about ultimate personal meaning or issues of teleological significance. Further, religious and spiritual issues may also be perceived as remnants of parental control that young adults may move against as the process of individuation unfolds. The higher scores on Religious Crisis may be a reflection of the more general feelings of emotional dysphoria that characterize this age group (Costa & McCrae, 1994). Young adults feel insecure and emotionally vulnerable as they interact with others and strive to find personal and social adequacy in their peer groups. These feelings of alienation and inadequacy begin to melt away as the person finds his or her place in the world.

Moving into middle adulthood is a time characterized by many firsts. People find love and marriage, begin a family, and undertake a vocational trajectory in the hope of building a life. Here the issues of meaning and community involvement become important. Building a future entails having a blueprint to follow. As such, the need to create ultimate meaning becomes more salient now because it helps to create an interpretive context for understanding the self. Having a broad sense of personal meaning provides emotional stability, which in turn enables one to make long-term commitments. It also helps one to find and develop a sense of community, within which social support and amity provide a focus and venue for ones identity and generativity needs. Thus, the middle adulthood group had higher levels of religious involvement and spiritual transcendence than the youngest age group.

Curiously, for those in the older adulthood group, their levels of spirituality were lower than those in the middle age group Although religious involvement remained at a comparable level. It seems odd that issues of meaning appear to be less salient at a time when many developmental theories claim that individuals are motivated to pull together a final, integrative sense of meaning that describes and characterizes the life that was led (e.g., Erikson, 1959). Thus, the findings for the older aged cohort appear incongruous with theory. From a cross-sectional perspective, this finding may just represent a cohort-specific effect: People of this generation always have been more focused on religious activities and involvements than on spiritual relationships. From a developmental perspective, lower scores on spirituality may represent a shifting focus toward the numinous as death becomes more salient. The greater emphasis on religious rituals and involvements may be providing individuals with greater confidence that they will find ultimate spiritual security in the next life. Marrow (1986) captured this motivation when explaining why St. Paul's ideas of salvation through faith have not been as persuasive as the need for good works, ". . . working to prescribed rules and earning quantifiable merit is more reassuring than belief . . . especially when the required faith remains refractory to our preferred methods of verification" (p. 106).

Thus, behavioral expressions of one's faith provide external "evidence" that one is committed to God and is actively working to perfect that relationship in concrete ways. Involvement in religious ritual may provide more psychological comfort to the elderly as they attempt to create the final synthesis of their lives. However, with age comes decreasing mobility and social contact, and therefore greater attention may need to be directed toward insuring the elderly's continued participation in social/religious activities.

Conclusions

Longitudinal research on spirituality and religiousness has clearly demonstrated that the numinous is an important part of most peoples' lives across their life span. These studies further demonstrated that the nature of peoples' involvements in the numinous do change over their life span, in that how it becomes expressed does vary over time, although no consistencies have yet been found across studies. Further, the spiritual experiences of men and women also vary. The results of this study provide support for these fundamental findings: Mean levels of spirituality and religiousness, as measured by the ASPIRES, do vary across age groups in nonlinear ways. In addition, mean levels on these dimensions are different for men and women, although these differences appear constant across age group. This study's significant contribution is that although the expression of spirituality and religious sentiments may vary across age and gender, the fundamental meaning of the construct remains constant. How people come to understand and experience the numinous, regardless of age and gender, is a unitary reality. Despite how it may be differently expressed by men and women, or by young and old, its underlying meaning is the same.

This finding explains why strong cross-observer validity is found with the ASPIRES scales both in the U.S. (Piedmont, 2010) and abroad (Piedmont, 2007). It also explains why the ASPIRES has been found both structurally and predictively valid across religious denominations, cultures, and languages (e.g., Chen, 2011; Piedmont & Leach, 2002; Rican & Janosova, 2010). The value of this finding is the parsimony it suggests to exist within the numinous domain. There is no need for a measure of spirituality for the elderly or one for the young nor is there a need for a female versus male measure of spirituality. The unitive nature of the construct provides additional evidence that religious and spiritual dynamics represent a cohesive, definable, and robust aspect of individual differences, qualities worthy of scientific examination.

Certainly more longitudinal research is needed in this area. Including standardized, validated measures of spiritual and religious qualities, such as the ASPIRES, that are relevant for all faith denominations and cultural contexts, is highly recommended. Use of such measures across time will provide better assessments of how numinous qualities may, or may not, be changing across the life span. The findings of this study represent one set of hypotheses that can be tested longitudinally. Replicating these findings within groups over time will provide a great foundation for constructing empirically informed developmental theories about how individuals create personal meaning and how aspects of the numinous become differentially salient as one deals with evolving life tasks.

References

Argue, A., Johnson, D. R., & White, L. K. (1999). Age and religiosity: Evidence from a three-wave panel analysis. *Journal for the Social Scientific Study of Religion, 38,* 423–435. doi:10.2307/1387762

Benson, P. L., Donahue, M. J., & Erickson, J. A. (1993). The Faith Maturity Scale: Conceptualization, measurement, and empirical validation. *Research in the Social Scientific Study of Religion, 5,* 1–26.

Brennan, M., & Mroczek, D. K. (2002). Examining spirituality over time: Latent growth curve and individual growth curve analyses. *Journal of Religious Gerontology, 14,* 11–29. doi:10.1300/J078v14n01_02

Buss, D. M. (2002). Sex, marriage, and religion: What adaptive problems do religious phenomena solve? *Psychological Inquiry, 13,* 201–203.

Chen, T. P. (2011). *A cross-cultural psychometric evaluation of the Assessment of Spirituality and Religious Sentiments Scale in Mainland China* (Unpublished doctoral dissertation). Loyola University Maryland, Baltimore, MD.

Costa, P. T., Jr., & McCrae, R. R. (1994). Stability and change in personality from adolescence through adulthood. In C. F. Halverson, G. A. Kohnstamm, & R. P. Martin (Eds.), *The developing structure of temperament and personality from infancy to adulthood* (pp. 139–150). Hillsdale, NJ: Lawrence Erlbaum Associates.

Dalby, P. (2006). Is there a process of spiritual change or development associated with ageing? A critical review of research. *Aging & Mental Health, 10,* 4–12. doi:10.1080/13607860500307969

Dillon, M., Wink, P., & Fay, K. (2003). Is spirituality detrimental to generativity? *Journal for the Scientific Study of Religion, 42,* 427–442. doi:10.1111/1468-5906.00192

Erikson, E. H. (1959). *Identity and the life cycle.* New York, NY: International Universities Press.

Fischer, C. S. (2010). *Made in America: A social history of American culture and character.* Chicago, IL: University of Chicago Press.

Gitlin, M. (2011). *The Baby Boomer encyclopedia.* Santa Barbara, CA: ABC-CLIO.

Gomez, R., & Fisher, J. W. (2005). The spiritual well-being questionnaire: Testing for model applicability, measurement and structural equivalencies, and latent mean differences across gender. *Personality and Individual Differences, 39,* 1383–1393. doi:10.1016/j.paid.2005.03.023

Good, M., Willoughby, T., & Busseri, M. A. (2011). Stability and change in adolescent spirituality/religiosity: A person-centered approach. *Developmental Psychology, 47,* 538–550. doi:10.1037/a0021270

Gorsuch, R. L. (1983). *Factor analysis* (2nd ed.). Hillsdale, NJ: Lawrence Erlbaum Associates.

Hill, P. C., & Pargament, K. I. (2008). Advances in the conceptualization and measurement of religion and spirituality: Implications for physical and mental health research. *Psychology of Religion and Spirituality, 5,* 3–17. doi:10.1037/1941-1022.S.1.3

Hill, P. C., Pargament, K. I., Hood, R. W., McCullough, M. E., Sawyers, J. P., Larson, D. B., & Zinnbauer, B. J. (2000). Conceptualizing religion and spirituality: Points of commonality, point of departure. *Journal for the Theory of Social Behavior, 30,* 51–77. doi:10.1111/1468-5914.00119

Ingersoll-Dayton, B., Krause, N., & Morgan, D. (2002). Religious trajectories and transitions over the life course. *International Journal of Aging & Human Development, 55,* 51–70. doi:10.2190/297Q-MRMV-27TE-VLFK

Isserman, M., & Kazin, M. (2011). *America divided: The civil war of the 1960s.* New York, NY: Oxford University Press.

Jones, R. P., Cox, D., & Banchoff, T. (2012). *A generation in transition: Religion, values, and politics among college-age Millennials. Finding from the 2012 Millennial Values Survey.* Washington, DC: Public Religion Research Institute, Inc. and Georgetown University's Berkley Center for Religion, Peace, and World Affairs.

Kapuscinski, A. N., & Masters, K. S. (2010). The current status of measures of spirituality: A critical review of scale development. *Psychology of Religion and Spirituality, 2,* 191–205. doi:10.1037/a0020498

Koenig, L. B., McGue, M., & Iacono, W. G. (2008). Stability and change in religiousness during emerging adulthood. *Developmental Psychology, 44,* 532–543. doi:10.1037/0012-1649.44.2.532

Marrow, S. B. (1986). *Paul: His letters and his theology: An introduction to Paul's epistles.* Mahwah, NJ: Paulist Press.

Maselko, J., & Kubzansky, L. D. (2006). Gender differences in religious practices, spiritual experiences and health: Results from the U.S. General Social Survey. *Social Science & Medicine, 62,* 2848–2860. doi:10.1016/j.socscimed.2005.11.008

Mattes, R. (2005). Spiritual need one: Spiritual development: The aging process: A journal of lifelong spiritual formation. *Journal of Religion, Spirituality, & Aging, 17,* 55–72. doi:10.1300/J496v17n03_06

McCullough, M. E., Enders, C. K., Brion, S. L., & Jain, A. R. (2005). The varieties of religious development in adulthood: A longitudinal investigation of religion and rational choice. *Journal of Personality and Social Psychology, 89,* 78–89. doi:10.1037/0022-3514.89.1.78

McCullough, M. E., & Laurenceau, J. P. (2005). Religiousness and the trajectory of self-rated health across adulthood. *Personality and Social Psychology Bulletin, 31,* 560–573. doi:10.1177/0146167204271657

McCullough, M. E., Tsang, J., & Brion, S. (2003). Personality traits in adolescence as predictors of religiousness in early adulthood: Findings from the Terman Longitudinal study. *Personality and Social Psychology Bulletin, 29,* 980–991. doi:10.1177/0146167203253210

Pew Research Center. (2007). *Trends in attitudes toward religion and social issues: 1987–2007.* Retrieved from http://pewresearch.org/pubs/614/religion-social-issues

Pew Research Center. (2010). *Millennials: A portrait of generation next.* Washington, DC: Author. Retrieved from http://

pewsocialtrends.org/files/2010/10/millennials-confident-connected-open-to-change.pdf

Piedmont, R. L. (1999). Does spirituality represent the sixth factor of personality? Spiritual transcendence and the five-factor model. *Journal of Personality, 67,* 985–1013. doi:10.1111/1467-6494.00080

Piedmont, R. L. (2004). Spiritual transcendence as a predictor of psychological outcome from an outpatient substance abuse program. *Psychology of Addictive Behaviors, 18,* 213–222. doi:10.1037/0893-164X.18.3.213

Piedmont, R. L. (2005). The role of personality in understanding religious and spiritual constructs. In R. F. Paloutzian & C. L. Park (Eds.), *Handbook of the psychology of religion and spirituality* (pp. 253–273). New York, NY: The Guilford Press.

Piedmont, R. L. (2007). Cross-cultural generalizability of the Spiritual Transcendence Scale to the Philippines: Spirituality as a human universal. *Mental Health, Religion, & Culture, 10,* 89–107. doi:10.1080/13694670500275494

Piedmont, R. L. (2010). *Assessment of Spirituality and Religious Sentiments (ASPIRES): Technical manual* (2nd ed.). Timonium, MD: Author.

Piedmont, R. L., Ciarrocchi, J. W., Dy-Liacco, G. S., & Williams, J. E. G. (2009). The empirical and conceptual value of the spiritual transcendence and religious involvement scales for personality research. *Psychology of Religion and Spirituality, 1,* 162–179. doi:10.1037/a0015883

Piedmont, R. L., Hassinger, C. J., Rhorer, J., Sherman, M. F., Sherman, N. C., & Williams, J. E. G. (2007). The relations among spirituality and religiosity and Axis II functioning in two college samples. *Research in the Social Scientific Study of Religion, 18,* 53–74. doi:10.1163/ej.9789004158511.i-301.24

Piedmont, R. L., & Leach, M. M. (2002). Cross-cultural generalizability of the Spiritual Transcendence Scale in India: Spirituality as a universal aspect of human experience. *American Behavioral Scientist, 45,* 1886–1899. doi:10.1177/0002764202045012011

Piedmont, R. L., & Nelson, R. (2001). A psychometric evaluation of the short form of the Faith Maturity Scale. *Research in the Social Scientific Study of Religion, 12,* 165–183.

Piedmont, R. L., Werdel, M. B., & Fernando, M. (2009). The utility of the Assessment of Spirituality and Religious Sentiments (ASPIRES) scale with Christians and Buddhists in Sri Lanka. *Research in the Social Scientific Study of Religion, 20,* 131–143. doi:10.1163/ej.9789004175624.i-334.42

Reich, K. H. (1997). Do we need a theory for the religiousness development of women? *International Journal for the Psychology of Religion, 7,* 67–86. doi:10.1207/s15327582ijpr0702_1

Rican, P., & Janosova, P. (2010). Spirituality as a basic aspect of personality: A cross-cultural verification of Piedmont's model. *The International Journal for the Psychology of Religion, 20,* 2–13. doi:10.1080/10508610903418053

Seifert, L. S. (2002). Toward a psychology of religion, spirituality, meaning-search, and aging: Past research and a practical application. *Journal of Adult Development, 9,* 61–70. doi:1068-0667/02/0100-0061/0

Slater, W., Hall, T. D., & Edwards, K. J. (2001). Measuring spirituality and religion: Where are we and where are we going? *Journal of Psychology and Theology, 29,* 4–21.

Strauss, W., & Howe, N. (1992). *Generations: The history of America's future, 1584 to 2069.* New York, NY: HarperCollins.

Van Wicklin, J. F. (1990). Conceiving and measuring ways of being religious. *Journal of Psychology and Christianity, 9,* 27–40.

Wink, P., & Dillon, M. (2002). Spiritual development across the adult life course: Findings from a longitudinal study. *Journal of Adult Development, 9,* 79–94. doi:10.1023/A:1013833419122

Wink, P., & Dillon, M. (2003). Religiousness, spirituality, and psychosocial functioning in late adulthood: Findings from a longitudinal study. *Psychology and Aging, 18,* 916–924. doi:1037/0882-7974.18.4.916

Wink, P., & Dillon, M. (2008). Religiousness, spirituality, and psychosocial functioning in late adulthood: Findings from a longitudinal study. *Psychology of Religion and Spirituality, 1,* 102–115. doi:10.1037/1941-1022.S.1.102

Critical Thinking

1. How has the concept of spirituality and religiousity evolved over the past 25 years in medicine?

2. How does spirituality and religiousity affect the resources provided by the health-care system?

3. Does the community play a role in the development and nurturing of spirituality and religion?

Create Central

www.mhhe.com/createcentral

Internet References

American Society on Aging: Forum on Religion, Spirituality and Aging (FORSA)
www.asaging.org/forum-religion-spirituality-and-aging-forsa

National Council on Aging
www.ncoa.org

Unit 3

UNIT

Prepared by: Elaina Osterbur, *Saint Louis University*

Societal Attitudes Toward Old Age

There is a wide range of beliefs regarding the social position and status of aging Americans today. Some people believe that the best way to understand the problems of older adults is to regard them as a minority group faced with difficulties similar to those of other minority groups. Discrimination against older people, like racial discrimination, is believed to be based on a bias against visible physical traits. Because the aging process is viewed negatively, it is natural that many older adults may try to appear and act younger. Some spend a tremendous amount of money trying to make themselves look and feel younger so they can blend in more readily with younger adults. Other older adults accept their position in an ageist society.

One theory suggests that older people are a weak minority group. However, this theory is questionable because too many circumstances prove otherwise. The U.S. Congress, for example, favors its senior members and delegates power to them by bestowing considerable prestige on them. Older adults vote and respect their position and rights as U.S. citizens. Furthermore, leadership roles in religious organizations are often held by older persons. Many older Americans are in good health, have comfortable incomes, and are treated with respect by friends and associates.

Perhaps the most realistic way to view people who are aged is as a status group, like other status groups in society. Every society has some method of "age grading" by which it groups together individuals of roughly similar age. ("Preteens" and "senior citizens" are some of the age-grade labels in U.S. society.) Because it is a labeling process, age grading causes members of the age group to be perceived by themselves as well as others in terms of the connotations of the label. Unfortunately, the tag "old age" often has negative connotations in U.S. society. Many of society's typical assumptions about the limitations of old age have been refuted. A major force behind this reassessment of the elderly is that so many people are living longer and healthier lives, and in consequence, playing more of a role in all aspects of our society. Older people can remain productive members of society for many more years than has been traditionally assumed.

The articles in this section attempt to explain a variety of social attitudes toward older adults such as biases and stereotypes. This section also includes issues related to technology use, friendships, sexuality, and societal issues related to ethnic minority groups.

Article   Prepared by: Elaina F. Osterbur, *Saint Louis University*

We Need to Fight Age Bias

Congress should act where the courts failed.

JACK GROSS

Learning Outcomes

After reading this article, you will be able to:

- Explain why younger adults often avoid spending time around older people.

- Describe how the media stereotype the image of older people.

- Discuss the different decisions that were made by the lower courts and the Supreme Court in the Jack Gross age discrimination in employment case.

- Explain how the Supreme Court's ruling in the Jack Gross case—that age had to be the exclusive factor in the business decision rather than just a motivating factor for age discrimination to have occurred—made it more difficult for demoted older workers to win their cases in court.

I never, never imagined when I was demoted seven years ago and then filed an age discrimination suit that I would end up in the U.S. Supreme Court, that I would testify before five congressional committees, or that my name would become associated with the future of age discrimination laws in our country. I do believe, however, that it happened for a reason.

This all began in January 2003. When my employer, Farm Bureau Financial Group (FBL) in Iowa, merged with the Kansas Farm Bureau, the company apparently wanted to purge claims employees who were over age 50. All the Kansas claims employees over 50 with a certain number of years of employment were offered a buyout, which most accepted. In Iowa, virtually every claims supervisor over 50 was demoted.

Being 54, I was included in that sweep, despite 13 consecutive years of top performance reviews. The company claimed this was not discrimination but simply a reorganization. In 2005, a federal jury spent a week hearing testimony and seeing the evidence. The jurors agreed with me, and determined that age was a motivating factor in my demotion. Since then, the case has taken on a life of its own, including an appeal to

the 8th Circuit Court and a U.S. Supreme Court hearing and decision.

Since the Age Discrimination in Employment Act was passed in 1967, courts had ruled consistently that the law protected individuals if their age was a factor in any employment decision. But in my case, the Supreme Court unexpectedly changed course and ruled that age had to be the exclusive reason for my demotion, even though that wasn't the question before them. They simply hijacked my case and used it as a vehicle to water down the workplace discrimination laws passed by Congress.

This new and much higher standard of proof is clearly inconsistent with the intent of the ADEA and four decades of precedent, and will affect millions of workers. A new trial was ordered and is scheduled for November, nearly eight years after my demotion.

I did not pursue this case just for myself. From my observation, discrimination victims are usually the most vulnerable among us, those who simply cannot fight back. Thanks to my attorneys, who believed in me, my case, and now our cause, I was able to take a stand against my unjust and unlawful treatment. Many of my friends are also farm or small-town "kids" who feel like they are the forgotten minority. Many have been forcibly retired or laid off. Some have been looking for work for months, only to find doors closed when they reveal the year they graduated. Others are working as janitors despite good careers and college degrees. They all know that age discrimination is very real and pervasive.

We now look to Congress to pass the Protecting Older Workers Against Discrimination Act (H.R. 3721), to provide the same protection for older people as protection given to people of color, women or people of different faiths.

While this ordeal has been stressful, observing all levels of our judicial and congressional processes "up close and personal" has been a real education. My faith in our judicial system was shattered by the Supreme Court's errant 5–4 decision. I believe Congress, as representatives of we, the people, will rectify it. You can help by contacting your own senators and representatives to encourage their support.

I am sincerely grateful for the assistance of people and groups truly dedicated to ending workplace discrimination of any kind in our great nation.

Critical Thinking

1. How did the Supreme Court's decision in the Jack Gross age discrimination case change the rules that determined if the employers had violated the Age Discrimination in Employment Act of 1967?
2. What bill now before Congress would give older workers the same protection as are given to people of color, women, or people of different faiths?
3. Does Jack Gross believe that the U.S. Congress will pass the new Protecting Older Workers Against Discrimination Act (H.R. 3721) which would re-establish the previous rules for judging age discrimination in employment which were established in 1967?

Create Central

www.mhhe.com/createcentral

Internet References

Adult Development and Aging: Division 20 of the American Psychological Association
    www.iog.wayne.edu/APADIV20/APADIV20.HTM
American Society on Aging
    www.asaging.org/index.cfm
Canadian Psychological Association
    www.cpa.ca

JACK GROSS was aided by AARP in the U.S. Supreme Court's precedent-setting age discrimination case.

Article   Prepared by: Elaina Osterbur, *Saint Louis University*

Older Adults and Technology Use

Aaron Smith

Learning Outcomes

After reading this article, you will be able to:

- Compare the two groups of older adults in terms of age and economic status and their technology usage.

- Identify barriers and challenges to adopting new technologies.

Main Findings

America's seniors have historically been late adopters to the world of technology compared to their younger compatriots, but their movement into digital life continues to deepen, according to newly released data from the Pew Research Center. In this report, we take advantage of a particularly large survey to conduct a unique exploration not only of technology use between Americans ages 65 or older and the rest of the population, but *within* the senior population as well.

Two different groups of older Americans emerge. The first group (which leans toward younger, more highly educated, or more affluent seniors) has relatively substantial technology assets, and also has a positive view toward the benefits of online platforms. The other (which tends to be older and less affluent, often with significant challenges with health or disability) is largely disconnected from the world of digital tools and services, both physically and psychologically.

As the internet plays an increasingly central role in connecting Americans of all ages to news and information, government services, health resources, and opportunities for social support, these divisions are noteworthy—particularly for the many organizations and individual caregivers who serve the older adult population. Among the key findings of this research:

Six in ten seniors now go online, and just under half are broadband adopters.

In April 2012 the Pew Research Center found for the first time that more than half of older adults (defined as those ages 65 or older) were internet users. Today, 59% of seniors report they go online—a six-percentage point increase in the course of a year—and 47% say they have a high-speed broadband connection at home. In addition, 77% of older adults have a cell phone, up from 69% in April 2012.

But despite these gains, seniors continue to lag behind younger Americans when it comes to tech adoption. And many seniors remain largely unattached from online and mobile life—41% do not use the internet at all, 53% do not have broadband access at home, and 23% do not use cell phones.

Younger, higher-income, and more highly educated seniors use the internet and broadband at rates approaching—or even exceeding—the general population; internet use and broadband adoption each drop off dramatically around age 75.

Seniors, like any other demographic group, are not monolithic, and there are important distinctions in their tech adoption patterns, beginning with age itself. Internet use and broadband adoption among seniors each fall off notably starting at approximately age 75. Some 68% of Americans in their early 70s go online, and 55% have broadband at home. By contrast, internet adoption falls to 47% and broadband adoption falls to 34% among 75–79 year olds.

In addition, affluent and well-educated seniors adopt the internet and broadband at substantially higher rates than those with lower levels of income and educational attainment:

- Among seniors with an annual household income of $75,000 or more, 90% go online and 82% have broadband at home. For seniors earning less than $30,000 annually, 39% go online and 25% have broadband at home.

- Fully 87% of seniors with a college degree go online, and 76% are broadband adopters. Among seniors who have not attended college, 40% go online and just 27% have broadband at home.

Older adults face a number of hurdles to adopting new technologies.

Older adults face several unique barriers and challenges when it comes to adopting new technologies. These include:

Physical challenges to using technology: Many seniors have physical conditions or health issues that make it difficult to use new technologies. Around two in five seniors indicate that they have a "physical or health condition that makes reading difficult or challenging" or a "disability, handicap, or chronic disease that prevents them from fully participating in many common daily activities." This group is significantly less likely than seniors who do not face these physical challenges to go online (49% vs. 66%), to have broadband at home (38% vs. 53%), and to own most major digital devices.

Skeptical attitudes about the benefits of technology: Older adults who do not currently use the internet are divided on the question of whether that lack of access hurts them or not. Half of these non-users (49%) agree with the statement that "people lacking internet access are at a real disadvantage because of all the information they might be missing," with 25% agreeing strongly. But 35% of these older non-internet users *disagree* that they are missing out on important information—and 18% of them strongly disagree.

Difficulties learning to use new technologies: A significant majority of older adults say they need assistance when it comes to using new digital devices. Just 18% would feel comfortable learning to use a new technology device such as a smartphone or tablet on their own, while 77% indicate they would need someone to help walk them through the process. And among seniors who go online but do not currently use social networking sites such as Facebook or Twitter, 56% would need assistance if they wanted to use these sites to connect with friends or family members.

Once seniors join the online world, digital technology often becomes an integral part of their daily lives.

Despite some of these unique challenges facing the older adult population when it comes to technology, most seniors who become internet users make visiting the digital world a regular occurrence. Among older adults who use the internet, 71% go online every day or almost every day, and an additional 11% go online three to five times per week.

These older internet users also have strongly positive attitudes about the benefits of online information in their personal lives. Fully 79% of older adults who use the internet agree with the statement that "people without internet access are at a real disadvantage because of all the information they

might be missing," while 94% agree with the statement that "the internet makes it much easier to find information today than in the past."

Seniors differ from the general population in their device ownership habits.

Device ownership among older adults differs notably from the population as a whole in several specific ways:

Few older adults are smartphone owners: More than half of all Americans now have a smartphone, but among older adults, adoption levels sit at just 18%. Additionally, smartphone ownership among older adults has risen only modestly in recent years, from 11% in April 2011. A significant majority of older adults (77%) do have a cell phone of some kind, but by and large these tend to be more basic devices.

Among older adults, tablets, and e-book readers are as popular as smartphones: Among the general public, smartphones are much more common than either tablet computers or e-book readers, such as Kindles or Nooks. But tablets, e-book readers, and smartphones are each owned by an identical 18% of older adults. In fact, the proportion of older adults who own *either* a tablet *or* an e-book reader is actually larger than the proportion owning a smartphone. Some 27% of seniors own a tablet, an e-book reader, or both, while 18% own a smartphone.

27% of older adults use social networking sites such as Facebook, but these users socialize more frequently with others compared with non-SNS users.

Today 46% of online seniors (representing 27% of the total older adult population) use social networking sites such as Facebook, and these social network adopters have more persistent social connections with the people they care about.

Some 81% of older adults who use social networking sites say that they socialize with others (either in person, online, or over the telephone) on a daily or near-daily basis. Among older adults who go online but do not use social networking sites, that figure is 71%; and for those who are not online at all, it is 63%.

Critical Thinking

1. How do older adults differ from younger adults in their technology usage?

2. Considering the websites that older adults frequent, in your opinion, why do older adults choose these sites?

Internet References

Eldercare.gov: Staying Connected Technology Options for Older Adults
    www.eldercare.gov/eldercare.net/public/Resources/Brochures/docs/N4A_Tech_Brochure_P06_high.pdf

Pew Research Center's Internet and American Life Project
www.pewinternet.org

Article   Prepared by: Elaina F. Osterbur, *Saint Louis University*

Health Disparities among Lesbian, Gay, and Bisexual Older Adults: Results from a Population-Based Study

KAREN I. FREDRIKSEN-GOLDSEN ET AL.

Learning Outcomes

After reading this article, you will be able to:

- Discuss the health outcomes of lesbian, gay, and bisexual older adults.

- Identify the health disparities among lesbian, gay, and bisexual older adults.

- Identify the methods to learn more about the health needs in the lesbian, gay, and bisexual communities.

Changing demographics will make population aging a defining feature of the 21st century. Not only is the population older, it is becoming increasingly diverse.[1] Existing research illustrates that older adults from socially and economically disadvantaged populations are at high risk of poor health and premature death.[2] A commitment of the National Institutes of Health is to reduce and eliminate health disparities,[3] which have been defined as differences in health outcomes for communities that have encountered systematic obstacles to health as a result of social, economic, and environmental disadvantage.[4]

Social determinants of health disparities among older adults include age, race/ethnicity, and socioeconomic status.[5] Centers for Disease Control and Prevention (CDC) and *Healthy People* 2020 identify health disparities related to sexual orientation as one of the main gaps in current health research.[6] The Institute of Medicine identifies lesbian, gay, and bisexual (LGB) older adults as a population whose health needs are understudied.[7] The institute has called for population-based studies to better assess the impact of background characteristics such as age on health outcomes among LGB adults. A review of 25 years of literature on LGB aging found that health research is glaringly sparse for this population and that most aging-related studies have used small, non-population-based samples.[8]

Several important studies have begun to document health disparities by sexual orientation in population-based data and have revealed important differences in health between LGB adults and their heterosexual counterparts, including higher risks of poor mental health, smoking, and limitations in activities.[9,10] Studies have found higher rates of excessive drinking among lesbians and bisexual women[9,10] and higher rates of obesity among lesbians[10,11] than among heterosexual women; bisexual men and women are at higher risk of limited health care access than are heterosexuals. In addition, important subgroup differences in health are beginning to be documented among LGB adults. For example, bisexual women are at higher risk than lesbians for mental distress and poor general health.[12] A primary limitation of most existing population-based research is a failure to identify the specific health needs of LGB older adults. Most studies to date address the health needs of LGB adults aged 18 years and older[9] or those younger than 65 years.[10] This lack of attention to older adult health leaves unclear whether disparities diminish or persist or even become more pronounced in later life.

A few studies have begun to examine health disparities among LGB adults aged 50 years and older.[13,14] Wallace et al. analyzed data from the California Health Interview Survey and found that LGB adults aged 50 to 70 years report higher rates of mental distress, physical limitations, and poor general health than do their heterosexual counterparts. The researchers also found that older gay and bisexual men report higher rates of hypertension and diabetes than do heterosexual men.[14] To better address the needs of an increasingly diverse older adult population and to develop responsive interventions and public health policies, health disparities research is needed for this at-risk group.

Examining to what extent sexual orientation is related to health disparities among LGB older adults is a first step toward developing a more comprehensive understanding of their health and aging needs. We analyzed population-based data from the Washington State Behavioral Risk Factor Surveillance System (WA-BRFSS) to compare lesbians and bisexual women and

Health Disparities among Lesbian, Gay, and Bisexual Older Adults by Karen Fredriksen-Goldsen et al.

63

gay and bisexual men with their heterosexual counterparts aged 50 years and older on key health indicators: outcomes, chronic conditions, access to care, behaviors, and screening. We also compared subgroups to identify differences in health disparities by sexual orientation among LGB older adults.

Methods

The BRFSS is an annual random-digit-dialed telephone survey of noninstitutionalized adults conducted by each US state. Each year, disproportionate stratified random sampling is used to select eligible households, and from each selected household 1 adult is randomly selected as the respondent.[15] Washington State began including a measure of sexual orientation in 2003. We aggregated the WA-BRFSS data collected from 2003 to 2010 for respondents aged 50 years and older (n = 96 992) and stratified by gender for further analyses. We selected 50 years as the lower age limit to be consistent with previous health studies focusing on sexual minority older adults,[13,14] as well as research addressing specific chronic health conditions[16,17] and older adult health and well-being, such as the Health and Retirement Study and other population-based studies.[18-20] Annual response rates to the WA-BRFSS range from 43% to 50%, calculated according to Council of American Survey and Research Organizations methods.[21] To adjust for unequal probabilities of selection resulting from nonresponse, sample design, and households without telephones, we applied sample weights provided by the WA-BRFSS.

According to weighted estimation, among women aged 50 years and older (n = 58 319), 1.03% (n = 562) identified as lesbian and 0.54% (n = 291) as bisexual; among men aged 50 years and older (n = 37 820), 1.28% (n = 463) identified as gay and 0.51% (n = 215) as bisexual. The age range in the sample for LGB older adults was 50 to 98 years (50–94 years for women and 50–98 years for men).

Measures

To measure sexual orientation, survey respondents were asked to select 1 of the following: heterosexual or straight, homosexual (gay or lesbian), bisexual, or something else. About 0.2% (n = 266) of the sample selected something else, and we excluded them from our analyses.

The background characteristics in this study were as follows: age, household income ($\leq$ 200% vs > 200% of the federal poverty level), education ($\leq$ high school vs $\geq$ some college), employment (part time or full time vs other), race/ethnicity (non-Hispanic White vs other), living arrangement (living alone vs other), and number of children in household. We categorized relationship status as married versus partnered (a member of an unmarried couple) versus other (divorced, widowed, separated, or never married).

Health outcomes (recommended and validated by CDC) in our study were poor physical health, disability, and poor mental health.[22] We defined poor physical health as 14 or more days of poor physical health during the previous 30 days and poor mental health as 14 or more days of poor mental health during the previous 30 days.[22] We defined disability as limitations in any activities because of physical, mental, or emotional

problems or any health problem that required the use of special equipment, as recommended by *Healthy People 2020*.[4]

The BRFSS asked respondents whether they had ever been told by a health professional they had arthritis, asthma, diabetes (not included if prediabetes or gestational diabetes alone), high blood pressure (not included if borderline or during pregnancy alone), or high cholesterol. As recommended by other health studies, we designated cardiovascular disease (CVD) as diagnosis by a physician of a heart attack, angina, or stroke.[23,24] We defined obesity as a body mass index score (defined as weight in kilograms divided by height in meters squared) of 30 or higher, as recommended by CDC.[25] The BRFSS measured health care access by asking whether respondents had insurance coverage, a personal doctor or provider, or a financial barrier to seeing a doctor in the past 12 months.

Health behaviors were (1) current smoking (defined, as suggested by CDC, as having ever smoked $\geq$ 100 cigarettes and currently smoking every day or some days[26]), (2) excessive drinking (defined, as suggested by National Institute of Alcohol Abuse and Alcoholism, as women having $\geq$ 4 and men having $\geq$ 5 drinks on 1 occasion during the past month[27]), and (3) physical activity (defined, as suggested by the US Department of Health and Human Services, as $\geq$ 30 minutes of moderate-intensity activity $\geq$ 5 days/week or $\geq$ 20 minutes of vigorous-intensity activity $\geq$ 3 days/week[28]). The BRFSS measured health screening, according to public health guidelines for older adults, by whether respondents received a flu shot in the past year,[29] an HIV test ever, a mammogram (for women) in the past 2 years,[30] and a prostate-specific antigen test (for men) in the past year.[31]

Statistical Analysis

We conducted analyses separately by gender. First, we described the weighted distribution of background characteristics by sexual orientation, comparing lesbians and bisexual women with heterosexual women aged 50 years and older and gay and bisexual men with heterosexual men aged 50 years and older, applying *t* tests or χ^2 tests as appropriate. We also tested statistical significance of differences in background characteristics between lesbians and bisexual women and between gay and bisexual men.

We then estimated weighted prevalence rates of health indicators, which were health outcomes, chronic conditions, access to care, behaviors, and screening, by sexual orientation (lesbian and bisexual vs heterosexual women; gay and bisexual vs heterosexual men). We conducted a series of adjusted logistic regressions, with control for sociodemographic characteristics (age, income, and education), to test associations between health-related indicators and sexual orientation. We also conducted adjusted logistic regression analyses to examine health disparities between lesbian and bisexual women and between gay and bisexual men. We used Stata version 11 (StataCorp LP, College Station, TX) for data analyses.

Results

Table 1 illustrates the weighted prevalence of background characteristics by sexual orientation among older adults. Lesbians

Table 1   Background Characteristics of Respondents Aged 50 Years and Older, by Sexual Orientation: Washington State Behavioral Risk Factor Surveillance System, 2003–2010

| | Women | | | | Men | | | |
| | | Lesbian and Bisexual | | | | Gay and Bisexual | | |
Characteristic	Heterosexual, % or Mean (SD)	Total, % or Mean (SD)	Lesbian, % or Mean (SD)	Bisexual, % or Mean (SD)	Heterosexual, % or Mean (SD)	Total, % or Mean (SD)	Gay, % or Mean (SD)	Bisexual, % or Mean (SD)
Age, y	63.82 (0.06)	58.63*** (0.37)	58.09 (0.40)	59.67 (0.78)	62.35 (0.07)	59.54*** (0.39)	59.26 (0.45)	60.22 (0.75)
≤ 200% poverty level	27.38	27.12	26.47	28.43	20.85	24.79	25.45	23.18
≤ high school	30.18	13.44***	13.83	12.69	24.96	14.57***	12.34	20.09
Employed	39.97	59.31***	63.07	52.08	51.17	55.30	55.25	55.43
Non-Hispanic White	91.79	90.31	89.86	91.23	90.40	93.22*	92.85	94.18
Relationship status								
Married	61.67	20.15***	9.57	40.44	77.60	20.83***	8.16	52.07
Partnered	1.59	27.83	36.96	10.31	1.50	20.27	27.30	2.96
Other	36.74	52.02	53.47	49.25	20.90	58.90	64.55	44.97
Children in household, no.	0.15 (0.00)	0.20 (0.04)	0.18 (0.05)	0.24 (0.06)	0.22 (0.00)	0.07*** (0.02)	0.03 (0.01)	0.15 (0.05)
Living alone	26.24	29.43	29.65	28.99	15.15	38.34***	40.66	32.59

Note. Estimates were weighted; significance tests were conducted to examine the association between background characteristics and sexual orientation (lesbians and bisexual women vs heterosexual women; gay and bisexual men vs heterosexual men).
*P < .05; ***P < .001.

and bisexual women were younger, had more education, and had higher rates of employment than did heterosexual women; income levels were similar. Lesbians and bisexual women were less likely to be married and more likely to be partnered than were their heterosexual counterparts, but the average number of children in the household and the likelihood of living alone were similar. Lesbians were more likely than bisexual women to be employed (P = .019) and less likely to be married, but more likely to be partnered (P < .001). We found no differences in other background characteristics.

Gay and bisexual men were significantly younger and more highly educated than were heterosexual men; income levels and employment rates were similar. Gay and bisexual men were less likely than heterosexual men to be married but more likely to be partnered; they also had fewer children in the household, were more likely to live alone, and were more likely to be non-Hispanic Whites. Gay men had more education (P = .037), were less likely to be married and more likely to be partnered (P < .001), and had fewer children in the household (P = .017) than did bisexual men.

Health Outcomes

Lesbians and bisexual women had higher odds than heterosexual women for disability (adjusted odds ratio [AOR] = 1.47) and poor mental health (AOR = 1.40), but not for poor physical health, after adjustment for age, income, and education (Table 2). Lesbians and bisexual women had similar rates of poor physical health, disability, and poor mental health.

In adjusted analyses, gay and bisexual men were more likely than heterosexual men to have poor physical health (AOR = 1.38), disability (AOR = 1.26), and poor mental health (AOR = 1.77). Although the unadjusted prevalence rates of disability were similar between sexual minority and heterosexual men, the analyses with adjustment for socio-demographic characteristics showed that gay and bisexual men were more likely than their heterosexual counterparts to have a disability. We did not observe differences in health outcomes between gay and bisexual men.

Chronic Conditions

Lesbians and bisexual women had greater adjusted odds of obesity (AOR = 1.42) relative to heterosexual women. Unadjusted odds of CVD were similar for sexual minority and heterosexual women, but after adjustment for sociodemographic characteristics, lesbians and bisexual women had significantly greater risk (AOR = 1.37). The unadjusted odds of asthma for lesbians and bisexual women were significantly higher than for heterosexual women, but the difference did not remain significant when the analyses adjusted for sociodemographic differences. We observed no significant differences in chronic conditions between lesbians and bisexual women in the adjusted analyses.

Gay and bisexual men had significantly lower odds of obesity than did heterosexual men (AOR = 0.72), after adjustment for sociodemographic factors. The unadjusted odds of asthma for gay and bisexual men were higher than for heterosexual men (OR = 1.41), but the difference did not remain significant after

Table 2   Weighted Prevalence Rates and Regression Analyses of Health Outcomes and Chronic Conditions among Respondents Aged 50 Years and Older: Washington State Behavioral Risk Factor Surveillance System, 2003–2010

| | Women | | | | Men | | | |
| | Lesbian and Bisexual | | | | | Gay and Bisexual | | |
Health Outcomes/ Conditions	Heterosexual, %	%	OR (95% CI)	AOR (95% CI)	Heterosexual, %	%	OR (95% CI)	AOR (95% CI)
Frequent poor physical health	15.47	15.79	1.02 (0.81, 1.30)	1.02 (0.80, 1.30)	12.88	16.79	1.36* (1.05, 1.78)	1.38* (1.04, 1.83)
Disability	36.87	44.27	1.36** (1.14, 1.62)	1.47*** (1.22, 1.77)	33.96	38.27	1.21 (0.98, 1.48)	1.26* (1.02, 1.56)
Frequent poor mental health	9.36	15.92	1.83*** (1.42, 2.37)	1.40* (1.07, 1.81)	6.88	13.09	2.04*** (1.51, 2.76)	1.77** (1.28, 2.45)
Obesity	25.93	36.27	1.63*** (1.36, 1.95)	1.42*** (1.18, 1.71)	27.07	22.57	0.79* (0.62, 0.99)	0.72* (0.56, 0.93)
Arthritis[a]	52.24	53.70	1.06 (0.83, 1.36)	1.29 (0.99, 1.67)	39.25	41.85	1.11 (0.84, 1.48)	1.19 (0.89, 1.60)
Asthma	15.89	20.57	1.37** (1.10, 1.70)	1.20 (0.96, 1.49)	11.56	15.52	1.41* (1.07, 1.85)	1.28 (0.95, 1.71)
Diabetes	11.87	13.59	1.17 (0.91, 1.51)	1.25 (0.96, 1.64)	13.96	12.44	0.88 (0.66, 1.17)	0.92 (0.67, 1.25)
High blood pressure[b]	43.33	36.02	0.74 (0.54, 1.00)	0.86 (0.62, 1.20)	44.35	40.59	0.86 (0.61, 1.21)	0.88 (0.61, 1.26)
High cholesterol[a]	47.13	44.10	0.88 (0.69, 1.14)	1.00 (0.77, 1.30)	50.21	51.66	1.06 (0.79, 1.42)	1.08 (0.80, 1.46)
Cardiovascular disease[c]	10.71	10.51	0.98 (0.73, 1.31)	1.37* (1.00, 1.86)	16.49	14.11	0.83 (0.62, 1.12)	1.04 (0.76, 1.43)

Note. AOR = adjusted odds ratio; CI = confidence interval; OR = odds ratio. Adjusted logistic regression models controlled for age, income, and education; heterosexuals were coded as the reference group.
[a]Questions were asked in 2003, 2005, 2007, and 2009.
[b]Question was asked in 2003, 2005, and 2009.
[c]Questions were asked in 2004 through 2010.
*P < .05; **P < .01; ***P < .001.

adjustment. The adjusted odds of diabetes were significantly higher for bisexual men (19.74%) than for gay men (9.50%; AOR = 2.33; *P* < .01). We detected no other significant differences in chronic conditions between gay and bisexual men.

Access to Care

As shown in Table 3, although we found no significant difference in the prevalence of having a health care provider, lesbians and bisexual women were less likely than heterosexual women to have health insurance coverage and more likely to experience financial barriers to health care. These differences, however, did not remain significant after adjustment for sociodemographic characteristics. We detected no significant differences in health care access indicators between lesbians and bisexual women.

In the unadjusted analyses, gay and bisexual men were less likely than heterosexual men to have health insurance coverage, but the difference did not remain significant after adjustment. No significant differences appeared in the indicators of health care access between gay and bisexual men.

Health Behaviors

Prevalence rates of physical activity were similar among all female respondents, but lesbians and bisexual women were more likely than heterosexual women to smoke (AOR = 1.57) and to drink excessively (AOR = 1.43; Table 3). Lesbians (9.95%) were significantly more likely than bisexual women (3.90%; AOR = 0.40) to drink excessively (*P* < .05).

Gay and bisexual men had higher adjusted odds of smoking (AOR = 1.52) and excessive drinking (AOR = 1.47) than did heterosexual men; prevalence rates of physical activities

were similar. We observed no differences in health behaviors between gay and bisexual men.

Health Screening

Sexual minority women were significantly less likely than heterosexual women to have had a mammogram (AOR = 0.71), more likely to have been tested for HIV (AOR = 1.80), and equally likely to have received a flu shot. We observed no significant differences in health screenings between older lesbians and bisexual women.

The adjusted analyses indicated that gay and bisexual men were more likely than heterosexual men to have received a flu shot (AOR = 1.47) and an HIV test (AOR = 7.91). In the initial analyses, sexual minority men were significantly less likely than heterosexual men to receive a prostate-specific antigen test, but the difference was not significant after adjustment for sociodemographic characteristics. Although we found no significant differences between gay and bisexual men in the prevalence of receiving a flu shot or a prostate-specific antigen test, bisexual men (60.33%) were less likely than gay men (82.59%) to have been tested for HIV (AOR = 0.31; *P* < .001).

Discussion

We conducted one of the first studies to comprehensively examine leading CDC-defined health indicators among LGB older adults in population-based data. Contrary to the myth that older adults will not reveal their sexual orientation in public health surveys, in this population-based survey we found that approximately 2% of adults aged 50 years and older self-identified as

Table 3 Weighted Prevalence Rates and Regression Analyses of Health Indicators among Respondents Aged 50 Years and Older: Washington State Behavioral Risk Factor Surveillance System, 2003–2010

| | Women | | | | Men | | | |
| | Heterosexual, | Lesbian and Bisexual | | | Heterosexual, | Gay and Bisexual | | |
Health Indicator	%	%	OR (95% CI)	AOR (95% CI)	%	%	OR (95% CI)	AOR (95% CI)
Access to care								
Insurance	94.56	91.24	0.60*** (0.44, 0.82)	0.79 (0.55, 1.13)	93.36	89.42	0.60** (0.43, 0.84)	0.71 (0.48, 1.04)
Financial barrier	8.26	13.05	1.67*** (1.29, 2.16)	1.25 (0.97, 1.62)	6.81	8.43	1.26 (0.86, 1.84)	0.97 (0.63, 1.50)
Personal provider	92.41	93.09	1.11 (0.76, 1.60)	1.43 (0.97, 2.11)	88.57	88.41	0.98 (0.73, 1.33)	1.16 (0.84, 1.60)
Behavior								
Smoking	11.61	18.33	1.71*** (1.36, 2.15)	1.57*** (1.22, 2.00)	13.15	20.04	1.66*** (1.30, 2.11)	1.52** (1.18, 1.96)
Excessive drinking	4.61	7.88	1.77** (1.27, 2.47)	1.43* (1.02, 2.00)	11.12	17.13	1.65** (1.24, 2.20)	1.47* (1.09, 1.98)
Physical activity[a]	49.02	51.92	1.12 (0.88, 1.01)	1.01 (0.78, 1.31)	51.23	53.04	1.08 (0.81, 1.43)	1.04 (0.78, 1.40)
Screening								
Flu shot	55.07	52.99	0.92 (0.77, 1.10)	1.20 (1.00, 1.44)	50.40	54.87	1.20 (0.98, 1.46)	1.47*** (1.18, 1.82)
Mammogram[b]	79.77	74.16	0.73* (0.54, 0.98)	0.71* (0.52, 0.97)	...	...	...	...
PSA test[b]	...	...	...	...	49.85	40.67	0.69* (0.51, 0.93)	0.81 (0.59, 1.10)
HIV test[c]	23.89	40.80	2.20*** (1.79, 2.70)	1.80*** (1.46, 2.23)	28.31	76.47	8.23*** (6.22, 10.88)	7.91*** (5.94, 10.54)

Note. AOR = adjusted odds ratio; CI = confidence interval; OR = odds ratio; PSA = prostate-specific antigen. Adjusted logistic regression models controlled for age, income, and education; heterosexuals were coded as the reference group.

[a]Questions were asked in 2003, 2005, 2007, and 2009.

[b]Questions were asked in 2004, 2006, and 2008.

[c]Question was asked only of those younger than 65 years.

*$P <.05$; **$P < .01$; ***$P <.001$.

lesbian, gay, or bisexual. The findings reveal significant health disparities among LGB older adults, with both strengths and gaps across the continuum of health indicators examined. Our results suggest that some health disparity patterns that have been found in LGB adults at younger ages[9,10] persist in later life, including higher likelihoods of disability, poor mental health, and smoking, and, among lesbians and bisexual women, excessive drinking and obesity. We also found some health disparities—heightened risks of CVD among lesbian and bisexual women and of poor physical health and excessive drinking among gay and bisexual men—that may emerge later in the life course. Such health disparities likely have detrimental consequences for the quality of life of these LGB older adults.[14,32,33]

According to the life course perspective, social context, cultural meaning, and structural location (in addition to time, period, and cohort) affect aging processes, including health.[34,35] Situating LGB older adults within the historical and social context of their lives may help us to better understand the health issues they face as they age.[36] LGB older adults came of age during a time when same-sex relationships were criminalized and severely stigmatized and same-sex identities were socially invisible.

Elevated risks of disability and poor mental health among LGB older adults may be linked with experiences of stigmatization[37–39] and victimization,[39;41] especially in light of the profound impact that events at a given stage of life can have on subsequent stages.[42] The social contexts in which they have lived may have exposed LGB older adults to multiple types of victimization and discrimination related to sexual orientation, disability, age, gender, and race/ethnicity.[41] D'Augelli and Grossman, for example, argue that lifetime experiences of victimization among sexual minority older adults because of their sexual orientation affects mental health in later life.[40] The evidence of physiological impact of chronic stressors on health[43] suggests that lifetime experiences of victimization may partially account for higher rates of disability among LGB older adults. Although our study was designed to identify health disparities among LGB older adults, further research is needed to compare LGB age cohorts and health changes over time.

Heightened risks of disability and poor physical and mental health among older gay and bisexual men may also be related to HIV.[44] Lacking information on HIV status in our data set, we could not explore this issue, but the disparity may be related to the prevalence of HIV among gay and bisexual men. With the advances in antiretroviral therapies, more adults with HIV are living into old age,[45,46] and older adults living with HIV have been found to be at increased risk of disability and poor physical and mental health.

Elevated risks of smoking and excessive drinking are of major concern among LGB older adults. Although smoking and excessive drinking are leading causes of preventable morbidity and mortality,[47] most prevention campaigns target only younger populations.[48,49] Intervention strategies that both identify and address distinctive cultural factors that may promote smoking and drinking among LGB older adults are desperately

Health Disparities among Lesbian, Gay, and Bisexual Older Adults by Karen Fredriksen-Goldsen et al.

67

needed. Previous research has found that LGB adults smoke at much higher rates than their heterosexual counterparts,[9,10,50] and our findings illustrate that such disparities persist among LGB older adults. We also found that older sexual minority women were more likely than older heterosexual women to drink excessively, which has also been documented in studies of younger sexual minority women.[9,10,50]

Existing research documents that drinking rates decline with age among older adults in general.[51] Although the prevalence rates of excessive drinking among younger gay, bisexual, and heterosexual adult men were similar in other population-based studies, we found higher rates among older gay and bisexual than heterosexual men. It may be that the rate of decline in drinking among older gay and bisexual men is slower than among older heterosexual men.[52] In addition, we found that older lesbians had higher rates of excessive drinking than did older bisexual women, which is also inconsistent with reports from population-based studies of younger lesbian and bisexual women.[10,50] A longitudinal study is warranted to better understand such changes in drinking behavior patterns among sexual minorities, and it will be important to examine how earlier experiences, such as frequent attendance at bars, clubs, and private house parties,[53] combined with minority stressors such as discrimination and victimization,[54] influence changes in drinking patterns over time among LGB older adults.

Older lesbians and bisexual women were more likely than their heterosexual counterparts to be obese and to have CVD; older gay and bisexual men were less likely than heterosexuals to be obese. The higher prevalence of obesity among lesbians and bisexual women than heterosexual women is well documented,[55] but increased risk of CVD has rarely been reported.[56] According to Conron et al., lesbian and bisexual adults may have a higher risk of CVD, possibly attributable to higher prevalence of obesity and smoking.[10] It is likely that disparities in obesity and smoking in early life influence disparities in CVD in later life among lesbians and bisexual women.[57,58]

Our subgroup analyses revealed that diabetes was more common in older bisexual than gay men, even though the obesity rates for the 2 groups were similar. The association between type 2 diabetes and obesity is well known.[59] Although previous studies found that among young adults, gay men were less likely to be obese than were heterosexual men, bisexual men were not.[10] Additional research is needed to investigate whether it is the duration of obesity among older bisexual men that increases their risk of diabetes,[60] as well as to further explore weight change and its impact on older gay men.

We observed some positive trends in preventive screenings, such as the higher likelihood of receiving a flu shot and an HIV test for gay and bisexual than for heterosexual men. Lesbians and bisexual women were more likely than their heterosexual peers to receive an HIV test. Yet we also found evidence of gaps and missed opportunities for prevention. For example, among sexual minority older men, bisexual men were less likely than gay men to obtain an HIV test. Older lesbians and bisexual women were less likely than heterosexual women to report having had a mammogram. Efforts to promote mammography screening among older lesbians and bisexual women

is particularly important, because higher risks of breast cancer have been documented among sexual minority women, attributable to elevated prevalence of obesity, substance use, and nulliparity.[61-63] Hart and Bowen suggest that lack of knowledge regarding breast cancer and the benefits of mammography combined with reluctance to use health services because of stigma likely prevent lesbians and bisexual women from receiving mammography in a timely manner.[64]

We observed several important differences in background characteristics by sexual orientation. Contrary to existing stereotypes, despite higher levels of education among LGB older adults, and the higher likelihood of employment among lesbians and bisexual women, LGB older adults do not have higher incomes than do heterosexuals, as observed in other population-based data.[65] In addition, LGB older adults are less likely than heterosexuals to be married but more likely to be partnered, which may have implications for health care advocacy, caregiving, and the availability of financial resources as they age. A recent study found that for gay men, being legally married is associated with mental health benefits.[38] Older gay and bisexual men have significantly fewer children in the household than do heterosexuals and are more likely to live alone, which corroborates findings in other population-based studies.[14] Higher rates of living alone may be related to the increased likelihood of the loss of a partner to AIDS.[66] It is also possible that structural factors do not support committed relationships or legal marriage among same-sex partners. LGB older adults who live alone are likely at risk for social isolation, which has been linked to poor mental and physical health, cognitive impairment, and premature morbidity and mortality in the general elderly population.[67]

Limitations

The cross-sectional nature of BRFSS data limits the ability to disentangle the temporal relationships between variables of interest. Although the purpose of the BRFSS is monitoring overall prevalence of health status, chronic conditions, and behaviors in the United States, and the measures are based on self-report, objective information such as symptoms and severity of health conditions is not available. We analyzed BRFSS data from only 1 state, limiting applicability to other state populations.

Our findings were limited with respect to the response rate of the BRFSS[68,69] and the self-identification of sexual orientation. The proportion of the older population that self-identified as sexual minorities in our data (~ 2%) was less than the 3.5% of adults aged 18 years and older who self-identified as LGB in most other population-based studies.[70] This may reflect the historical context in which today's LGB older adults came of age; these cohorts may be less likely than younger age groups to identify themselves as a sexual minority in a telephone-based survey.

Conclusions

More research with a life-course perspective is needed to examine how age and cohort effects may differentiate the experiences of younger and older LGB adults. Studies that examine the interplay between resilience and the stressors associated with aging and living as a sexual minority would likely help us better understand the mechanisms through which social contexts directly and indirectly affect the health of LGB older adults. Further research, especially a longitudinal study of health among LGB older adults that directly tests the relationships between transitions and trajectories through the life course and investigates the role of human agency in adapting to structural and legal constraints, would provide a greater understanding of how life experiences and shifting social contexts affect health outcomes in later life. Because LGB older adults may rely less on partners, spouses, and children, future research needs to investigate how differing types of social networks, support, and family structures influence health and aging experiences.[71] Although the sample size in our data did not allow for direct comparisons across different birth cohorts of LGB older adults, they are needed. The oldest-old LGB population, for example, may have experienced greater challenges in disclosing their sexual orientation; they may also have faced more barriers to social resources affecting health outcomes.

Our findings document population-based health disparities among LGB older adults. Early detection and identification of factors associated with such at-risk groups will enable public health initiatives to expand the reach of strategies and interventions to promote healthy communities. It is imperative that we understand the health needs of older sexual minorities in general as well as those specific to subgroups in this population to develop effective preventive interventions and services tailored to their unique needs. It is imperative that we begin to address healthy aging in our increasingly diverse society.

Human Participant Protection

The institutional review board of the University of Washington approved this study.

References

1. Vincent GA, Velkoff VA. *The Next Four Decades, The Older Population in the United States: 2010 to 2050.* Washington, DC: US Census Bureau; 2010.

2. Centers for Disease Control and Prevention, Merck Company Foundation. The state of aging and health in America. 2007. Available at: www.cdc.gov/aging/pdf/saha_2007.pdf. Accessed October 26, 2011.

3. *Biennial Report of the Director, National Institutes of Health, Fiscal Years 2008 & 2009.* Washington, DC: National Institutes of Health; 2010.

4. Disparities. HealthyPeople.gov. Available at: www.healthypeople.gov/2020/about/disparitiesAbout.aspx#six. Accessed October 26, 2011.

5. MacArthur Foundation Research Network on an Aging Society. Facts and fictions about an aging America. *Contexts.* 2009;8(4):16–21.

6. Truman BI, Smith KC, Roy K, et al. Rationale for regular reporting on health disparities and inequalities—United States. *MMWR Suveill Summ.* 2011;60(suppl):3–10.

7. Institute of Medicine. *The Health of Lesbian, Gay, Bisexual, and Transgender People: Building a Foundation for Better Understanding.* Washington, DC: National Academies Press; 2011.

8. Fredriksen-Goldsen KI, Muraco A. Aging and sexual orientation: a 25-year review of the literature. *Res Aging.* 2010;32(3):372–413.

9. Dilley JA, Simmons KW, Boysun MJ, Pizacani BA, Stark MJ. Demonstrating the importance and feasibility of including sexual orientation in public health surveys: health disparities in the Pacific Northwest. *Am J Public Health.* 2010;100(3):460–467.

10. Conron KJ, Mimiaga MJ, Landers SJ. A population-based study of sexual orientation identity and gender differences in adult health. *Am J Public Health.* 2010;100(10):1953–1960.

11. Boehmer U, Bowen DJ, Bauer GR. Overweight and obesity in sexual-minority women: evidence from population-based data. *Am J Public Health.* 2007;97(6):1134–1140.

12. Fredriksen-Goldsen KI, Kim H-J, Barkan SE, Balsam KF, Mincer S. Disparities in health-related quality of life: a comparison of lesbian and bisexual women. *Am J Public Health.* 2010;100(11):2255–2261.

13. Valanis BG, Bowen DJ, Bassford T, Whitlock E, Charney P, Carter RA. Sexual orientation and health: comparisons in the Women's Health Initiative sample. *Arch Fam Med.* 2000;9(9):843–853.

14. Wallace SP, Cochran SD, Durazo EM, Ford CL. *The Health of Aging Lesbian, Gay and Bisexual Adults in California.* Los Angeles: University of California, Los Angeles Center for Health Policy Research; 2011.

15. Centers for Disease Control and Prevention. Behavioral Risk Factor Surveillance System operational and user's guide. Available at: ftp://ftp.cdc.gov/pub/Data/Brfss/userguide.pdf. Accessed July 10, 2012.

16. Levin B, Lieberman DA, McFarland B, et al. Screening and surveillance for the early detection of colorectal cancer and adenomatous polyps, 2008: a joint guideline from the American Cancer Society, the US Multi-Society Task Force on Colorectal Cancer, and the American College of Radiology. *CA Cancer J Clin.* 2008;58(3):130–160.

17. AgePage. Menopause. National Institute on Aging. Available at: www.nia.nih.gov/healthinformation/publications/menopause.htm. Accessed June, 24, 2011.

18. Alexander CM, Landsman PB, Teutsch SM, Haffner SM, Third National Health and Nutrition Examination Survey (NHANES III), National Cholesterol Education Program (NCEP). NCEP-defined metabolic syndrome, diabetes, and prevalence of coronary heart disease among NHANES III participants age 50 years and older. *Diabetes.* 2003;52(5):1210–1214.

19. Office of Applied Studies. *The NSDUH Report—Serious Psychological Distress Among Adults Aged 50 or Older: 2005 and 2006.* Rockville, MD: Substance Abuse and Mental Health Services Administration; 2008.

20. Bowen ME, González HM. Racial/ethnic differences in the relationship between the use of health care services and functional disability: the health and retirement study (1992–2004). *Gerontologist.* 2008;48(5):659–667.

21. 2003–2010 Behavioral Risk Factor Surveillance System summary data quality reports. Centers for Disease Control and Prevention. Available at: www.cdc.gov/brfss/annual_data/annual_data.htm#2001. Accessed July 10, 2012.

Health Disparities among Lesbian, Gay, and Bisexual Older Adults by Karen Fredriksen-Goldsen et al.

69

22. *Measuring Healthy Days*. Atlanta, GA: Centers for Disease Control and Prevention; 2000.

23. Fan AZ, Strine TW, Jiles R, Berry JT, Mokdad AH. Psychological distress, use of rehabilitation services, and disability status among noninstitutionalized US adults aged 35 years and older, who have cardiovascular conditions, 2007. *Int J Public Health*. 2009;54(suppl 1):100–105.

24. Shankar A, Syamala S, Kalidindi S. Insufficient rest or sleep and its relation to cardiovascular disease, diabetes and obesity in a national, multiethnic sample. *PLoS ONE*. 2010;5(11):e14189.

25. Overweight and obesity: defining overweight and obesity. Centers for Disease Control and Prevention. Available at: www.cdc.gov/obesity/defining.html. Accessed April 10, 2012.

26. Centers for Disease Control and Prevention. Vital signs: current cigarette smoking among adults aged ≥ 18 years– United States, 2005–2010. *MMWR Morb Mortal Wkly Rep*. 2011;60(35):1207–1212.

27. National Institute of Alcohol Abuse and Alcoholism. NIAAA council approves definition of binge drinking. *NIAAA Newsletter*. 2004;3:3.

28. Objectives 22-2 and 22-3. *Healthy People 2010* (conference ed, 2 vols). Washington, DC: US Department of Health and Human Services; 2000.

29. Key facts about seasonal flu vaccine. Centers for Disease Control and Prevention. Available at: www.cdc.gov/flu/protect/keyfacts.htm. Accessed December 13, 2011.

30. National Cancer Institute fact sheet: mammograms. National Cancer Institute. Available at: www.cancer.gov/cancertopics/factsheet/detection/mammograms. Accessed December 13, 2011.

31. National Cancer Institute fact sheet: prostate-specific antigen (PSA) test. National Cancer Institute. Available at: www.cancer.gov/cancertopics/factsheet/detection/PSA. Accessed December 13, 2011.

32. Fried LP, Guralnik JM. Disability in older adults: evidence regarding significance, etiology, and risk. *J Am Geriatr Soc*. 1997;45(1):92–100.

33. Fredriksen-Goldsen KI, Kim H-J, Emlet CA, et al. The aging and health report: disparities and resilience among lesbian, gay, bisexual, and transgender older adults. 2011 Available at: http://caringandaging.org. Accessed December 13, 2011.

34. Mayer KU. New directions in life course research. *Annu Rev Sociol*. 2009;35:413–433.

35. Elder GH., Jr. Time, human agency, and social change: perspectives on the life course. *Soc Psychol Q*. 1994;57(1):4–15.

36. Clunis DM, Fredriksen-Goldsen KI, Freeman PA, Nystrom N. *Lives of Lesbian Elders: Looking Back, Looking Forward*. Binghamton, NY: Haworth Press; 2005.

37. Meyer IH. Prejudice, social stress, and mental health in lesbian, gay, and bisexual populations: conceptual issues and research evidence. *Psychol Bull*. 2003;129(5):674–697.

38. Wight RG, LeBlanc AJ, de Vries B, Detels R. Stress and mental health among midlife and older gay-identified men. *Am J Public Health*. 2012;102(3):503–510.

39. Fredriksen-Goldsen KI, Emlet CA, Kim HJ, et al. The physical and mental health of lesbian, gay male, and bisexual (LGB) older adults: the role of key health indicators and risk and protective factors. *Gerontologist*. Epub ahead of print October 3, 2012.

40. D'Augelli AR, Grossman AH. Disclosure of sexual orientation, victimization, and mental health among lesbian, gay, and bisexual older adults. *J Interpers Violence*. 2001;16(10):1008–1027.

41. Fredriksen-Goldsen KI, Kim H-J, Muraco A, Mincer S. Chronically ill midlife and older lesbians, gay men, and bisexuals and their informal caregivers: the impact of the social context. *Sex Res Social Policy*. 2009;6(4):52–64.

42. Marmot MG, Wilkinson RG. *Social Determinants of Health*. 2nd ed. New York, NY: Oxford University Press; 2006.

43. Juster RP, McEwen BS, Lupien SJ. Allostatic load biomarkers of chronic stress and impact on health and cognition. *Neurosci Biobehav Rev*. 2010;35(1):2–16.

44. Jia H, Uphold CR, Zheng Y, et al. A further investigation of health-related quality of life over time among men with HIV infection in the HAART era. *Qual Life Res*. 2007;16(6):961–968.

45. Justice AC. HIV and aging: time for a new paradigm. *Curr HIV/AIDS Rep*. 2010;7(2):69–76.

46. Brennan DJ, Emlet CA, Eady A. HIV, sexual health, and psychosocial issues among older adults living with HIV in North America. *Ageing Int*. 2011;36(3):313–333.

47. Center for Substance Abuse Treatment. *Substance Abuse Among Older Adults*. Rockville, MD: Substance Abuse and Mental Health Services Administration; 1998. Treatment Improvement Protocol (TIP) Series 26.

48. Backinger CL, Fagan P, Matthews E, Grana R. Adolescent and young adult tobacco prevention and cessation: current status and future directions. *Tob Control*. 2003;12(suppl 4):iv46–iv53.

49. Wakefield MA, Loken B, Hornik RC. Use of mass media campaigns to change health behaviour. *Lancet*. 2010;376(9748): 1261–1271.

50. Burgard SA, Cochran SD, Mays VM. Alcohol and tobacco use patterns among heterosexually and homosexually experienced California women. *Drug Alcohol Depend*. 2005;77(1):61–70.

51. Kanny D, Liu Y, Brewer RD. Centers for Disease Control and Prevention. Binge drinking–United States, 2009. *MMWR Surveill Summ*. 2011;60(suppl):101–104.

52. Green KE, Feinstein BA. Substance use in lesbian, gay, and bisexual populations: an update on empirical research and implications for treatment. *Psychol Addict Behav*. 2012;26(2):265–278.

53. Trocki KF, Drabble L, Midanik L. Use of heavier drinking contexts among heterosexuals, homosexuals and bisexuals: results from a National Household Probability Survey. *J Stud Alcohol*. 2005;66(1):105–110.

54. Brubaker MD, Garrett MT, Dew BJ. Examining the relationship between internalized heterosexism and substance abuse among lesbian, gay, and bisexual individuals: a critical review. *J LGBT Issues Couns*. 2009;3(1):62–89.

55. Bowen DJ, Balsam KF, Ender SR. A review of obesity issues in sexual minority women. *Obesity (Silver Spring)* 2008;16(2):221–228.

56. Roberts SA, Dibble SL, Nussey B, Casey K. Cardiovascular disease risk in lesbian women. *Womens Health Issues.* 2003;13(4):167–174.

57. Hubert HB, Feinleib M, McNamara PM, Castelli WP. Obesity as an independent risk factor for cardiovascular disease: a 26-year follow-up of participants in the Framingham Heart Study. *Circulation.* 1983;67(5):968–977.

58. He J, Ogden LG, Bazzano LA, Vupputuri S, Loria C, Whelton PK. Risk factors for congestive heart failure in US men and women: NHANES I epidemiologic follow-up study. *Arch Intern Med.* 2001;161(7):996–1002.

59. Nguyen NT, Nguyen XM, Lane J, Wang P. Relationship between obesity and diabetes in a US adult population: findings from the National Health and Nutrition Examination Survey, 1999–2006. *Obes Surg.* 2011;21(3):351–355.

60. Lee JM, Gebremariam A, Vijan S, Gurney JG. Excess body mass index-years, a measure of degree and duration of excess weight, and risk for incident diabetes. *Arch Pediatr Adolesc Med.* 2012;166(1):42–48.

61. Case P, Austin SB, Hunter DJ, et al. Sexual orientation, health risk factors, and physical functioning in the Nurses' Health Study II. *J Womens Health (Larchmt)* 2004;13(9):1033–1047.

62. Cochran SD, Mays VM, Bowen D, et al. Cancerrelated risk indicators and preventive screening behaviors among lesbians and bisexual women. *Am J Public Health.* 2001;91(4):591–597.

63. Dibble SL, Roberts SA, Nussey B. Comparing breast cancer risk between lesbians and their heterosexual sisters. *Womens Health Issues.* 2004;14(2):60–68.

64. Hart SL, Bowen DJ. Sexual orientation and intentions to obtain breast cancer screening. *J Womens Health (Larchmt)* 2009;18(2):177–185.

65. Albelda R, Badgett MVL, Schneebaum A, Gates GJ. *Poverty in the Lesbian, Gay, and Bisexual Community.* Los Angeles, CA: Williams Institute; 2009.

66. Cochran SD, Mays V, Corliss H, Smith TW, Turner J. Self-reported altruistic and reciprocal behaviors among homosexually and heterosexually experienced adults: implications for HIV/AIDS service organizations. *AIDS Care.* 2009;21(6):675–682.

67. Cornwell EY, Waite LJ. Measuring social isolation among older adults using multiple indicators from the NSHAP Study. *J Gerontol B Psychol Sci Soc Sci.* 2009;64B(suppl 1):i38–i46.

68. Schneider KL, Clark MA, Rakowski W, Lapane KL. Evaluating the impact of non-response bias in the Behavioral Risk Factor Surveillance System (BRFSS). *J Epidemiol Community Health.* 2012;66(4):290–295.

69. Keeter S, Kennedy C, Dimock M, Best J, Craighill P. Gauging the impact of growing nonresponse on estimates from a national RDD telephone survey. *Public Opin Q.* 2006;70(5):759–779.

70. Gates GJ. *How Many People Are Lesbian, Gay, Bisexual, and Transgender?* Los Angeles, CA: Williams Institute; 2011.

71. Muraco A, Fredriksen-Goldsen K. "That's what friends do": informal caregiving for chronically ill lesbian, gay, and bisexual elders. *J Soc Pers Relat.* 2011;28(8):1073–1092.

Critical Thinking

1. Do you think that the attitudes of professionals and others influence service delivery to the lesbian, gay, and bisexual population?

2. How do you think some of the gaps in health disparities can be closed, or even shortened?

Create Central

www.mhhe.com/createcentral

Internet References

The LGBT Aging Project
www.lgbtagingproject.org

National Resource Center on LGBT Aging
www.lgbtagingcenter.org

KAREN I. FREDRIKSEN-GOLDSEN, HYUN-JUN KIM, SUSAN E. BARKAN, AND CHARLES P. HOY-ELLIS are with the School of Social Work, University of Washington, Seattle. ANNA MURACO is with the Department of Sociology, Loyola Marymount University, Los Angeles.

Fredriksen-Goldsen et al., Karen. From *American Journal of Public Health,* October 2013, pp. 1802–1809. Copyright © 2013 by American Public Health Association. Reprinted by permission via Sheridan Reprints.

Unit 4

UNIT

Prepared by: Elaina Osterbur, *Saint Louis University*

Problems and Potentials of Aging

Aging is part of every aspect of the life cycle. Aging begins the day we are born. Every aspect of lifespan transitions includes aging at its core. Theories abound within these transitions that help to explain the problems and potentials along the lifespan. Developmental psychologists and psychoanalysts explain the development of attachment, psychosexual development, cognitive development, and much more. Many of these theorists explain development from birth to death. Other theorists concentrate on biological aging.

American society is often concerned with the biology of aging because of the potential for disability at older ages. Diseases such as cancer and heart disease not only cause disability, but can also cause death. Stroke, diabetes, and arthritis are among the top 10 chronic diseases of aging. These diseases can cause disability that affects older adults' activities of daily living, as well as the instrumental activities of daily living. The prevention of chronic disease in older adults is a major priority of healthcare systems and institutions.

The maintaining of health is also important to older adults because many older Americans try to remain masters of their own destinies for as long as possible. They fear dependence and try to avoid it. Many are successful at maintaining independence and the right to make their own decisions. Others are less successful and must depend on their families for care and making critical decisions. However, some older people are able to overcome the difficulties of aging and to lead comfortable and enjoyable lives.

The articles in this section explain age-associated diseases and their impact on policy, medical technology, and population health.

Article   Prepared by: Elaina Osterbur, *Saint Louis University*

Peripheral Arterial Disease and Exercise for Older Adults

How a walking regimen improves fitness and reduces pain caused by poor blood flow in the legs.

SALLY PAULSON AND JOOHEE SANDERS

Learning Outcomes

After reading this article, you will be able to:

- Describe the pathophysiology of peripheral arterial disease.

- Discuss the impact of exercise on the treatment of peripheral arterial disease.

- Identify the types of exercise that benefit older adults with peripheral arterial disease.

Peripheral arterial disease (PAD) occurs when plaque accumulates in the arteries of the legs. Reduced blood flow and loss of oxygen in the tissues beyond the obstruction cause localized muscular pain, or **claudication,** especially during exercise (Bulmer & Coombes 2004; Womack & Gardner 2003).

PAD decreases the functional capacity of older adults, who during physical activity often experience intermittent claudication, which can impair their ability to do everyday tasks. Exercise can be an effective, drug-free treatment that enhances functional capacity by altering hemo-dynamic and metabolic efficiencies.

Peripheral arterial disease decreases the functional capacity of older adults, who during physical activity often experience intermittent claudication, which can impair their ability to do everyday tasks.

Pathophysiology of Peripheral Arterial Disease

PAD affects more than 8 million Americans (Rosamond et al. 2008) and is associated with a high risk of cardiovascular death because narrowed arteries limit blood flow to the limbs. Risk factors for PAD include hypertension, diabetes mellitus, hyperlipidemia, premature atherosclerosis and smoking.

Limb **ischemia** (reduced blood flow) in turn triggers muscle pain (especially in the legs) during weight-bearing exercises; rest usually brings relief. This chronic vascular insufficiency can lead to significant functional impairment (Regensteiner et al. 1993a). As the disease progresses, people may become increasingly incapacitated and lose the ability to perform simple tasks like walking without becoming fatigued. This may lead to muscle fiber denervation, atrophy and altered metabolism (Regensteiner et al. 1993b; Kemp et al. 2001). Thus, it is thought that PAD is a disease characterized not only by hemodynamic insufficiency but also by subsequent metabolic and mechanical impairments.

Claudication Pain Levels

1. minimal pain
2. moderate pain
3. intense pain
4. maximal pain

Source: ACSM 2013.

Sample Exercise Prescription

Aerobic Training
Mode: intermittent walking
Frequency: 2–3 days per week, progressing up to
    5 days
Duration: 20–50 minutes, not including rest
Intensity: 40% of heart rate reserve, gradually progress-
    ing up to 70%

Resistance Training
Mode: all major muscle groups
Frequency: 2–3 days per week
Duration: 8–10 reps, progressing up to 3 sets
Intensity: easy to moderate

In healthy people, blood flow is by far the most important determinant of aerobic capacity. In people with PAD, the contribution of O_2 extraction to the aerobic capacity may be more even. The ischemic muscle must work harder to compensate for inadequate blood supply for a given power output. Consequently, the lack of O_2 supply favours anaerobic metabolism, leading to an early accumulation of lactate and ending exercise prematurely (Kemp et al. 1995).

It is clear there is a mismatch in O_2 delivery and utilization in individuals with PAD. Although revascularization surgery can improve calf-muscle blood flow, studies have not found consistent evidence of an increase in exercise performance (Regensteiner et al. 1993a). Thus, engaging in a long-term, continuous exercise training program to improve metabolic capacity is recommended.

Exercise Testing and Prescription

Older adults with PAD should obtain medical clearance and complete an exercise test before participating in an exercise program. Evaluation protocols include a graded treadmill test and a 6-minute walk test (Womack & Gardner 2003). The degree of claudication pain and time of onset should be recorded during the exercise test. The test should be terminated if a client experiences intense pain or if a cardiovascular abnormality is observed. Questionnaires (such as the Walking Impairment Questionnaire, Physical Activity Recall or Medical Outcomes Study) can be used if a treadmill or walking test cannot be performed (Womack & Gardner 2003).

Exercise can significantly improve functional capacity in older adults with PAD and is therefore considered one of the best ways to treat limb ischemia. The exercise program should aim to relieve symptoms, reduce pain and improve functional performance and quality of life (Wang et al. 2010).

Chronic exercise has been shown to increase walking distance before the onset of leg pain (McDermott et al. 2008). Furthermore, 3 months of exercise has been shown to improve maximum walking distance by as much as 80% (Tan et al. 2000). Even 14 days of physical exercise enhanced blood flow enough to induce improvements in claudication in study participants (Arosio et al. 1999). Aerobic adaptation can also play a significant role in improving functional performance. Exercise training may augment metabolic activity by improving oxidative metabolism and O_2 extraction, thus reducing O_2 tension and the cost of exercise—and lessening cardiac burden.

Aerobic Training

Exercise sessions for older adults with PAD mainly focus on aerobic training to optimize functional performance. The preferred training method is walking, because it improves gait patterns and quality of life (Womack & Gardner 2003). Aerobic training is performed in intervals because older adults may be able to walk for only a short time before claudication pain begins. For most, the pain subsides in 5 minutes and the activity can resume (Bulmer & Coombes 2004). This cycle of walking until pain and then resting should continue until the person has achieved the desired duration. For instance, an older adult with PAD may be able to walk for only 5 minutes before the onset of mild to moderate claudication pain. The individual should rest until the pain subsides (about 5 minutes) and then complete another bout of walking. Thus, 20 minutes of exercise will require a 40-minute timeframe.

The recommended frequency for aerobic training is 2–3 days per week (Bulmer & Coombes 2004), with 3 being ideal. Initially, the session should last 20 minutes, at ~40% of heart rate reserve (HRR), and should progress toward 50 minutes with an increase in intensity, up to 70% of HRR. Walking speed is determined by the point where moderate claudication pain occurs within 5 minutes (Womack & Gardner 2003). The grade or speed of the treadmill is increased once a client can complete 8–10 minutes of pain-free walking. If the speed is under 2 miles per hour, then speed is increased. If the speed is over 2 mph, then the grade is increased.

The overall goal is to reach 35–50 minutes of continuous pain-free walking (Lampman & Wolk 2009). Intensity will be gradually advanced as functional performance improves and pain decreases. Peak walking ability should occur after 12–24 weeks of continuous training (Bulmer & Coombes 2004).

Resistance Training

While the benefits of aerobic training have been clearly documented to improve functional performance in PAD clients, there is little information on resistance training. Some research has shown that people with PAD lose muscular strength in their lower extremities (McDermott et al. 2008; Wang et al. 2010). Investigators have found that resistance training can increase walking performance (Hiatt et al. 1990), leg strength and rate of force development in people with PAD (Wang et al. 2010). Therefore, older adults with PAD can benefit from resistance training in addition to intermittent walking.

Resistance training should initially focus on major muscle groups in the legs and should progress to including the arms to help with activities of daily living. Intensity should be easy to moderate. Duration should start with 1 set of 8–10 repetitions and gradually progress to 3 sets. Frequency should be 2–3 days per week, and 1 day should be added every 2–3 weeks, as tolerated, to progress toward 5 days of combined aerobic and resistance training (Lampman & Wolk 2009).

Conclusion

Older adults with PAD have reduced functional capacity because of claudication. Thus, health and fitness professionals need to recognize the basic physiological phenomenon behind PAD and develop exercise programs to improve quality of life. Intermittent exercise 2–3 days per week is recommended to achieve 35–50 minutes of continuous pain-free walking.

Older adults should walk until the onset of moderate claudication, then rest and resume activity once the pain subsides. The primary goal is to improve walking efficiency through aerobic training. Resistance training should be a complement to aerobic training and not a substitute.

References

ACSM (American College of Sports Medicine). 2013. *ACSM's Guidelines for Exercise Testing and Prescription*. Baltimore: American College of Sports Medicine.

Arosio, E., et al. 1999. Increased endogenous nitric oxide production induced by physical exercise in peripheral arterial occlusive disease patients. *Life Sciences, 65* (26), 2815–22.

Bulmer, A.C., & Coombes, J.S. 2004. Optimising exercise training in peripheral arterial disease. *Sports Medicine, 34* (14), 983–1003.

Hiatt, W.R., et al. 1990. Benefit of exercise conditioning for patients with peripheral arterial disease. *Circulation, 81* (2), 602–609.

Kemp, G.J., et al. 1995. Calf muscle mitochondrial and glycogenolytic ATP synthesis in patients with claudication due to peripheral vascular disease analysed using 31P magnetic resonance spectroscopy. *Clinical Science, 89* (6), 581–90.

Kemp, G.J., et al. 2001. Mitochondrial function and oxygen supply in normal and in chronically ischemic muscle: A combined 31P magnetic resonance spectroscopy and near infrared spectroscopy study in vivo. *Journal of Vascular Surgery, 34* (6) 1103–10.

Lampman, R.M., & Wolk, S.W. 2009. Peripheral arterial disease. In: J. Ehrman et al. (Eds.), *Clinical Exercise Physiology* (2nd ed.). Champaign, IL: Human Kinetics.

McDermott, M.M., et al. 2008. Associations between lower extremity ischemia, upper and lower extremity strength, and functional impairment with peripheral arterial disease. *Journal of the American Geriatrics Society, 56* (4), 724–29.

Regensteiner, J.G., et al. 1993a. Functional benefits of peripheral vascular bypass surgery for patients with intermittent claudication. *Angiology, 44* (1), 1–10.

Regensteiner, J.G., et al. 1993b. Chronic changes in skeletal muscle histology and function in peripheral arterial disease. *Circulation, 87* (2), 413–21.

Rosamond, W., et al. 2008. Heart disease and stroke statistics—2008 update: A report from the American Heart Association Statistics Committee and Stroke Statistics Subcommittee. *Circulation, 117* (4), e25–146.

Tan, K.H., et al. 2000. Exercise training for claudicants: Changes in blood flow, cardiorespiratory status, metabolic functions, blood rheology and lipid profile. *European Journal of Vascular and Endovascular Surgery, 20* (1), 72–78.

Wang, E., et al. 2010. Maximal strength training improves walking performance in peripheral arterial disease patients. *Scandinavian Journal of Medicine & Science in Sports, 20* (5), 764–70.

Womack, C.J., & Gardner, A.W. 2003. Peripheral arterial disease. In J.L. Durstine & G.E. Moore (Eds.), *ACSM's Exercise Management for Persons with Chronic Diseases and Disabilities* (2nd ed.). Champaign, IL: Human Kinetics.

Critical Thinking

1. What are claudication pain levels and how do they affect an older person's function?

2. Compare and contrast each exercise prescription and its effects on function.

Internet References

American College of Sports Medicine
http://www.acsm.org

Centers for Disease Control and Prevention (CDC): How Much Physical Activity Do Older Adults Need?
http://www.cdc.gov/physicalactivity/everyone/guidelines/olderadults.html

SALLY PAULSON, PhD, is an associate professor in the department of exercise science at Shippensburg University, Shippensburg, Pennsylvania. She is a certified athletic trainer and strength and conditioning specialist. She has worked with various populations, including obese adults and adults with developmental disabilities. **JOOHEE SANDERS**, PhD, is an associate professor in the department of exercise science at Shippensburg University, Shippensburg, Pennsylvania. She has served as a sport physiologist at the U.S. Olympic Training Center, in Lake Placid, New York. Her doctoral research studied mitochondrial function and blood flow of muscle tissue in diseased populations.

Article   Prepared by: Elaina F. Osterbur, *Saint Louis University*

The Worst Place to Be If You're Sick

Hospital errors cause 100,000 deaths yearly. These are preventable deaths. What's wrong, and can it be made right?

KATHARINE GREIDER

Learning Outcomes

After reading this article, you will be able to:

- Describe the mistakes that were identified as causing serious health problems for patients in hospitals throughout the country.
- Explain how 100 Michigan hospital intensive care units managed to reduce patient infections by two-thirds.

American hospitals are capable of great medical feats, but they also are plagued by daily errors that cost lives. No one knows that better than Ilene Corina. In the 1990's, she saw a medical team rescue her fragile premature newborn, but she also endured the death of another son—a healthy 3-year-old—when, she says, doctors failed to attend to complications from a routine tonsillectomy.

When a family member dies because of a hospital's mistake, "what do we care about the excellence in the system?" says Corina, 51, of Long Island, N.Y., founder and president of a patient safety advocacy group. "We have to voice our anger about the problems we see in the health care system."

Corina had already joined the patient safety movement when, in 1999, the Institute of Medicine's now-famous report, *To Err Is Human,* burst into public consciousness with its startling announcement: Each year as many as 100,000 Americans die in hospitals from preventable medical mistakes.

Today, more than a decade into the fight against medical errors, there's little reason to believe the risks have declined substantially for the 37 million people hospitalized each year. In fact, recent studies suggest a problem that's bigger and more complex than many had imagined. A report released in January on Medicare patients found that hospital staff did not report a whopping 86 percent of harms done to patients. If most errors that harm patients aren't even reported, they can never be tracked or corrected, the Health and Human Services Department report pointed out.

The number of patients who die each year from hospital errors is equal to 4 jumbo jets crashing each week.

This latest study built on an earlier HHS study of Medicare patients that found one in seven suffered serious or long-term injuries, or died, as a result of hospital care. Researchers said about 44 percent of the problems were preventable.

In another key study published last spring in the journal *Health Affairs,* researchers examined patient charts at three of America's leading hospitals and found that an astounding one in three admissions included some type of harm to the patient.

Mistakes run the gamut. The surgeon nicks a healthy blood vessel; a nurse mistakenly administers a toxic dose of medicine; the staff fails to adequately disinfect a room, and a patient contracts a dangerous "superbug."

The number of patients who die each year from preventable hospital errors is equal to four full jumbo jets crashing each week. If airline tragedies of that magnitude were occurring with such frequency, no one would tolerate the loss.

One study of Medicare patients found that 1 in 7 died or were harmed by their hospital care.

"At its deepest level, what we're now having trouble with is the enormous complexity of medicine," says Atul Gawande, a surgeon, Harvard associate professor and author who promotes the use of medical checklists to save lives. "We now have 13,600 diagnoses, 6,000 drugs, 4,000 medical and surgical procedures," he says. And yet "we have not paid attention to the nuts and bolts of what's required to manage complexity." Experts like Gawande say one reason medical errors continue at such high rates is that hospitals have only recently begun to copy aviation's decades-long effort to create safety procedures that take into account human fallibility—often using only simple checklists.

There has been some progress, to be sure. Around the country, safety innovators have introduced promising ways to minimize slipups—from using checklists to reporting hospital infection rates on state websites. Last spring the Obama administration announced it would spend $1 billion to fund safety measures by hospitals, with the ambitious goal of reducing preventable patient injuries by 40 percent by the end of next year.

Still, the question of how close hospitals can ever come to being error-free is controversial. It seems fair to expect them to reduce the number of times—as many as 40 per week—that U.S. surgeons operate on the wrong person or body part. But what about other procedures?

Patient safety advocates have been able to raise the bar on hospitals in some key areas, showing that they *can* prevent harm to even the most vulnerable patients. A case in point: bloodstream infections that result from inserting a tube into a large vein near the heart to deliver medication. For years, these infections, which resulted in some 30,000 deaths annually, were viewed as largely unavoidable.

But then, in a program launched in 2004, more than 100 Michigan intensive care units managed to reduce these infections by two-thirds—and save some 1,500 lives in just 18 months—using a short checklist of practices for handling the catheters, and a culture change aimed at getting all staff on board. Hospitals around the country then took up the challenger, and the results were impressive.

The trouble is, there are plenty of other problems that may not be susceptible to an approach that tests a simple process that can then be used nationwide. A recent program looking at lapses that could lead to surgery on the wrong section of the patient found that errors can creep in just about anywhere, from scheduling to the marking of the surgical site. A couple of hospitals, for example, were using pens those ink washed off during surgical prep, making the marks useless. Flaws in this process vary from one hospital or surgery center to another, says Mark Chassin, M.D., president of the Joint Commission, the major accrediting organization for hospitals.

1,500 lives were saved in 18 months when Michigan ICUs began using a checklist of practices for handling catheters.

Other, apparently straight-forward problems—like health care workers not washing their hands—have proved surprisingly stubborn. Only about half of hospital workers follow hand washing guidelines, despite excellent staff training and ubiquitous hand sanitizer dispensers at many hospitals, says Robert Wachter, M.D., a patient safety expert at the University of California, San Francisco. He points out an airline pilot would be disciplined or fired for ignoring safety rules. But while penalizing careless individuals remains controversial—and largely untried—in health care, activities have made hospitals more accountable.

Public reporting of hospital performance, more or less unheard of a decade ago, has been an important strategy. Twenty-nine states now require public reporting of hospital infection rates, and 28 require some information on medical errors. The HHS website has now added a key catheter infection rate, along with other results.

There are hundreds of ways to measure safety performance, from death rates after heart surgery to whether doctors gave the right antibiotic. What to report has been a major debate. Infection rates, initially resisted by hospitals, are now generally regarded as some of the most reliable data available to the public, since in most cases reports are made through a standard system developed by the U.S. Centers of Disease Control and Prevention.

Money may be another motivator for hospitals. In 2008 Medicare took the small step of restricting payments to hospitals for extra costs associated with 10 hospital-acquired conditions. This year it will begin giving extra money to hospitals that score the highest on a set of standards linked to better results for patients.

Naturally, many patients want to compare the safety records of their local hospitals before checking in. But that's still tough to do. "There are no existing data that can allow you to be confident you've picked the safest, highest-quality place to get care," says Chassin, who helped prepare the seminal *To Err is*

Protect Yourself from Hospital Errors

Advocates agree that patients can minimize their risks by keeping a close eyes on their care. Hospitals are busy places with lots of moving parts. "You cannot assume that people in the hospital have a really clear idea of who you are or why you're there," says Jean Rexford, director of the Connecticut Center for Patient Safety. Here are some tips on how to protect yourself:

- Bring an advocate—a friend or family member—especially for check-in and discharge. Many hospitals have a patient advocate or staff person you can consult. Or you can hire your own advocate, but be aware that the profession lacks licensing requirements, so get referrals and check credentials.
- Bring a notebook. Write down all your medications, why you take them and who prescribed them. Include phone numbers of key personal and medical contacts (and don't forget your cellphone and charger). In the hospltal, when questions arise, write them down.
- Bring a big bottle of hand sanitizer. Put it by your bed to remind you and the staff to keep hands clean.

For More:

- Hospitalcompare.hhs.gov
- Agency for Healthcare Research and Quality, ahrq.gov
- Consumers Union, consumerreports.org
- Connecticut Center for Patient Safety ("5 Things to Know"), ctcps.org

Human report "One reason is that safety and quality varies even within health systems. Just because they're great in one area doesn't mean that they're great in another."

Critical Thinking

1. Twenty-nine states now require what kind of public reporting on medical problems?

2. What financial measures has Medicare taken to force hospitals to comply with safer procedures and results?

3. Why is there no data available that allows the patients to be sure they are choosing the best hospital?

Create Central

www.mhhe.com/createcentral

Internet References

AARP Health Information
www.aarp.org/bulletin

Alzheimer's Association
www.alz.org

A.P.T.A. Section on Geriatrics
http://geriatricspt.org

Caregiver's Handbook
www.acsu.buffalo.edu/~drstall/hndbk0.html

Caregiver Survival Resources
www.caregiver.com

International Food Information Council
www.ifi c.org

University of California at Irvine: Institute for Brain Aging and Dementia
www.alz.uci.edu

Article   Prepared by: Elaina F. Osterbur, *Saint Louis University*

Poll: Upbeat Baby Boomers Say They're Not Old Yet

Learning Outcomes

After reading this article, you will be able to:

- Describe how the baby boomers' views of aging differ from those of younger adults.

- Cite what factors baby boomers consider to be the most undesirable aspects of getting older.

Baby boomers say wrinkles aren't so bad and they're not that worried about dying. Just don't call them "old."

The generation that once powered a youth movement isn't ready to symbolize the aging of America, even as its first members are becoming eligible for Medicare. A new poll finds three-quarters of all baby boomers still consider themselves middle-aged or younger, and that includes most of the boomers who are ages 57–65.

Younger adults call 60 the start of old age, but baby boomers are pushing that number back, according to the Associated Press-LifeGoesStrong.com poll. The median age they cite is 70. And a quarter of boomers insist you're not old until you're 80.

"In my 20s, I would have thought the 60s were bad, but they're not so bad at all," says 64-year-old Lynn Brown, a retired legal assistant and grandmother of 11 living near Phoenix in Apache Junction, Ariz.

The 77 million boomers are celebrating their 47th through 65th birthdays this year.

Overall, they're upbeat about their futures. Americans born in the population explosion after World War II are more likely to be excited about the positive aspects of aging, such as retirement, than worried about the negatives, like declining health. A third of those polled feel confident about growing older, almost twice as many as find it frustrating or sad. Sixteen percent report they're happy about aging, about equal to the number who say they're afraid. Most expect to live longer than their parents.

"I still think I've got years to go to do things," says Robert Bechtel, 64, of Virginia Beach, Va. He retired last year after nearly four decades as a retail manager. Now Bechtel has less stress and more time to do what he pleases, including designing a bunk bed for his grandchildren, remodeling a bathroom and teaching Sunday school.

A strong majority of baby boomers are enthusiastic about some perks of aging—watching their children or grandchildren grow up, doing more with friends and family, and getting time for favorite activities. About half say they're highly excited about retirement. Boomers most frequently offered the wisdom accumulated over their lives as the best thing about aging.

"The older you get, the smarter you get," says Glenn Farrand, 62, of Ankeny, Iowa.

But, he adds, "The physical part of it is the pits."

Baby boomers most often brought up failing health or fading physical abilities when asked to name the worst thing about getting older.

Among their top worries: physical ailments that would take away their independence (deeply worrisome to 45 percent), losing their memory (44 percent), and being unable to pay medical bills (43 percent). Many also fret about running out of money (41 percent).

Only 18 percent say they worry about dying. Another 22 percent are "moderately" concerned about it. More than two-thirds expect to live to at least age 76; 1 in 6 expects to make it into the 90s.

About half predict a better quality of life for themselves than their parents experienced as they aged.

"My own parents, by the time they were 65 to 70, were very, very inactive and very much old in their minds," says Brown. So they "sat around the house and didn't go anywhere."

"I have no intentions of sitting around the house," says Brown, whose hobbies include motorcycle rides with her husband. "I'm enjoying being a senior citizen more than my parents did."

But a minority of boomers–about a fourth–worry things will be harder for them than for the previous generation.

"I think we'll have less," said Vicki Mooney, 62, of Dobbs Ferry, N.Y., who fears older people will be pinched by cuts to Social Security and Medicare and rising health care costs. "The main difference in the quality of life is wondering if we will have a safety net."

Baby boomers with higher incomes generally are more optimistic about aging than their poorer peers. Women tend to feel sunnier than men; college graduates are more positive than those without a degree.

A third of baby boomers say their health has declined in the last five years, and that group is more likely to express fear or frustration about aging. Still, most boomers rate themselves in good or even excellent health overall, with less than 1 in 10 doing poorly.

Looking older is seriously bugging just 12 percent of baby boomers. The vast majority say they wouldn't get plastic surgery. That includes Johanna Taisey, 61, of Chandler, Ariz., who says aging is "no problem at all . . . it's just nature."

"Age with dignity," Taisey advises.

Among the 1 in 5 who have had or would consider cosmetic surgery, about half say they might improve their tummy or eyes. A sagging chin is the next biggest worry—nearly 40 percent would consider getting that fixed.

Only 5 percent of baby boomers say they might use the chemical Botox to temporarily smooth away wrinkles; 17 percent would consider laser treatments to fix varicose veins.

But boomers, especially women, are taking some steps to look younger. A majority of the women—55 percent—regularly dye their hair, and they overwhelmingly say it's to cover gray. Only 5 percent of the men admit using hair color.

A quarter of the women have paid more than $25 for an anti-aging skincare product, such as a lotion or night cream. Just 5 percent of the men say they've bought skincare that expensive.

Almost all baby boomers—90 percent—have tried to eat better. Three-quarters say they're motivated more by a desire to improve their health than their appearance. Most boomers—57 percent—say in the past year they've taken up a regular program of exercise. About the same number do mental exercises, such as crossword puzzles or video games, to stay sharp.

Sixty-four-year-old Loretta Davis of Salem, W.Va., reads and plays games on her computer and takes walks. Diabetes and hypertension keep her focused on her diet these days. "I wish I had been more conscious of what I was eating earlier in life," said Davis, who worked in a grocery store, a factory and an ice cream shop before being disabled by polio in the 1980s.

But Davis says getting older doesn't bother her: "I'm just glad to still be here."

The AP-LifeGoesStrong.com poll was conducted from June 3 to June 12 by Knowledge Networks of Menlo Park, Calif., and involved online interviews with 1,416 adults, including 1,078 baby boomers born between 1946 and 1964. The margin of sampling error for results from the full sample is plus or minus 4.4 percentage points; for the boomers, it is plus or minus 3.3 percentage points.

Knowledge Networks used traditional telephone and mail sampling methods to randomly recruit respondents. People selected who had no Internet access were given it free.

Critical Thinking

1. When considering getting older, what are the things that worry the baby boomers the most?

2. What did boomers consider to be the best thing about aging?

3. How do most of the boomers rate their overall health at their current age in life?

Create Central

www.mhhe.com/createcentral

Internet References

AARP Health Information
   www.aarp.org/bulletin

Alzheimer's Association
   www.alz.org

A.P.T.A. Section on Geriatrics
   http://geriatricspt.org

Caregiver's Handbook
   www.acsu.buffalo.edu/~drstall/hndbk0.html

Caregiver Survival Resources
   www.caregiver.com

International Food Information Council
   www.ific.org

University of California at Irvine: Institute for Brain Aging and Dementia
   www.alz.uci.edu

Unit 5

UNIT

Prepared by: Elaina Osterbur, *Saint Louis University*

Retirement: American Dream or Dilemma?

Since 1900, the number of people in America who are 65 years or more of age has been increasing steadily, but a decreasing proportion of that age group remains in the workforce. In 1900, nearly two-thirds of those over the age of 65 worked outside the home. By 1947, this number had declined to about 48 percent, and in 1975, about 22 percent of men age 65 and over were still in the workforce. The long-range trend indicates that fewer and fewer people are employed beyond the age of 65. Some choose to retire at age 65 or earlier; for others, retirement is mandatory. A recent change in the law, however, allows individuals to work as long as they want with no mandatory retirement age.

Gordon Strieb and Clement Schneider (Retirement in American Society, 1971) observed that for retirement to become an institutionalized social pattern in any society, certain conditions must be present. A large group of people must live long enough to retire; the economy must be productive enough to support people who are not in the workforce; and there must be pensions or insurance programs to support retirees.

Retirement is a rite of passage. People can consider it either as the culmination of the American Dream or as a serious problem. Those who have ample incomes, interesting things to do, and friends to associate with often find the freedom of time and choice that retirement offers very rewarding. For others, however, retirement brings problems and personal losses. Often, these individuals find their incomes decreased; they miss the status, privilege, and power associated with holding a position in the occupational hierarchy. They may feel socially isolated if they do not find new activities to replace their previous work-related ones. Additionally, they might have to cope with the death of a spouse and/or their own failing health.

Older persons approach retirement with considerable concern about financial and personal problems. Will they have enough retirement income to maintain their current lifestyle? Will their income remain adequate as long as they live? Given their current state of health, how much longer can they continue to work? The articles in this unit deal with changing Social Security regulations and changing labor demands that are encouraging older people to work beyond the age of 65.

Article

Prepared by: Elaina F. Osterbur, *Saint Louis University*

Will Baby Boomers Phase into Retirement?

Julie I. Tacchino

Learning Outcomes

After reading this article, you will be able to:

- Define phased retirement.
- Understand the challenges that phased retirement presents.
- Understand the benefits of phased retirement for employees and employers.

Introduction and Overview

For a long time the approach to retirement was very standard—work to a specified age and then jump off the cliff into retirement. Today there is no one standard retirement approach. Given the different needs of the aging workforce and the companies that employ them, the importance of adaptive and innovative retirement strategies for both employees and employers has become critical. One such strategy is phased retirement. Currently, there is no standard legal or agreed-on definition of phased retirement.[1] Phased retirement can be thought of as a broad variety of employment arrangements allowing retirees to continue working reduced workloads while gradually shifting from full-time work to full-time retirement.

A large majority of baby boomers intend to continue working after they reach traditional retirement age, and a majority of those individuals want to work part-time in different fields from their previous careers.[2] This most likely means that phased retirement will grow in the future. In fact, while only 21% of surveyed companies believe that phased retirement is critical to their company's Human Resources strategy today, over 60% believe it will be critical in five years.[3] Of the retirees working in retirement, Rappaport reported that one study found that 31% were working for the same employer as before retirement, 40% worked for a different company, and 27% became self-employed.[4] Further, 45% of working retirees were doing the same type of work they did prior to retirement, 26% were doing different work but using the same skills they had before retirement, and 33% were doing work that was entirely different from the work

they did before retirement.[5] Given the demands of an aging workforce, employers need to come up with formal solutions to retain their older workers and guide them toward their intended retirement goals.

Phased retirement is a great solution to the worker population issue because it comes in many varieties. Phased retirement can be used in jobs that require the same work, jobs that require different work, or jobs that require skills similar to those developed at the full-time job. Through phased retirement employees can stay with their current companies to transfer knowledge to the younger workforce, they can also utilize their skills and abilities at different companies, start their own businesses, or start on completely new "career paths." Phased retirement offers so many different routes providing a variety of exciting choices for retirement-aged workers.

Phased retirement supports different lifestyles—whether it's a client who wants to travel or one who is sick and can no longer work full time. Phased retirement can be a positive option for clients who do not want to, or cannot yet, fully retire. One paradox of phased retirement is that those employees management most wants to retain are more likely to find it hard to limit themselves to part-time work.[6] This is no surprise given that while the younger workers are expected to have a multitude of jobs during their careers, the aged workforce is more likely to have been with the same company throughout their careers. The historical knowledge and skills that the aging workers have accumulated throughout their careers with a given company are invaluable and companies do not want to part with them.

Additionally, people who choose phased retirement are better educated, more likely to have a positive view of work (for example, believe that work is by itself important apart from a means of acquiring money), have greater household wealth and income, and are often in white-collar positions. In other words, they are the same type of people who are more likely to seek the aid of a financial planner.[7] This is also a good description of the baby boomer. Boomers with such characteristics are significant assets for employers, which is why having a formalized phased retirement program is an important tool for companies.

Characteristics of Phased Retirement

Phased retirement is a great retirement option because it can take employees and employers in so many different directions. With the plethora of phased retirement options available, it can be overwhelming to determine which choices are right for employees to follow and for employers to offer. Phased retirement often has one or more of the following characteristics.

Full-Time to Part-Time Employment

The most common characteristic of phased retirement is going from full-time to part-time employment. This can be done in different ways. The employee or former employee can reduce the number of hours worked. For example, the phased retiree cuts back from eight hours per day to four-to-six hours per day. Or the employee or former employee can reduce the amount of days per week worked. For example, the phased retiree cuts back from five days a week to three days per week. The employee or former employee may even reduce the number of weeks worked. This can be done through a variety of methods. For example, the phased retiree could take extended vacation time or limit the work period to seasonal work. Another example of cutting back on the time worked would be having the employee or former employee limit work to projects engaged in on a full-time basis but for a limited period of time.

Other Characteristics

Other characteristics of phased retirement may include the employee or former employee engaging in a job-sharing program, or entering into a contract that provides flexibility in setting hours, or negotiating reduced job duties. Another common characteristic would be doing some sort of consulting work for an ex-employer, another employer, or multiple employers as an independent contractor. For example, a phased retiree who was formerly a tax accountant could work part-time during tax season. With today's technology, engaging in telecommuting or working remotely is a useful tool for phased retirement programs. As phased retirement grows in popularity, the characteristics and options will most likely expand.

Different Approaches to Phased Retirement

With the various characteristics of phased retirement plans, a good way to group phased retirement options is by win-win, where not just the employee but also the employer "wins out" or is favored by the phased retirement option, and employee-favored, where the employee is favored in the phased retirement decision and the employer is most likely not impacted.

Win-Win Phased Retirement Options

Formal and Informal Phased Retirement

One type of phased retirement is the formal phased retirement. Formal phased retirement occurs when formal workplace policies exist that allow an employee to continue working with his or her current employer at a reduced schedule. At the same time, the employee may or may not be receiving retirement benefits. If they exist, formal phased retirement policies often are contained in the personnel policies of the employer. They tend to be most commonly available from large employers.[8] Sponsors of formal phased retirement programs have noted that they do not expect retirees to stay active for very long. One manager said, "Although there are some exceptions, most people work about three years in our program."[9] A formal phased retirement program can be a useful tool for companies. Having a formal program shows the company has an innovative and adaptive style, creates a culture that values employees, and places value on age at a time when many companies devalue age by encouraging early retirement. Companies are used to staying innovative and creative to attract new employees, but it is now crucial they stay innovative to retain all employees, especially those employees nearing retirement age. With the increasing need for phased retirement options, formal phased retirement will most likely grow among companies.

Informal phased retirement is a type of phased retirement in which informal workplace arrangements and practices exist that allow an employee to continue working with his or her current employer at a reduced schedule. At the same time, the employee may or may not be receiving retirement benefits. Informal phased retirement is more common than formal phased retirement. It is often done on a case-by-case basis. Traditionally, employers have been more inclined to accommodate informal phased retirement requests from high-performing workers who require little supervision.[10]

Both formal and informal phased retirements create win-win situations for employers and employees. Employers keep their hard-working "golden" employees longer, possibly allowing them to impart their wisdom to the younger workforce; and employees are able to enjoy their work, while easing into their new lives as retired persons. However, a formal plan is recommended over an informal plan. Standard policies and procedures let employees know their options, and keep employers prepared, structured, and honest when setting up phased retirement plans.

Retire and Rehire

Once an employee has retired, the former employer may rehire him or her for part-time work or a consulting job. In order for the employer's retirement system to be unaffected, there must be a bona fide termination of employment. However, there is no specific legal definition of bona fide termination of employment.[11] This is a definite win-win scenario. Employees who are hired back as consultants for their companies are often paid large amounts for short periods of work, and when an employer needs a consultant, who better to hire than a former employee who already possesses knowledge pertaining to the company and does not require formal training?

Phasing

Phasing a little, or working close to a full-time schedule by only making a modest change in work schedule and conditions, is another win-win phased retirement scenario. When phasing a little, clients typically keep their benefits but they are unlikely to be drawing retirement benefits from the employer. Clients who are phasing a little are often thought of as phasing preretirement.[12] Another strategy is phasing a lot, or work that is dramatically different from a full-time schedule. When phasing a lot, employees will probably lose their employer-provided benefit eligibility. Clients who are phasing a lot are often thought of as phasing postretirement.[13] All of these phasing options are extremely beneficial to the employee, providing flexibility and the ability to retire at his or her own pace. At the same time, employers are able to retain skilled employees who contribute experienced knowledge to the organization. Employers should be prepared to allow flexibility when employees are phasing a little or a lot. Allowing employees to set their own reduced schedules for their convenience (e.g., taking Fridays off), will be more attractive to employees when deciding which phased retirement option is best for them.

Employee-Favored Retirement Options

To reiterate, employers don't necessarily lose in these scenarios, they are just not directly involved with their former employees. In these situations, from the original employer's perspective the employee has completely retired. These scenarios require significant effort on the part of employees, but are a great way to phase into retirement.

Bridge Jobs

Bridge jobs are jobs selected by the employee without the support of a formal employer program. These jobs occur immediately or shortly after the employee has left his or her long-time employer and the employee may or may not yet have started receiving retirement benefits from the prior employer. Bridge jobs spanning a period from the end of work with a full-time employer to full-time retirement out of the labor force are becoming more common.[14] This scenario "bridges" the gap between full-time employment and full-time retirement, allowing employees to hold off on collecting retirement benefits. This is a great retirement savings strategy for two reasons. First, the longer the employee's retirement fund remains untouched, the better. Second, bridge jobs will more than likely pay less than what the employee was paid in his or her previous job. This drop in income, which occurs in many phased retirement plans, is positive because it allows the employee to adapt to a reduced income instead of going from the full-time salary that he or she is used to, to a significantly lower retirement income. Phased retirement is typically a white-collar phenomenon, as evidenced by better education and greater household wealth.[15] Although it is easy to argue that finding a job with a different employer when nearing retirement age is next to impossible, employers in industries similar to that of the retiree's former employer may well value the wisdom and knowledge that comes with the retirement age, making bridge jobs a viable option for retirement-aged individuals. Although it may not be common now, recruiting retirement-aged employees from similar industries will most likely grow

as a competitive strategy for companies as phased retirement grows in popularity.

Wisdom Careers

Another phased retirement program that utilizes one's skills encompasses wisdom careers, which are follow-up careers that capitalize on the retired employee's wisdom, skills, and abilities. Wisdom careers are great options for clients who have been in the same profession or industry for the majority of their careers. The retiree can become a self-employed consultant who uses his or her past experiences to help other companies. Knowledge transfer is invaluable for many industries and career paths. Utilizing the business and/or field wisdom of retired persons is important for employers looking to grow and develop in their industries.

Encore Careers

An encore career is one in which a client retires and starts a new career in a different industry. According to AARP, "Encore careers are increasingly common among Americans 50+. An estimated nine million boomers have found their second acts, and more than 30 million others say they would like to make a career change."[16] Occasionally clients may retire at an early age to "double dip" and get a second pension. They may also retire to start an entrepreneurial venture. No matter what the case, an encore career is an important form of phased retirement to consider. Again, this shows the importance of destandardization of retirement. Retirement age has always been seen as the time to stop working. This adaptive approach makes retirement age a time to start a new career path, showing a complete, 180-degree change in perception.

These are just some phased retirement options that employees can consider and employers can take advantage of or capitalize on. The changing face of retirement requires employers to be innovative and think ahead to create phased retirement programs that entice employees to stay with the company so both the employee and employer can win. While most employers focus on being competitive to recruit those younger in their careers, the need for competitive recruiting and retaining of older workers is becoming essential.

Why Employees Choose Phased Retirement

There are several reasons employees may opt for phased retirement. One reason phased retirement is a growing trend is that continued work is more feasible. Some of today's physically easier, technology-aided jobs make phased retirement more attainable. Advancements in technology have lessened the importance of age as a factor of work and allow retirement-aged employees to continue working and retire at their own leisure. Not only is phased retirement more feasible, it is also more necessary. Pensions are becoming less and less common and employees are in control of their own retirement incomes. There are no guarantees. The reality is that employees need to work longer to ensure they can sustain their retirement incomes, and phased retirement increases retirement income. It allows clients to continue to contribute to their retirement plans; when a client is not satisfied with his or her retirement income, he or she can supplement it with additional income from a phased retirement option. The client may opt for part-time work to correct the situation. With increasing options for sustaining retirement income, what better way to take action and control over one's own retirement bank than to have a phased retirement income?

Phased retirement is also a growing choice among retirees because of the cohort effect. Today's retirees have greater longevity, higher levels of education, and greater occupational profiles, the combination of which provides a basis for staying employed longer.[17] Education and career status are valued in America. People work their entire lives to reach their career goals and often find it is incredibly difficult to leave their careers behind. As we continue to recognize the importance of sustaining a career that was years in the making, more and more employees are feeling comfortable with the decision to work longer periods and extend the "normal" career span.

Additionally, phased retirement allows employees to "try out" leisure activities that could eventually be part of full-time retirement. Retirement is a major life change and phased retirement allows employees to ease into an unfamiliar retirement in their own time and at their own leisure. The ability to negotiate the transition a step at a time allows for better emotional preparation.[18] If we fail to recognize the emotions that come with retirement, then we fail to do our jobs as financial planners. Retirement is not a black and white subject where the only goal is to have enough money to live out one's final years; there is so much more to it. People put their lives into building their careers; phased retirement not only permits acknowledgement of that effort but also allows our clients to adapt to the emotional significance of both having a career and retiring from it.

Phased retirement is a great option also because part-time work allows employees to adjust for age-related changes in stamina or ability. A desire to continue working may not equate to a wish to work full time.[19] Phased retirement allows employees to continue active involvement in the workforce at a pace with which they can be more comfortable.[20] With modern medicine, everything possible is done to keep people alive; why wouldn't the same mentality apply to people's careers? Just because agility declines between the beginning of one's career and what is currently known as the retirement age, does not mean that one has to stop working. Additionally, employees may have more to give. When traditional retirement age arrives, some clients still have plenty of energy and desire to contribute.[21]

In fact, probably the most important, yet most overlooked, reason phased retirement is increasing in popularity is that people want to work. Retirement may be great for some individuals, but how many of us really want to go from working eight hours each day to spending eight hours each day watching TV? Work keeps life interesting and fresh. Employees nearing retirement age won't necessarily want to throw away their careers and embark full time on their hobbies, making phased retirement a great option for the aging workforce.

Employees may be bored in their current careers and they may want to try new work activities. Semiretirement may be a good opportunity to double back and travel down the road not taken. It may allow clients to follow their hearts and passions, and not their wallets, or it may tap into a client's entrepreneurial spirit.[22] Again, it is crucial to adjust our perceptions and recognize that retirement age does not have to mean the end of a career; it might mean the beginning of one. With age and experience come opportunities and options. Phased retirement may be an opportunity to jettison the boring and burdensome projects at work and to choose only those projects that stimulate the client.

Phased retirement also allows for a better work-life balance. Many professional and white-collar jobs have become very demanding, often requiring 50- to 60-hour work weeks. Phased retirement may allow for the intervention of sanity into the client's world by enabling him or her to have some flexibility with how time is spent.[23] Along with achieving a better work-life balance, a person may want to spend some more time with his or her spouse. Phased retirement may be a great option for a client with that desire.[24] Many people have accepted that when in the prime of their careers, work-life balance is at times unachievable. Instead of viewing retirement as a hobby-life balance, why not look at it as a work-life balance in which the life side of the balance finally outweighs the work?

Phasing into retirement can also allow employees to retain benefits. With the rising costs of health care, phased retirement might be necessary to keep employer-provided health insurance, a potentially significant benefit. As people age they are more likely to need better health care. Under the right set of circumstances, phased retirement may allow the client to continue to have employer-sponsored health care; however, this is not always the case. Having a formalized phased retirement plan that allows benefits will certainly put companies at a competitive advantage when recruiting experienced, retirement-aged personnel.

Why Employers Should Encourage Phased Retirement

As discussed earlier, several phased retirement strategies are win-win, where both the employee and employer come out with a winning hand, so to speak. First, these strategies enable employers to retain and recruit older workers who have unique skills and talents.[25] In one survey, 72% of companies said that phased retirement is important for retaining the experience, knowledge, and skills of older workers.[26] This is especially useful for employers whose employees have been with the company for most of their careers. When employees spend their careers in one company, their skills grow and adapt to the company's needs. In addition, older workers who have been with the same company throughout their careers often retain useful, historical knowledge of the company that others may not have. Further, experienced employees often understand the corporate culture and environment. This knowledge is a valuable resource for any company, making phased retirement programs an important offering for employers.

Phased retirement can create effective knowledge-sharing relationships between older mentors and younger protégés.[27] Given all the experience, knowledge, and skills boomers have attained and retained, mentor relationships can help ease the blow that will be sustained when boomers retire. Knowledge transfer is a powerful tool that can help companies retain relevant historical information and useful skills and abilities that are significant to the role the retiree may have. This retention can only occur if the older workforce is able to take the time to share its knowledge with younger protégés. Whenever possible, management should make sure that returning retirees know that an important part of their role is to transfer their critical knowledge to the next generation of employees.[28] It will certainly be an adjustment for current employees who are headed for retirement and retirees who are returning to the workplace to be charged with sharing this knowledge with the younger workforce. Employees are often territorial about their work and having older employees share knowledge with younger employees is rarely welcomed with open arms. It is important to be open and honest with employees about the goal of knowledge sharing. This is often a delicate situation and being open and honest will make them feel important and useful rather than threatened by the idea of sharing their skills and abilities with their potential successors.

Another reason employers should encourage phased retirement is that it accommodates special projects or time-shortened scenarios because retirees comprise a good resource for these contingencies. Again, retirees or employees nearing retirement have accumulated or developed a skill set that makes them effective in their positions. They are already trained so when an employer is in a time-sensitive situation, it is a clear win-win to offer retirees a phased retirement option. Retirees can continue working while employers have the needed human capital on their teams without having to train a new or existing employee. In addition, phased retirement preserves human capital and lowers training costs.[29]

This innovative approach to retirement gives employers a competitive edge in attracting and retaining desirable employees. Having a formalized phased retirement program shows that the company is pioneering a revolutionary change in a transforming workplace. If a company is adapting to one change, it is most likely aware of other needed changes and is willing to make the changes. Employees do not want to work for a company that is antiquated in its policies and procedures. Companies that do not adapt will fail in today's work environment. Additionally, phased retirement programs show employers value their employees because they are looking to retain them past retirement age. Seeing and responding to employee and societal needs by having a formalized phased retirement program gives companies a competitive advantage.

Lastly, another relevant reason employers should encourage phased retirement is that it addresses the potential labor shortage that will occur when boomers retire.[30] "While the percentage of adults ages 65 and older will increase from 17% today to 27% in 30 years—an increase from 37 million to 77 million people—there will not be enough members of the baby bust generation to fill their shoes."[31] This void in human capital that

employers will inevitably experience shows the true value of phased retirement. Having a formal phased retirement policy in place now will help employers avoid the labor shortage as their boomer workforce heads for retirement.

Challenges of Phased Retirement

Although phased retirement programs are a great solution for retirement income gaps for employees and knowledge gaps for employers, there are several challenges associated with phased retirement. As discussed earlier, there is no legal definition of bona fide termination of employment, something that is necessary to terminate and rehire employees without affecting their retirement plans. The lack of legal guidance can pose a barrier for employers who would like to use a retire and rehire program as a phased retirement option.

The type of retirement plan your client has may pose challenges to phasing into retirement—especially if he or she wants to phase before full retirement age. Because defined-benefit plans do not typically allow distributions until age 62, phasing into retirement beforehand could subject the plan to tax consequences.[32] According to Moran, ". . . the IRS has consistently emphasized that a plan cannot allow participants to 'retire' or 'terminate employment,' receive a pension, and then immediately return to work. . ."[33] This creates barriers for clients who would like to phase into retirement before the "normal" or acceptable age of 62, and for companies providing defined-benefit plans, that would like to implement a formalized phased retirement plan.

In addition to legal challenges, there are emotional barriers to phased retirement for your client. While it is a benefit that your client does not have to jump off the cliff to full-time retirement, but instead can climb down at his or her own leisure, it is not easy to release the control to coworkers. This can be especially true of the mentor and protégé relationships. While training and transferring work to the protégé, it is more than likely that the protégé will want to make his or her mark on the work and change it up. It can be quite difficult to watch someone else take something you've been doing one way and flip it upside down. It is important for both employers who support mentor-protégé relationships and employees who take advantage of them to be aware of this emotional barrier.

Although there are challenges to phased retirement, the barriers do not outweigh the positive impact phased retirement can have on employers and employees.

The Future of Retirement

A standard approach to retirement is a thing of the past. It's time to look to the future. It is our responsibility to think ahead and prepare innovative ideas about and creative approaches to the changing face of retirement. Employers need to accommodate employee needs by staying current on retirement trends. Phased retirement plans can be a winning situation for both the employee and employer, allowing employees to ease into one of the biggest changes in life, while allowing employers to retain vital skills and knowledge important for their companies. When companies foresee and adapt to the ever-evolving retirement needs of their employees, talented employees are retained and employers keep a competitive edge, creating a win-win situation.

References

1. Anna Rappaport, "Phased retirement—An important part of the evolving retirement scene." *Benefits Quarterly* 25, no. 2 (2009): 38–50.
2. The New Retirement Survey, Merrill Lynch, 2005.
3. Stephen Miller, "Retiring boomers spark phased retirement interest." *HR Magazine* 53, no. 9 (2008): 32.
4. Rappaport 2009, 41.
5. *Ibid*, 42.
6. David Delong, MetLife Mature Market Institute. "Searching for the Silver Bullet: Leading Edge Solutions for Leveraging an Aging Workforce." November 2007. https://www.metlife.com/assets/cao/mmi/publications/studies/mmi-searching-silver-bullet.pdf.
7. Yung-Ping Chen and John C. Scott, "Phased retirement: Who opts for it and toward what end." *AARP Public Policy Institute.* (2005). http://assets.aarp.org.rgcenter.econ/inb113_retire.pdf.
8. Robert Hutchens, "Phased retirement: Problems and prospects." *Retirement Income Reporter* 14, no. 6 (2008): 6–12.
9. DeLong, 2007.
10. Hutchens, 2008, 9.
11. Rappaport, 2009, 39.
12. *Ibid*, 40–42.
13. *Ibid.*
14. Chen and Scott, 2005, 5.
15. Hutchens, 2008, 7.
16. "Encore career strategies: Finding a career change that suits you for the second half of life." AARP, *Inside E Street*, Feb. 13, 2012. http://aarp.org/work/job-hunting/info-2-2012/encore-career-strategies-inside-estreet.html.
17. Neal E. Cutler, "Working *in* retirement: The longevity perplexities continue." *Journal of Financial Service Professionals* 65, no. 4 (2011): 19–22.
18. Hutchens, 2008, 6.
19. Chen and Scott, 1.
20. Hutchens, 2008, 6.
21. Edelstein, "Choosing a second career over traditional retirement." *RetirementAdvice.com* February 18, 2011. http://retirementadvice.com/choosing-a-second-career-over-retirement/.
22. *Ibid.*
23. Rappaport 2009, 44.
24. *Ibid.*
25. DeLong, 2007.
26. Miller, 2008, 32.
27. DeLong, 2007.
28. *Ibid.*, 24.
29. Tomeka M. Hill, "Why doesn't every employer have a phased retirement program?" *Benefits Quarterly* 26, no. 4 (2010): 29–39.
30. F. Pierce Noble and Erica Harper, "Strategy and policy for phased retirement." *Benefits Quarterly* 26, no. 3 (2010): 11–14.
31. "Time to Develop a Phased Retirement Program?" *Design Firm Management & Administration Report 5,* no. 12 (2005): 2–3. *ProQuest.*Web. Oct. 8, 2012. http://0-search.proquest.com.libcat.widener.edu/docview/223213655/13CDEF825BC5A9483F3/1?accountid=29103.
32. Anne E. Moran, "Phased retirement: Challenges for employers." *Employee Relations Law Journal* 38, no. 2 (2012): 68–74.
33. *Ibid.*

Critical Thinking

1. What is phased retirement?
2. What kind of challenges does phased retirement present?
3. What are the benefits of phased retirement for employees and employers?

Create Central

www.mhhe.com/createcentral

Internet References

AARP
www.aarp.org
Health and Retirement Study (HRS)
www.umich.edu/~hrswww

JULIE I. TACCHINO, MSTFP, graduated in December 2012 from Widener University's Master of Taxation and Financial Planning program. She currently works as a Human Resources Analyst.

Article

Prepared by: Elaina F. Osterbur, *Saint Louis University*

Live for Today, Save for Tomorrow

What if working longer meant more fun, not less—and a bigger nest egg, too? You can make it happen if you start planning now.

CARLA A. FRIED

Learning Outcomes

After reading this article, you will be able to:

- Discuss the advantages to older workers of working beyond the anticipated retirement age.

- Explain how working beyond retirement age causes preretirement savings to grow.

- Explain why waiting until your late 70s or early 80s is the best time to begin buying or cashing in on a monthly annuity.

As a senior financial planner, Christine Fahlund is not in the habit of telling people to stop saving for retirement. You wouldn't expect her employer, T. Rowe Price, to be wild about the idea, either. They are in the business of gathering investors' money into mutual funds and 401(k) plans. (Disclosure: Among those plans is the one for employees of AARP.) But in a new strategy that the company has been promoting this year, not only do Fahlund and T. Rowe Price suggest that you stop saving for retirement once you hit age 60; they encourage you to take the money you were previously putting into your 401(k) or other retirement account and—brace yourself—spend it. On fun stuff. "Your 60s should be a time when you start to enjoy yourself more," Fahlund says. "Take more trips. Spend time with the grandkids. Buy the boat or put in the pool you've been dreaming of."

And here's the kicker: If you follow their advice, you could end up with a higher income in retirement than you might have otherwise.

Is this a joke? Did Fahlund and company just snooze through the Great Recession? It's not, and they didn't. What T. Rowe Price calls "practice retirement" could, in fact, be a realistic option for you. But there's a big catch. Two catches, in fact. You have to have significant savings by the time you hit 60. And you have to commit to working well past your early 60s, because you're going to live off that income while your savings and your Social Security benefits sit untouched, gaining in value.

You may already be postponing your retirement: More than 60 percent of workers say they expect to retire at age 65 or later, according to the most recent survey by the Employee Benefit Research Institute, up from 45 percent in 1991. But few view the prospect with enthusiasm. Working longer is Plan B, a sign that something went wrong in your retirement schedule.

"Practice retirement" operates from a different set of assumptions. Steven Sass, director of the Financial Security Project at the Center for Retirement Research at Boston College, says most people think the point of working longer is to

Table 1   How Much You Need to Save

Your Retirement Will be More Comfortable if You Work Well into Your 60s		
If You Plan to Retire at Age 62		
And your total household income is	$50,000	$75,000	$100,000
You'll need this much in savings by age 60	$600,000	$975,000	$1.4 million
If You Plan to Retire at Age 65		
And your total household income is	$50,000	$75,000	$100,000
You'll need this much in savings by age 60	$450,000	$825,000	$1.1 million
If You Plan to Retire at Age 70		
And your total household income is	$50,000	$75,000	$100,000
You'll need this much in savings by age 60	$250,000	$525,000	$700,000

Notes: T. Rowe Price assumes you will want to replace 75 percent of your income and that you will not make any withdrawals from your retirement account, or initiate your Social Security payout, until you retire. The calculation also assumes a portfolio will earn 7 percent before retirement and 6 percent after.

Source: T. Rowe Price.

sacrifice and save. That's not it. "The payoff of working longer," says Sass, who coauthored *Working Longer: The Solution to the Retirement Income Challenge*, "is that you can preserve your retirement savings and delay taking Social Security." Medical researchers have long known that staying on the job pays benefits to the mind and body. By protecting your nest egg, enhancing your benefits, and limiting the number of years your stash needs to support you, working longer has a similar effect on your financial health.

And that creates some opportunities, including the one at the heart of Fahlund's suggestion: Put yourself in a position where you can afford to stop saving, or at least slow down, when you reach 60. Then: Live a little. "Get back to looking forward to your 60s as a time to be enjoyed," she says. "You are delaying retirement, but you don't have to delay enjoyment."

Still sound too good to be true? Here are some answers to your probable concerns:

You'd Need to Save a Fortune to Take "Practice Retirement" at Age 60

Obviously, you can't stop saving at age 60 if you never really started. You need a healthy sum of money in the bank. But the required amount may be less than you're probably thinking.

The table estimates how much you need to squirrel away by age 60 to be able to turn off the savings spigot at that point. What you'll need depends on your current income, as well as the date when you expect to start tapping your savings and collecting Social Security. Bottom line: The longer you keep your hands off the retirement cookie jar, the less you'll need to have saved up by age 60. *Dramatically* less.

For example, a couple with $75,000 in joint household income who want to retire at 62 and have 75 percent of their preretirement income would need $975,000 in savings by age 60. But if they're willing to keep working until age 67, T. Rowe Price estimates they'd need $675,000. Those five extra years on the job cut the amount needed at age 60 by almost one-third. And if the couple don't touch their savings until 70, they need to set aside an even lower amount—$525,000. Hello, mission possible.

One assumption is critical: This model assumes your portfolio will earn 7 percent before you retire and 6 percent in retirement. That might seem too optimistic. To build in a margin of safety, you could assume a 5 percent preretirement return and 4 percent afterward. (By comparison, AARP's financial-planning tool assumes a 6 percent return preretirement, 3.6 percent afterward.) If the more cautious assumption proves accurate, you'd need to work one more year than you anticipated. But even that scenario is probably more affordable than you guessed. That's because the key ingredient in the recipe isn't the rate of return. It's your intention to keep working. "The investment earnings on your contributions at this later stage are less important," says Sass. "The value is that you have a job that supports you and helps you preserve your retirement security by not beginning to draw down your savings. We're talking about a few extra years of working to secure your finances for decades."

Come On—Decades? Working a Few Years More Can't Possibly Make That Much Difference

Most retirement experts say that it does. The Retirement Policy Center at the Urban Institute, for example, estimates that for every year you work past age 62, you increase your eventual retirement income by an average of 9 percent. At that rate, working eight years longer would double your retirement income. Here's why:

- Working longer means your retirement savings need not stretch over so many years. You've probably already heard this longevity riff: A 65-year-old man today has an average life expectancy of 17 years; a woman, 20 years. So you figure, "Okay, if I make it to 65, I will die at 82 or 85."

  But that's not necessarily correct. Your life expectancy isn't a calculation of when you will die; it's the age at which 50 percent of your age group will still be alive. So if you're 65 today, you've got even odds of making it into your mid-80s and beyond. It's even trickier if you're married. There's a better than 60 percent chance that one spouse of a 65-year-old couple today will still be alive at age 90. In other words, if you don't delay retirement—the average American man leaves the workforce at age 64; the average woman, at 62—the chances are good that your nest egg will have to stretch for 30 years.

  That can spread your savings thin. You can see the effect by plugging numbers into AARP's retirement calculator (aarp.org/retirementcalculator). Based on AARP's assumptions, a 60-year-old woman making $75,000 a year who retires at age 62 with a nest egg of $250,000 can sustain an annual income of about $31,000 through age 91. That same nest egg could support a healthier income of nearly $41,000 if she didn't touch her savings and delayed retiring until age 70.

- You give your savings more time to grow. If you work until age 70, your nest egg will be bigger than at 62 because it has eight more years to incubate. As long as you have a respectable amount saved by 60, letting that money grow undisturbed matters more to your financial security than does your adding new cash each year. If you have $250,000 in your 401(k) at age 60, the 7 percent annual rate of return assumed by T. Rowe Price would add $17,500 to your account in the first year alone. That's probably more than you'd contribute to a 401(k) or IRA. Over 10 years that 7 percent rate would lift your savings from $250,000 up to $500,000 by the time you retire, even if you never saved another penny.

- You can delay claiming your Social Security. Individuals can begin receiving benefits as early as age 62. But as the table shows, you'll lock in a higher payout if you hold off. "People's jaws drop when I tell them how much bigger their benefit will be if they wait," says Sass.

What It Takes to Keep Working

Even before the Great Recession triggered massive layoffs, older workers often faced unique job disruption. About one-third of workers ages 51 through 55 in 1992 were involuntarily bounced from their jobs by the time they reached their mid to late 60s, according to a 2009 Urban Institute study. One-fourth lost their jobs because of a layoff or business closing; another 12 percent were forced to stop working because of illness.

But the upside to working through your 60s is so strong that it's worth fighting back to stay on the job, if you can. These principles should help.

Move the Goalposts

If you're still harboring thoughts that retiring at 62 is "right," you risk mentally retiring at 60 or so. That makes you easier pickings if the boss decides to cut overhead. Plan to work until at least your late 60s and you will stay more engaged in your work.

Quitting Is Not an Option

Don't think you can give full retirement a whirl at age 62 and then just go back to work if your new life doesn't shake out as expected. "Retirement is a bit of a black hole," says *Working Longer* coauthor Sass. "It's habit-forming."

Be a Problem Solver

"Look around and see what holes your employer needs to fill, then offer to step in," says Sass. "The more flexible you are, the more valuable you are."

If You Have to Switch Jobs, Plan on Making Less

Some good news: If you've been at your job for a long time, you're in a better position than colleagues with less tenure. "Older workers are better protected from losing a job, but once they lose that job, they have a much harder time [than younger workers] finding a new job," says Richard Johnson, an Urban Institute retirement-policy expert. And the next job will likely be at a lower salary, so don't hold out for a fatter paycheck. Remember, though, that the main goal is to earn enough to cover your living costs.

Take Care of Yourself

A healthier you increases the odds you'll be able to keep working. It also makes it likelier you'll enjoy your 60s—and beyond.

Michael Wilson, a financial planner in Orland, Indiana, notes that the financial crisis makes it crucial to consider delaying. "If your 401(k) tanked, you will be leaning on Social Security even more."

- Finally, you reduce your out-of-pocket health care costs. Not many employers still offer retirement health coverage, so if you retire before 65 you may face stiff private insurance costs until Medicare kicks in. "The longer you can hold on to employer health benefits, the more you'll help preserve your retirement savings," says Richard Johnson of the Urban Institute's Retirement Policy Center.

It's Crazy Not to Save during Your 60s. What if the Market Collapses? What if You Get Sick? What if You Lose Your Job?

Working longer gives you the chance for some immediate gratification in your 60s, but it's not a free ticket to fiscal irresponsibility. Don't stop contributing to your 401(k) if your employer provides a match, for example; instead, dial back your contributions but keep saving enough to qualify for the maximum match. Otherwise you're essentially passing up free money. Don't drag debt into retirement. If you carry credit card balances, pay them off before you get into practice retirement's live-it-up mode. (Then keep them paid off.) Fahlund also recommends making big-ticket purchases while you have the income to cover them. And stay alert to market headwinds. If T. Rowe Price's 7 percent preretirement and 6 percent postretirement return assumptions look dicey after a few years, you may have to adjust by diverting more of your income into savings again, or trimming your expenses, or even delaying retirement by a year or more.

Can you really count on keeping your current job all the way to 70? Even if your employer is willing, your health may have other ideas. If you think that you're hale enough to go the distance, and secure in your position, practice retirement could be a possibility. "You have to take a look at your current job circumstances and ask yourself what is the likelihood you will be with that employer at age 67," Sass says. "If you do change jobs, you will probably lose money."

But don't forget that you can safely earn less than you once did. Since you are no longer diverting 10 or 15 percent of your salary into savings, you can bring home 10 or 15 percent less and still maintain the same quality of life. The aim is simply to resist tapping your savings and Social Security benefits until you are deep in your 60s.

Which brings us to the true benefit of working to a later age: options. One option is to have fun and spend more in a practice retirement. Another is to earn less money and take your foot off the career gas—or do work that's more meaningful to you. As long as you're still earning your living, the choice is yours. And with a Plan B like that, who really misses Plan A?

Social Security: Patience Pays

Your Social Security benefits revolve around your Normal Retirement Age (NRA)—the age at which you are entitled to 100 percent of your benefit. If you were born in 1960 or later, your NRA is 67. If you were born from 1943 to 1954, your NRA is 66, and if you were born from 1955 to 1959 your NRA is somewhere between 66 and 67. If you wait until your NRA or later to claim your benefit, you'll receive much higher monthly payments.

	How much bigger your benefit will be if you defer claiming your benefit until your NRA	Additional annual benefit increase between your NRA and 70	How much bigger your benefit will be if you wait until 70 to start receiving Social Security, compared with taking payouts at 62
If your NRA is 66 . . .	25%	8%	76%
If your NRA is 67 . . .	30%	8%	77%

A new AARP online calculator will give you a personalized snapshot of how waiting can balloon your Social Security benefit. Go to **aarp.org/socialsecuritybenefits.**

Critical Thinking

1. What critical factors should a person consider before deciding to work beyond their anticipated retirement age?
2. If the individual works into their late 60s or early 70s, are they likely to be more or less engaged in their work?
3. In terms of a worker's knowledge and skill in their present job or their flexibility in assuming a new job, what is the biggest advantage in terms of the worker's ability to continue being employed in their later years?

Create Central

www.mhhe.com/createcentral

Internet References

AARP
www.aarp.org
Health and Retirement Study (HRS)
www.umich.edu/~hrswww

Article   Prepared by: Elaina Osterbur, *Saint Louis University*

5 Ways to Make Your Retirement Not Suck

ANN BRENOFF

Learning Outcomes

After reading this article, you will be able to:

- List the five ways that the effects of retirement can be eased.
- Discuss the future standard of living of most retirees.

By most indicators, there is a Silver Tsunami coming—millions of people who will enter retirement without enough money to house and feed themselves for the rest of their lives. Need evidence?

As *The New York Times* reported, "The Center for Retirement Research at Boston College said in 2013 that more than half of working-age households faced a deteriorating standard of living in retirement. A Pew Research Center survey published in 2012 found that the percentage of people ages 55 to 64 who doubt that they will have enough to live on during retirement rose to 39 percent in 2012 from 26 percent in 2009. And the number of seniors experiencing hunger rose 200 percent between 2001 and 2011, according to a report by the Meals on Wheels Research Foundation."

So are we all headed for cat food in a can? Here are five ways to make sure your retirement doesn't suck.

1. Figure out where you will live.

Housing is everyone's big ticket item. Maintaining a home or apartment in cities like New York, Los Angeles and San Francisco can be super-expensive. There are many places where you can pay far less for rent or home ownership. Getting a handle on just this one monthly expense can totally shape your retirement life.

The Internet is filled with Most Affordable Places To Retire lists. The are generally based on median home prices and take things into consideration like weather and crime rate. What most of them ignore is the desire and need to be near family and friends. If uprooting is indeed the path you chose, it makes sense to visit some of these places before you commit to living in them. And that's something you can and should do before you retire.

2. It's not too late to start saving.

Many of us haven't yet figured out that saving can feel as good as spending. What we do is spend to our earning capacity; the more we earn, the more we purchase. AARP says that three out of five households headed by someone 65 or older have no money in retirement savings accounts. That's none, as in zero.

To not be lumped in that group, there are small things you can be doing now that will help later. It may not feel extravagant to eat lunch out every day or stop for take-out food when you're too wiped out to fix dinner when you get home after work, but it all adds up. Think about how many hundreds of dollars you spend each year making your morning coffee run. There is going to come a day when you wish you had put that money in your IRA or 401k.

3. Learn to live on a budget.

Retired people live on fixed incomes that generally are a combination of Social Security and a company pension and/or withdrawals from their 401k or IRA. They may have some passive investment income, but that's not most of us. Today's job market isn't a happy place for most post-50s. They are met with rejection and told that their skills are out-of-date. So if you are entertaining a fantasy of being able to pick up a little supplemental income from a part time job when you retire, well, you might want to change the channel to some reality TV. It's smarter to practice living on a budget—because that's what you will be doing in retirement.

4. **Prepare your home for the long run.**

If you own your home and plan on staying in it, now is a good time to make sure it can accommodate you as you get older. Think about things like steps, first floor master bedrooms, cabinets that you can reach. And think hard whether you will still need the space. Even if your home is paid off, houses are expensive to heat and cool. We know a woman who wound up selling her house after she realized she only went up to her second floor to clean the dust bunnies once a month.

Also, look for ways whether your home can provide some income for you. Is it big enough to rent a room to a college student or another retired person? Investigate whether the garage can be converted into a guest house and become a good source of rental income for you. If any remodeling or updating needs to be done, do it while you are still working. Keeping your home in tip-top shape also ensures that if you do wind up selling it, it is less likely to linger on the market long.

5. **Lower your expectations.**

Sorry, but this is a reality many will face. You will not have your parents' retirement, nor will you even have the one you were expecting 10 years ago. What you can realistically expect is to work longer, be forced to be creative about reducing housing expenses and ways to do the traveling you hope to, and accept the fact that your retirement may look very different than the one you dreamed about.

Critical Thinking

1. Discuss the resources that are available to older adults heading for retirement.

2. What do you think the statement "lower your expectations" can explain?

Internet References

AARP: AARP Retirement Calculator: Are You Saving Enough?
http://www.aarp.org/work/retirement-planning/retirement_calculator.html

Social Security Administration: Retirement Benefits
http://www.ssa.gov/retirement/retirement.htm

Ann Brenoff, "5 Ways to Make Your Retirement Not Suck," *Huffington Post*, May 5, 2014.

Article   Prepared by: Elaina Osterbur, *Saint Louis University*

Recordkeeping for Retirement Starts with MySSA

KENN BEAM TACCHINO

Learning Outcomes

After reading this article, you will be able to:

- List the reasons that older adults need to provide documentation of income, as well as a Social Security statement, when planning for retirement.
- Discuss the contents of a retirement file.

Vacation time, when clients look to tackle personal projects that they have put off during the work year, may be a good time to assemble all the documentation needed to plan retirement. Every client should have a retirement file that contains the following:

- The retirement plan itself, as well as the summary plan description provided by his/ her employer.
- Benefit statements from IRAs, 401(k) plans, and other plans that show how his/her funds are invested, as well as the current value of these funds.
- Information about the client's health and long-term care policies.
- The will.
- Any living wills or durable powers of attorney for health care.
- Investment policy statements and withdrawal policy statements.
- Any other relevant investment, tax, or legal documents.

For many, a crucial item that is too often missing from the file is their Social Security statement. Clients might ask: "Didn't I used to receive something in the mail from Social Security every year about three months prior to my birthday?" Yes, but . . . .

What Happened and What Now

It used to be the client could request a Social Security statement in the mail by filing the form SSA-7004. However, this option no longer exists. Then from 1999 to 2011 the Social Security Administration mailed Social Security statements to anyone who was 25 or older. In May of 2012 they stopped these automatic mailings and went online to save money. The online statement is created by your clients at the website of the Social Security Administration, using the tab "MySSA." The automated future we all expected for the new millennium had arrived. However, in response to criticism that only a small percentage of people created their accounts online, (about 6 percent), another change was mandated. Starting in September of 2014, the Social Security Administration will resume mailings of the Social Security statement at 5-year intervals to workers who have not made their own accounts on MySSA. The statement will be sent to workers at ages 25, 30, 35, 40, 45, 50, 55, and 60.

Most experts believe that record-keeping would be best served by creating an online account at MySSA and checking it annually (rather than waiting every 5 years for a mailing). Fortunately, accounts are created in three easy steps. First, clients will need to go to www.socialsecurity.gov/myaccount and select "create an account." Second, they will need to provide some personal information to verify their identity. This information includes Social Security number, mailing address, email address, birth date, phone number, and some pesky security questions (such as the name of a bank where (s)he applied for a home equity loan, or the name of his/her high school). And third, your client will need to choose a username and password. Planners need to know that not everyone is eligible to set up an account. To create an account the client must be at least 18 years old, have a valid e-mail address, have a Social

Security number, and have a U.S. mailing address. Some of your clients may be wondering if they are eligible to receive a statement about an ex-spouse so they can tell how much they might receive based on the ex-spouse's Social Security record. If the former spouse is still living, privacy rules prohibit the Social Security Administration from giving out the ex-spouse's statement. However, a visit or call to Social Security can tell the client what to do and know in order to claim any spousal or survivor benefits to which (s)he is entitled.

How Does MySSA Help Plan for Retirement?

One benefit of the Social Security statement is that it can determine whether your client's earnings are accurately posted. Assessing this is crucial because the client's Social Security benefit is based on the amount (s)he earns each year of his/her career. If there is an error in posting earnings, the amount of benefits (s)he receives may be compromised. The sooner your client finds an error, the more documentation (s)he will have available to verify that the Social Security system has it wrong and (s)he actually earned more than (s)he has been given credit for. If your client uncovers an issue, (s)he can go in to the local Social Security office (it might be best to make an appointment to avoid having to sit and wait) or call the Social Security helpline at 800-772-1213, Monday through Friday from 7 A.M. to 7 P.M. In either case, your client should have his/her documents ready when (s)he speaks to the representative. If your client is going into the Social Security office, (s)he should have two copies of his/her benefit statement and two copies of the evidence that supports his/her claim to the higher income. This way the client can leave a copy with the Social Security representative. One important thing for your client to consider when perusing his/her statement is that Social Security has a taxable wage base (e.g., in 2010 and 2011 it was $106,800; in 2012 it was $110,100; in 2013 it was $113,700; and in 2014 it is $117,000), and earnings above that amount will not be shown in his/her earnings history.

Another thing the statement will tell your clients is their full retirement age. Spoiler alert—for anyone born between 1943 and 1954 the full retirement age is 66. For anyone born in 1960 or later the full retirement age is 67. For those in between, add two months per year (e.g., for those born in 1955 it will be 66 and 2 months, and for those born in 1957 it will be 66 and 6 months).

Another crucial element of the statement is that it contains an estimate of the client's retirement benefits. More specifically, the statement contains an estimate of the monthly retirement benefit that (s)he will receive at age 62, full retirement age, and age 70. The estimated benefits take into account certain assumptions such as the fact that for the current year and the

years up to retirement, the individual will continue to work and make about the same as the latest earnings shown on record. If your client earns more or less than is projected, his/her benefits could be higher or lower accordingly. Another consideration regarding these estimates is that the current year's benefit formula is used in the benefit computations. In future years it is likely that this formula will be changed to reflect inflation, and therefore your clients are looking at an estimate of the current projection of their benefits; not the inflated future value of their benefit. Finally, remember that Social Security benefits are inflated after the client retires so the benefit (s)he receive in the first year of retirement will increase every time Social Security gives an annual cost of living adjustment (although purchasing power will remain the same). For a personalized benefit that allows the client to run alternative scenarios based on different future earnings or different future retirement dates the client can go to www.socialsecurity.gov/estimator.

Since Social Security is not just about retirement your client can find out about any disability benefits that might be coming his/her way. In addition, the statement indicates any survivor benefits to which the client's family may be entitled. Other useful information includes:

- An estimate of the Social Security benefits that your client has paid.
- Information about whether your client qualifies for Medicare and how to sign up for it.
- Information about the windfall elimination and government-pension-offset provisions.
- Links to some useful resources.

How Does MySSA Help after Receiving Social Security or Medicare Benefits?

The MySSA site is also useful if your client is already retired. It provides information about benefits and payments. If (s)he needs proof of receiving Social Security benefits, Supplemental Security Income (SSI), and/or Medicare, the client can request a benefit verification letter online. This letter is sometimes called a "budget letter," a "benefits letter," a "proof of income letter," or a "proof of award letter." This tool is an official letter from Social Security that can be used as proof of:

- Income when (s)he applies for a loan or mortgage.
- Income for assisted housing or other state or local benefits.
- Current Medicare health insurance coverage.
- Retirement status.
- Disability.

Clients can select the information they want to be included, or left out of, their online benefit verification letters.

Your client can also use MySSA if (s)he wants to change address or phone number or if (s)he wants to start or change direct deposits of benefit payments.

Marketing Yourself with Full-Service Planning

The MySSA website, the Social Security statement, and the other documents in the client's retirement file provide a number of opportunities for a planner to market himself or herself with clients and provide full-service planning. Here are a dozen services that planners should consider providing:

1. Review the summary plan description with the client to explain the options under the plan and clarify any issues that cause the client confusion.
2. Analyze benefit statements to assess if the client's asset allocation model is optimal for his/her situation. Remember to include "outside" investments and human capital opportunities in your analysis.
3. Review the long-term care policy and health policies to discern if there are gaps in, or duplication of, coverage.
4. Make sure beneficiary designations are up-to-date.
5. Verify that the client has a living will or a durable power of attorney for health care.
6. Review the investment policy statement and withdrawal policy statements.
7. Coordinate the disability benefits provided by Social Security with the client's long-term disability policy. In other words, make sure (s)he has enough disability insurance outside the Social Security system; however, don't double count the private long-term disability policy and Social Security disability when assessing needs.
8. Coordinate the Social Security survivor's benefits with other life insurance benefits.
9. Help the client to create a Social Security account if (s)he needs your assistance.
10. Make sure the client verifies earnings on the Social Security statement and help him/her to make corrections if earnings are misstated.
11. Point out the full retirement age as illustrated in the Social Security statement and review with the client the proper time to retire. Make sure the client realizes that Social Security claiming and retirement can be two different events. Also use the Social Security statement to focus on the replacement ratio provided at age 70 by Social Security.
12. Use the Social Security Estimator to run alternative projections of Social Security based on "what if" scenarios.

Help with these and other record-keeping tasks can engender trust and help the client to think with better clarity about his/her retirement. This creates a win/win scenario for both you and your client.

Critical Thinking

1. How does the MySSA site assist older adults in their retirement planning process?
2. How does the MySSA site assist older adults who are already retired?

Internet References

my Social Security
  http://www.ssa.gov/myaccount/
U.S. Social Security Administration
  http://www.ssa.gov/1

KENN BEAM TACCHINO, JD, LLM, RICP, is a professor of taxation and financial planning at Widener University in Chester, PA. Professor Tacchino has won awards for both his teaching and his scholarly writing. Among other consulting activities, he conducts retirement planning seminars for employee groups.

Unit 6

UNIT

Prepared by: Elaina Osterbur, *Saint Louis University*

The Experience of Dying

Modern science has allowed individuals to have some control over many aspects of life including the ability to prolong life. Medical technology can keep people alive, cause disability, and cure disease. The ability of technology to prolong life has prompted several growing social issues such as physician-assisted suicide, hospice, and palliative care. Three states (Oregon, Vermont, and Washington) have passed legislation that legalizes physician-assisted suicide. The state of Montana has legal physician-assisted suicide via court ruling. The rise of the hospice movement and palliative care is another response to the growing number of both young and old patients who have been diagnosed with a terminal disease who wish to live out the rest of their days in comfort.

The experience of dying not only affects the person who is dying but also caregivers, family members, and friends who are left behind. Grieving is an important response to the loss of a loved one. Much research has been done in this area and suggests that the emotional and psychological response to the loss of a spouse is similar between men and women. The five stages of grief (denial, anger, bargaining, depression, and acceptance) are universal and are experienced by all walks of life. During times of mourning, people grieve not only for the loss of a loved one, but also for themselves and for the finiteness of life.

However, life and death defy scientific explanation or reason.

The fear of death leads people to develop defense mechanisms to insulate themselves psychologically from the reality of their own death. The individual knows that someday he or she must die, but this event is nearly always thought to be likely to occur in the far distant future. The individual does not think of himself or herself as dying tomorrow or the next day but years from now. In this way, people are able to control their anxiety about death.

The readings in this unit address bereavement, grief, hospice, and palliative care.

Article

Prepared by: Elaina F. Osterbur, *Saint Louis University*

A Longitudinal Analysis of Social Engagement in Late-Life Widowhood

LINDA M. ISHERWOOD, DEBRA S. KING, AND MARY A. LUSZCZ

Learning Outcomes

After reading this article, you will be able to:

- Describe the role that social activities and contact with children has on the adjustment to late-life widowhood.

- Identify the group of individuals who were found to have low levels of social engagement in widowhood.

Widowhood is one of the major transitions faced in older age (McCallum, 1986) and is considered part of the normative aging process (Baltes & Baltes, 1990). Widowhood engenders a far greater impact on an individual than purely an emotional loss; the transition to widowhood also involves the adjustment to a new role as a single person and the subsequent changes in life that this entails (Carr & Utz, 2002). Social engagement—having close relationships and participating in social activities—strongly influences the ability of the widowed spouse to successfully adapt to widowhood (Bennett, Gibbons, & Mackenzie-Smith, 2010). Therefore, it is important to understand how relationships and social activities change as a consequence of widowhood, and the potential role that social engagement has in protecting widowed people from the strain of bereavement and promoting healthy aging.

Active social engagement has been shown to play an important role during later life and in models of healthy aging. Continuing active engagement in life, along with the avoidance of disease and disability, and the maintenance of cognitive and physical functioning, has been proposed as a vital component of healthy aging (Rowe & Kahn, 1998). With ageing, undesirable changes (or losses) relating to physical, psychological, and social domains become more prevalent (Baltes & Baltes, 1990). The more resources an individual has, including ongoing social resources such as strong social networks and opportunities for social activity, the better their ability to cope with the losses associated with older age (Baltes & Lang, 1997).

By definition, those who have been widowed have lost a key figure in their network of social partners, with potentially an associated reduction in social engagement. The central purpose of this article is to examine the changes in social engagement which occur over time among widowed older adults. Social contact during the earlier stages of bereavement tends to be focused on adult children (Guiaux, van Tilburg, & van Groenou, 2007) and is an important source of emotional support (Ha, 2010). Friends play a more important role in terms of contact and support later in widowhood (Guiaux et al., 2007; Ha, 2008) and this contact is often centered around social activities (Chambers, 2005). Our study examines two key aspects of social engagement: the extent of contact with children and participation in social activities during late-life widowhood.

It is particularly important to understand the social engagement experiences of older widowed men and women for their experiences are likely to be different from that of those widowed at younger ages. Unlike their younger counterparts, the older widowed person is more likely to also be coping with other concurrent stressors such as health concerns, reduced mobility, financial pressures, relocation, cognitive decline, and loss of friends or family members (Carr, 2006). The life-span developmental perspective—which provided the theoretical grounding for this study—emphasizes that transitions during the life course are shaped by contextual factors (Baltes, 1987). Therefore, concomitant changes relating to aging may also have implications for social engagement, and hence the experience of social engagement during late-life widowhood must be viewed against this background.

Relationships with family, friends, and the wider social network take on increased significance following the death of a spouse (Feldman, Byles, & Beaumont, 2000). Social contact with network members during widowhood is an important factor in the facilitation or impediment of successful adjustment to spousal bereavement (van Baarsen, van Duijm, Smit, Snijders, & Knipscheer, 2002). Frequency of contact with others has been associated with well-being in widowhood (Bisconti, Bergeman, & Boker, 2006; Lund, Caserta, & Dimond, 1993) and a lack of social contact identified as a major risk factor for post-bereavement loneliness (Pinquart, 2003).

Two previous studies have examined longitudinal change in contact with the social network during widowhood. These studies produced equivocal results possibly due to methodological differences in their design. Guiaux and colleagues (2007) explored changes in contact and support with the social network before and after widowhood over a 10-year period with outcome data collected every 3 years. Immediately following their loss, widowed individuals reported higher levels of contact with their social network than their still-married peers, with contact peaking at 2.5 years after widowhood. In a study of 108 bereaved spouses interviewed six times in the first 2 years of widowhood, Lund and colleagues (1990) found that contact with family and close friends reached its highest point at 2 months post-bereavement; contact with the primary social network then fell after this point (particularly for older widowed males).

Social activities may also play an important role in the process of adaptation to widowhood. Social activities are those activities which are performed with others and, more than any other activity domain, have been associated with physical and emotional well-being (Adams, Leibbrandt, & Moon, 2011). Kleiber and colleagues (2002) propose that social activities have four different functions during negative life events: activities may act as a buffer; generate hope for the future; provide continuity; and play a central role in personal transformations. Participation in social activities during widowhood has been associated with lower levels of loneliness (Pinquart, 2003), guilt and sadness (Sharp & Mannell, 1996), enhanced morale and reduced stress (Patterson & Carpenter, 1994), and better physical and mental health (Janke, Nimrod, & Kleiber, 2008a). Older widowed individuals may be at risk of lower levels of social participation as significant declines in activity levels have been associated with aging (Bennett, 2005), in particular due to reduced financial status, shrinking of social networks owing to deaths of friends, deterioration in physical health (Bennett, 1997), and poorer perceived health status (Patterson, 1996).

There have been no consistent findings regarding the impact of widowhood on levels of social activity. Previous studies examining participation in social activities have differed considerably in their design, in particular in the timing of measurements, the use of a married control group, and whether pre-loss measures were collected. These studies also measured social activity in very different ways, which could account for the disparate findings. In a comparison of married and widowed older adults and their participation in 20 different activities (solitary as well as social), Bennett (2005) found that widowhood (and especially recent bereavement) led to a decrease in overall levels of activity. Likewise, a study exploring patterns of leisure activity in a sample of recently widowed older adults (Janke, Nimrod, & Kleiber, 2008b) found that the majority of participants reduced their involvement in activities following widowhood.

Meanwhile, other studies have reported increased participation in social activities during widowhood. A study by Utz and colleagues (2002) comparing levels of formal and informal social participation of recently widowed and married participants found that frequency of informal activities increased after widowhood; widowed and married participants reported similar levels of formal activities. Donnelly and Hinterlong (2010), however, in a quasi-replication of the study by Utz et al., found that widowed individuals tended to increase participation in both informal and formal activities. A study examining leisure activity in a female sample aged 50 years or older (Janke et al., 2008a) found that while widowed women increased their involvement in all activities (except gardening) over time, married participants decreased their participation in most leisure activities.

The main purpose of this study was to explore the changes and continuities which occur in social engagement during late-life widowhood. Previous widowhood research has recommended the use of prospective longitudinal data, married control groups, and collecting data prior to widowhood to ensure that pre-loss characteristics and resources can be controlled (Carr & Utz, 2002). This study follows these recommendations. Previous longitudinal studies have reported differing findings with regard to trajectories of change in social engagement in late-life widowhood. To date, there has been no consensus regarding the relationship between widowhood and the frequency of contact and social activities in later life. Contact in widowhood (particularly during the early stages) tends to be focused on adult children (Guiaux et al., 2007). To our knowledge, there have been no previous studies examining trajectories of change in contact with children during widowhood.

The majority of longitudinal studies of bereavement have focused on the earlier stages of the widowhood transition and used data drawn over two or three occasions. Very little is known of the longer-term outcomes of widowhood with regard to changes in social contact and activities. This study provides an opportunity for an extended longitudinal investigation of social engagement in late-life widowhood as data are available from five occasions over a 16-year period, enabling an examination of social engagement in early and later widowhood.

The particular aspects of social engagement focused on in this study were personal and phone contact with children and participation in social activities. Two primary research questions were developed:

1. Do widowed and married participants exhibit different levels of contact with children and participation in social activities over time?
2. What are the predictors of contact with children and participation in social activities during late-life widowhood?

Method
Participants

Participants were drawn from the Australian Longitudinal Study of Ageing (ALSA). Commenced in 1992, the ALSA aims to enhance understanding of biological social, and psychological factors associated with age-related changes in the health and well-being of older people (aged 65 years and over). To date, the ALSA has collected 11 waves of data: six major waves comprised of in-depth face-to-face interviews, clinical assessments, and self-completed questionnaires; and five waves utilizing shorter telephone interviews. Data on personal and phone contact with children and participation in social activities collected over the first five major waves (T1 = 1992 − 1993, T3 = 1994 − 1995, T6 = 2000 − 2001, T7 = 2002 − 2003, T9 = 2007 − 2008) of the ALSA were used for the longitudinal analyses.

A Longitudinal Analysis of Social Engagement in Late-Life Widowhood by Linda M. Isherwood, Debra S. King, and Mary A. Luszcz

105

ALSA participants who, at baseline, were married and had at least one living child were included in the sample for this study ($N = 1,266$). The widowed sub-sample was comprised of 344 participants who experienced spousal loss after baseline. The married participant group ($N = 922$) were continuously married throughout their participation in the ALSA. On average, 2.27 observations were available for each married participant. Widowed participants had an average of 3.69 observations each, representing 9.38 years in study.

Measures
Dependent Variables

Personal contact with children—The frequency of personal contact with children was determined by the question "Think of your children and/or children-in-law who do not live with you. In the past 12 months, how often did you have personal contact with at least one of them?" Frequencies were coded never (0), less than once a month (1), almost once a month (2), two or three times a month (3), once a week (4), and more than once a week (5).

Phone contact with children—The frequency of phone contact with children was ascertained by the question "Again, think of your children and/or children-in-law who do not live with you. In the past 12 months, how often did you have phone contact with at least one of them?" Frequencies were again coded never (0), less than once a month (1), almost once a month (2), two or three times a month (3), once a week (4), and more than once a week (5).

Social Activities—Questions regarding participation in social activities in the ALSA were derived from the Adelaide Activity Profile (AAP). The AAP is an instrument for the measurement of lifestyle activities of older people relating to domestic chores, household maintenance, service to others, and social activities (Clark & Bond, 1995). Participants were asked about their frequency of participation in eight social activities over the previous 3 months: voluntary or paid employment; inviting people to the home; telephone calls to friends or family; social activities at a center or club; attendance at religious services or meetings; outdoor social activities; recreational or sporting activities; going for a drive or outing. The scores from the individual questions were summed to create a total social activities score (0 to 24).

Predictor variables and covariates—A number of variables identified in previous widowhood studies were used as either predictors or control variables at different stages in the analyses. These variables included socio-demographic (sex, age, marital status, household income, education), physical health (number of chronic conditions, self-rated health), psychological health (cognitive impairment, depression), and social network variables (number of children, child in close proximity). Sex, age, and education (time-invariant predictors) were based on self-reported data at baseline. All other covariates (time-varying predictors) used in this study were measured at each of the five major waves. The coding for these variables is outlined in Table 1.

Statistical Analysis

Multi-level modeling (MLM) was used to investigate longitudinal change in contact with children and in social activities.

MLM has several advantages over repeated measures statistical models: both within-individual change and between-individual differences can be modeled; the number of observations can vary across participants thus allowing for missing data; occasions of measurement do not need to be fixed but can vary in their timing; and both time-varying (measures collected repeatedly over time) and time-invariant (attributes which are stable and measured only once) predictors can be included in the model (Singer & Willett, 2003). MLM enables both fixed and random effects to be modeled. Fixed effects describe the average patterns of change within a population, while random effects enable within- and between-person variance to be accounted for in the model.

Hox (2010) recommends that if categorical data has at least five categories and the distributions are symmetric, then the potential bias introduced to the model is small and multi-level modeling can be used. The outcome variables for contact with children were therefore treated as linear dependent variables in the multilevel analysis. All the MLM analyses were conducted using SPSS Version 17.0 Linear Mixed Models program.

Comparison of Widowed and Married Participants

In order to ascertain whether widowed and married participants exhibited different levels of contact with children and participation in social activities over time, a series of multi-level models were developed. A forward modeling approach was used with predictors added to the model in subsequent steps. Predictors were retained in the model if overall model fit was improved. In order to ascertain the model of best fit for each of the outcome variables, the deviance statistic (-2LL) of the current model was compared to that of the previous model.

An unconditional growth model (Singer & Willett, 2003) was initially developed containing the random and fixed effects of "time in study." Hence, both the average rate of change over time in social engagement and the between-person variability in this change could be modeled. "Time in study," which was 0 for each participant at baseline, enabled exploration of changes in social engagement with each additional year in study. The fixed effects of "widowed status" at each wave were then added into the model enabling comparisons in levels of social engagement of widowed and married participants over time. Dummy variables for marital status (Married = 0, Widowed = 1) were created for each occasion of measurement. A fixed quadratic function of time in study explored whether change was better represented using a more complex polynomial function of time rather than a linear model (Singer & Willett, 2003). A final model controlled for socio-demographic, health, and network variables in order to ascertain whether marital status was a significant predictor of social engagement.

Predictors of Change for Widowed Participants

The predictors of change in contact with children and participation in social activities during late-life widowhood were then explored. The analysis again began with an unconditional

Table 1 Descriptive Statistics for Participants at Baseline

Variable	Classification	Widowed (n = 344)		Married (n = 922)	
		n	(%)	n	(%)
Sex	Male	113	32.8	571	61.9
	Female	231	67.2	351	38.1
Age	65-74	5	48.1	372	40.3
	75-84	222	42.0	444	48.2
	85 +	95	9.9	106	11.5
	Mean (SD)	76.25	(5.79)	76.96	(5.84)
Household income	≤ $12,000	61	17.7	144	15.6
	$12,000-$30,000	234	68.0	623	67.6
	> $30,000	30	8.7	91	9.9
	Missing	19	5.5	64	6.9
Education (age left school)	≤ 14 years	176	51.2	522	56.6
	> 14 years	164	47.7	394	42.7
	Missing	4	1.2	6	0.6
Chronic conditions	0-1	251	73.0	633	68.5
	2-3	85	24.7	278	30.1
	4 +	8	2.3	13	1.4
	Mean (SD)	1.03	(0.97)	1.14	(0.99)
Self-rated health	Excellent/very good	153	44.5	315	34.2
	Good	107	31.1	277	30.0
	Fair/poor	84	24.4	325	35.2
	Missing	0	0.0	5	0.5
CES-D	No depression (<16/40)	307	89.2	789	85.6
	Depression (≥ 16/60)	36	10.5	119	12.9
	Missing	1	0.3	14	1.5
	Mean	7.42	(7.14)	7.58	(7.15)
MMSE	No cognitive impairment (>23/30)	294	85.5	708	76.8
	Cognitive impairment (≤ 23/30)	47	13.7	197	21.3
	Missing	3	0.9	17	1.8
	Mean	27.04	(3.19)	26.06	(4.32)
Number of children	1	56	16.3	132	14.3
	2	112	32.6	329	35.7
	3	93	27.0	238	25.8
	4 +	83	24.1	223	24.1
	Mean (SD)	2.74	(1.32)	2.79	(1.46)
Child in close proximity	0 children	27	7.8	83	9.0
	≥ 1 child	317	92.2	839	91.0
	Missing	0	0.00	1	0.1

growth model containing the fixed and random effects of "time in study." However, in this analysis, "time in study" was centered on widowhood (where time = 0 was the date of widowhood for each participant) enabling changes in the social engagement variables for each additional year in study before and after widowhood to be identified. Predictors (fixed effects only) were then added to the model in order to ascertain whether they had a significant relationship with levels of social engagement during widowhood. The predictors were added individually beginning with the time-variant predictors (Hox, 2010). Finally, fixed quadratic functions of time in study were added to the model. Using the date of widowhood as a breakpoint, "quadratic time before widowhood" and "quadratic time after widowhood" were calculated at each wave (Guiaux et al., 2007).

Results

Descriptive statistics for the widowed and married participants at baseline are presented in Table 1. The distribution of men and women according to marital status varied. Females comprised the majority (67.2%) of the widowed sub-sample while males formed the majority (61.9%) of the married participants, $\chi^2(1, 1266) = 84.14$, $p < .001$, $phi = .26$. Although small, significant differences were found between the married and subsequently widowed participants at baseline. Widowed participants were significantly younger, $t = 2.73$ (618.28), $p = .006$, reported better self-rated health, (χ^2 (5, 1262) = 26.58, $p < .001$, $phi = .15$, and exhibited higher cognitive performance, $t = -4.34$ (809.24), $p = <.001$.

The results from the multi-level models of best fit for each of the social engagement variables are reported in Table 2.

Personal Contact with Children
Comparison of Widowed and Married Participants

Preliminary models suggested that widowed participants had higher levels of personal contact with their children than their married counterparts. However, once the final quadratic model of best fit controlled for psychological and physical health, social network variables, and socio-demographic factors, the difference between widowed and married participants, $\gamma = 0.117$, $p = .099$, was no longer significant, indicating that marital status is not predictive of personal contact with children in later life. For the average participant, personal contact with children decreased significantly over time, $\gamma = -0.044$, $p = .002$, reaching a low point at 11.0 years in study after which contact began to increase.

Predictors of Change for Widowed Participants

The model of best fit introduced health, social network, and socio-demographic predictors into the linear multi-level model. Controlling for all the predictors in this model, the average participant had 4.145 units ($p < .001$) of personal contact with their children at the time of widowhood (where a score of 4 indicates weekly contact and 5 is more than once a week). This frequent level of personal contact did not change significantly over time, $\gamma = -0.002$, $p = .783$, suggesting that fact-to-face contact with children does not vary with the length of widowhood.

Close proximity to children, $\gamma = -1.869$, $p < .001$, was the only predictor significantly related to personal contact with children. Hence widowed participants with at least one child living within an hour's travel had considerably higher levels of personal contact with their children.

Phone Contact with Children
Comparison of Widowed and Married Participants

After controlling for health, socio-demographic, and network variables, the quadratic model of best fit showed a small but significant difference between widowed and married participants in level of phone contact, $\gamma = 0.154$, $p = .024$, indicating that widowhood is associated with more phone contact with children than remaining married. The trajectories of change in phone contact for married and widowed participants are shown in Figure 1. Phone contact with children significantly decreased over time ($\gamma = -0.068$, $p < .001$), reaching a low-point for the average participant at 8.5 years in study, after which contact started to increase again.

Predictors of Change for Widowed Participants

Controlling for the predictors in the linear model of best fit, the average participant had 4.336 units ($p < .001$) of phone contact with their children at the time of widowhood. Change in phone contact over time was not significant, $\gamma = -0.009$, $p = .125$, suggesting that the frequency of phone contact does not change during the different phases of widowhood.

Income, $\gamma = 0.100$, $p = .047$, and sex, $\gamma = -0.438$, $p = < .001$, were found to be significant predictors of phone contact with children during widowhood. Having a higher income or being female were both predictive of higher levels of phone contact with children.

Social Activities
Comparison of Widowed and Married Participants

The model of best fit suggested that the average married participant had a social activities score of 6.517 ($p < .001$) at baseline, reducing by 0.059 ($p = .001$) with each passing year. Widowed participants on average scored 1.376 ($p < .001$) higher on the social activities scale compared to married participants, suggesting that widowhood is associated with more participation in social activities in older age.

Predictors of Change for Widowed Participants

Controlling for the predictors in the quadratic model of best fit, the average participant had a social activities score of 7.357 ($p < .001$) at the time of widowhood. With each additional year after widowhood, social activities increased by 0.197 ($p < .001$). The quadratic parameters for time before and after widowhood were both significant, $\gamma = 0.020$, $p = .001$; $\gamma = -0.017$, $p = .009$, indicating that the increase in social activities tapered off with time after widowhood. Figure 2 illustrates the average trajectory in social activities score during the transition to widowhood. Before widowhood, social activities were lowest at 4.9 years prior to bereavement. Activities then increased until 5.8 years after widowhood when participation began to decrease again.

Table 2 Social Engagement—Multi-Level Models of Best Fit

Parameters	Comparison between widowed and married participants		
	Personal contact[a]	Phone contact[a]	Social activities[b]
Fixed effects			
Intercept	3.913***	4.213***	6.517***
Time in study	−0.044**	−0.068***	−0.059**
Widowed status	0.117	0.154*	1.376***
Quadratic time in study	0.002*	0.004***	—
Random effects			
Variance residual	0.611***	0.663***	5.177***
Variance intercept	0.747***	0.731***	6.953***
Variance slope	0.004***	0.001	0.027***
Covariance	−0.026***	−0.014*	−0.148**
Model fit			
-2LL	7335.420	7342.084	12700.735
df	18	18	17

Parameters	Predictors of change for widowed participants		
	Personal contact[c]	Phone contact[c]	Social activities[d]
Level-1 fixed effects			
—Intercept	4.145***	4.336***	7.357***
Time in study	−0.002	−0.009	0.197***
Cognitive impairment	0.067	−0.150	−0.969*
Depression	−0.078	0.026	−0.856*
Self-rated health	—	—	−0.464**
Chronic conditions	—	—	—
Close proximity to children	−1.869***	—	—
Number of children	—	—	—
Income	−0.031	0.100*	0.025
Quadratic time before widowhood	—	—	0.020**
Quadratic time after widowhood	—	—	−0.017**
Level-2 fixed effects			
Sex	—	−0.438***	−0.529
Age	—	—	−0.115***
Education	−0.093	0.047	0.955**
Random effects			
Variance residual	0.643***	0.599***	5.751***
Variance intercept	0.555***	0.618***	5.954***
Variance slope	0.004**	0.001	0.021*
Covariance	−0.007	−0.003	−0.052
Model fit			
-2LL	2723.162	2616.007	4718.699
df	11	11	15

Note: *df* indicates the number of parameters used in the model.

[a] Model included the fixed and random effects of time in study, the fixed effects of widowed status and quadratic time in study, and also controlled for socio-demographic, health, and network variables.

[b] Model included the fixed and random effects of time in study, the fixed effects of widowed status and also controlled for socio-demographic, health, and network variables.

[c] Model included the fixed and random effects of time in study and the fixed effects of socio-demographic, health, and network predictors.

[d] Model included the fixed and random effects of time in study, the fixed effects of quadratic time before and after widowhood, and the fixed effects of socio-demographic, health, and network predictors.

*$p < .05$, **$p < .01$, ***$p < .001$.

A Longitudinal Analysis of Social Engagement in Late-Life Widowhood by Linda M. Isherwood, Debra S. King, and Mary A. Luszcz

109

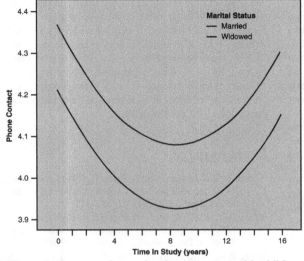

Figure 1 Average change in phone contact with children for married and widowed participants.

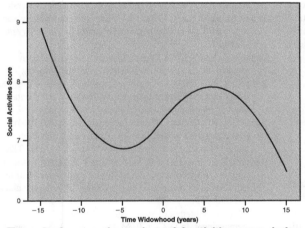

Figure 2 Average change in social activities score during widowhood.

Cognitive impairment, $\gamma = -0.969$, $p = .013$, depression, $\gamma = -0.856$, $p = .010$, self-rated health, $\gamma = -0.464$, $p = .002$, age, $\gamma = -0.115$, $p < .001$, and education, $\gamma = 0.955$, $p = .004$, were all found to be significant predictors of participation in social activities during widowhood. Thus, having an absence of cognitive impairment and depressive symptomatology, better self-rated health, being younger, and having a higher level of education were associated with greater levels of social activity during widowhood.

Discussion

This study explored the levels and predictors of social engagement during late-life widowhood. As the results indicate, levels of social engagement remain high during older age and the

transition to widowhood served to enhance phone contact with children and participation in social activities.

Contact with Children

Comparisons between widowed and married participants indicated that frequency of phone contact with children was greater for the widowed participants. Both married and widowed participants were found to have similarly high levels of face-to-face contact with their children. These results concur with the findings or Guiaux and colleagues (2007) that widowed individuals have higher levels of overall contact with their children compared to married older adults. However, Guiaux et al. used a measure of total contact with children in their study and did not differentiate between personal and phone contact. The current study, while showing that contact with children may increase overall with widowhood, also suggests that there are differences in the trajectories of personal and phone contact in later life. Hence, it is important to distinguish the nature of the contact.

Around the time of widowhood, participants reported on average high levels of both personal and phone contact with their children. Neither type of contact was shown to change significantly over time, indicating that the length of widowhood does not have an impact on the intensity of contact with children. The consistency of contact with children during widowhood found in this study differs from the findings or previous studies which have shown increased levels of contact with the social network during widowhood (Lund et al., 1990; Guiaux et al., 2007). However, it is difficult to fully compare the results of the current study with these previous studies given the methodological differences between them. Socio-emotional selectivity theory proposes that older adults place an increasing focus on close relationships (Carstensen, 1992). Our findings of sustained high levels of contact with children throughout widowhood confirm the importance of the parent-child relationship during this transition.

Nonetheless, these average effects varied as a function of other individual difference factors which were shown to influence the amount or type of contact. Living in close proximity to at least one child was found to significantly predict the level of personal contact with children, while having a higher income and being female were significant predictors of higher levels of phone contact. Previous research with an older cohort has suggested that wives tend to act as "kin-keeper" during a marriage facilitating social interactions for the couple and that widowed men may consequently be at more risk of social isolation (Chipperfield & Havens, 2001). Our findings concur that males, as well those from lower socio-economic groups, and individuals who do not have a child living nearby may experience lower levels of social contact during widowhood.

Social Activities

Longitudinal comparisons of married and widowed individuals revealed that becoming widowed leads to a significant increase in the extent of participation in social activities. This confirms the results of previous studies (Donnelly & Hinterlong, 2010; Janke et al., 2008a; Utz et al., 2002) which also found that widowed individuals had higher levels of participation in social activities. However, these studies only examined social activities during earlier stages of widowhood (18 months and up to 3 years and 5 years post-bereavement respectively); moreover, the study by Janke and colleagues (2008a) used an exclusively female sample. The current study, by examining the experiences of older widowed males and females up to 15 years post-widowhood, enables a longer-term view of social activity following spousal bereavement.

Participation in social activities during widowhood was shown to increase initially with each year after bereavement, reaching a peak at 5.8 years after which time participation began to fall. Age, poorer self-rated health, cognitive impairment, depression, and lower levels of education were all found to be detrimental to participation rates in social activities. Hence, as Bennett (2005) suggests, the very old (who are more likely to be suffering from cognitive decline and physical and mental health problems) may be less able to participate in social activities with others during widowhood.

The results should be interpreted in the context of several limitations. Timing between data collection was not uniform and varied between 2 to 6 years. The larger time intervals may have masked shorter-term fluctuations in social engagement, particularly during the initial stages of widowhood. This study focused on contact with children following spousal bereavement; contact with members of the wider social network was unable to be ascertained as the relevant data was not collected at all time points of the ALSA. An overall measure of social activity was used in the study. We were therefore unable to differentiate whether change occurred in the frequency of particular social activities over time, that is, between levels of participation in formal and informal activities.

These limitations are counterbalanced by the strengths of the study. The data on social engagement was drawn from a population-based study over a 16-year period which, to our knowledge, provides the longest exploration of social engagement in widowhood. Our findings thus enhance understanding of the longer-term impact of widowhood on levels of social engagement. Trajectories of change in contact with children during the transition to widowhood were examined for the first time, differentiating between personal and phone contact. By only including participants who were married at baseline, the study was able to control for pre-loss characteristics. A large sample of older adults was used with a wide age range (65-94 years at baseline) and length of widowhood (up to 15 years).

The results of this study showed that the transition to widowhood is characterized by enhanced levels of social engagement. Frequency of phone contact with children and participation in social activities were shown to be higher for the widowed participants in this study; and social participation increased during the first 6 years of widowhood. High levels of social engagement during widowhood may not only assist individuals in successfully overcoming the challenges of spousal bereavement but may also enhance healthy aging.

However, opportunities for social engagement in widowhood were not found to be uniform. In particular, the very-old, males,

and those in lower socio-economic groups, in poorer health, or without a child living nearby may have restricted opportunities for social contact and activities in widowhood and thus be more vulnerable to social isolation. It is important that practitioners identify those bereaved individuals who may be more at risk of lower levels of social engagement. Promoting opportunities for contact and social activity could have a positive impact on older adults' adjustment to widowhood and provide enhanced opportunities for healthy aging.

References

Adams, K. B., Leibbrandt, S., & Moon, H. (2011). A critical review of the literature on social and leisure activity and wellbeing in later life. *Ageing & Society, 31,* 683–712.

Baltes, P. B. (1987). Theoretical proposition of life-span developmental psychology: On the dynamics between growth and decline. *Developmental Psychology, 23,* 611–626.

Baltes, P. B., & Baltes, M. M. (1990). Psychological perspectives on successful aging: The model of selective optimization with compensation. In P. B. Baltes & M. M. Baltes (Eds.), *Successful aging: Perspectives from the behavioral sciences* (pp. 1–34). Cambridge: The Press Syndicate of Cambridge University.

Baltes, M. M., & Lang, F. R. (1997). Everyday functioning and successful aging: The impact of resources. *Psychology and Aging, 12,* 433–443.

Bennett, K. M. (1997). A longitudinal study of wellbeing in widowed women. *International Journal of Geriatric Psychiatry, 12,* 61–66.

Bennett, K. M. (2005). Psychological wellbeing in later life: The longitudinal effects of marriage, widowhood and marital status change. *International Journal of Geriatric Psychiatry, 20,* 280–284.

Bennett, K. M., Gibbons, K., & Mackenzie-Smith, S. (2010). Loss and restoration in later life: An examination of dual process model of coping with bereavement. *Omega, 61,* 315–332.

Bisconti, T. L., Bergeman, C. S., & Boker, S. M. (2006). Social support as a predictor of variability: An examination of the adjustment trajectories of recent widows. *Psychology and Aging, 21,* 590–599.

Carr, D. (2006). Methodological issues in studying late life bereavement. In D. Carr, R. M. Nesse, & C. B. Wortman (Eds.), *Spousal bereavement in late life* (pp. 19–48). New York: Springer.

Carr, D., & Utz, R. (2002). Late-life widowhood in the United States: New directions in research and theory. *Ageing International, 27,* 65–88.

Carstensen, L. (1992). Social and emotional patterns in adulthood: Support for socioemotional selectivity theory. *Psychology and Aging, 7,* 331–338.

Chambers, P. (2005). *Older widows and the lifecourse: Multiple narratives of hidden lives.* Aldershot: Ashgate Publishing Ltd.

Chipperfield, J. G., & Havens, B. (2001). Gender differences in the relationship between marital status transitions and life satisfaction in later life. *Journal of Gerontology: Psychological Sciences, 56B,* 176–186.

Clark, M. S., & Bond, M. J. (1995). The Adelaide Activities Profile: A measure of the lifestyle activities of elderly people. *Aging: Clinical & Experimental Research, 7,* 174–184.

Donnelly, E. A., & Hinterlong, J. E. (2010). Changes in social participation and volunteer activity among recently widowed older adults. *The Gerontologist, 50,* 158–169.

Feldman, S., Byles, J. E., & Beaumont, R. (2000). 'Is anybody listening?' The experiences of widowhood for older Australian women. *Journal of Women & Aging, 12,* 155–176.

Guiaux, M., van Tilburg, T., & van Groenou, M. B. (2007). Changes in contact and support exchange in personal networks after widowhood. *Personal Relationships, 14,* 457–473.

Ha, J. (2008). Changes in support from confidants, children, and friends following widowhood. *Journal of Marriage and Family, 70,* 306–318.

Ha, J. (2010). The effects of positive and negative support from children on widowed older adults' psychological adjustment: A longitudinal analysis. *The Gerontologist, 50,* 471–481.

Hox J J. (2010). *Multilevel analysis: Techniques and application.* New York: Routledge.

Janke, M. C, Nimrod, G., & Kleiber, D. A. (2008a). Leisure activity and depressive symptoms of widowed and married women in later life. *Journal of Leisure Research, 40(2),* 250–266.

Janke, M. C, Nimrod, G., & Kleiber, D. A. (2008b). Reduction in leisure activity and well-being during the transition to widowhood. *Journal of Women and Aging, 20,* 83–98.

Kleiber, D. A., Hutchinson, S. L., & Williams, R. (2002). Leisure as a resource in transcending negative life events: Self-protection, self-restoration, and personal transformation. *Leisure Sciences: An Interdisciplinary Journal, 24,* 219–235.

Lund, D., Caserta, M., & Dimond, M. (1993). The course of spousal bereavement in later life. In M. Stroebe, W. Stroebe, & R. Hansson (Eds.), *Handbook of bereavement: Theory, research and intervention.* Cambridge: Cambridge University Press.

Lund, D. A., Caserta, M. S., van Pelt, J., & Gass, K. A. (1990). Stability of social support networks after late-life spousal bereavement. *Death Studies, 14,* 53–73.

McCallum, J. (1986). Retirement and widowhood transitions. In H. Kendig (Ed.), *Ageing and families: A support networks perspective.* Sydney: Allen & Unwin.

Patterson, I. (1996). Participation in leisure activities by older adults after a stressful life event: The loss of a spouse. *International Journal of Aging & Human Development, 42,* 123–142.

Patterson, I., & Carpenter, G. (1994). Participation in leisure activities after the death of a spouse. *Leisure Sciences, 16,* 105–117.

Pinquart, M, (2003). Loneliness in married, widowed, divorced, and never-married older adults. *Journal of Social and Personal Relationships, 20,* 31–53.

Rowe, J. W., & Kahn, R. L. (1998). *Successful aging.* New York: Pantheon Books.

Sharp, A., & Mannell, R. C. (1996). Participation in leisure as a coping strategy among bereaved women. In D. Dawson (Ed.), *Proceedings of the Eighth Canadian Congress on Leisure Research.* Ottawa, ON: University of Ottawa.

Singer, J. D., & Willett, J. B. (2003). *Applied longitudinal data analysis: Modeling change and event occurrence.* Oxford: Oxford University Press.

Utz, R. L., Carr, D., Nesse, R., & Wortman, C. B. (2002). The effect of widowhood on older adults' social participation: An evaluation of activity, disengagement, and continuity theories. *The Gerontologist, 42,* 522–533.

van Baarsen, B., van Duijn, M. A. J., Smit, J. H., Snijders, T. A. M., & Knipscheer, K. P. M. (2002). Patterns of adjustment to partner loss in old age: The widowhood adaptation longitudinal study. *Omega, 44,* 5–36.

Critical Thinking

1. How did the transition to widowhood affect the levels of social engagement of these individuals?

2. How did the social activities of widowed persons compare to those of married persons?

3. What is a major problem the older persons may experience if their level of social engagement declines during widowhood?

Create Central

www.mhhe.com/createcentral

Internet References

Agency for Health Care Policy and Research
www.ahcpr.gov

Growth House, Inc.
www.growthhouse.org

Hospice Foundation of America
www.HospiceFoundation.org

Article   Prepared by: Elaina Osterbur, *Saint Louis University*

Finding Common Ground to Achieve a "Good Death"

Family Physicians Working with Substitute Decision-makers of Dying Patients. A Qualitative Grounded Theory Study

AMY TAN AND DONNA MANCA

Learning Outcomes

After reading this article, you will be able to:

- Identify the process of finding common ground to achieve a "good death" for the patient.

- Explain the components of the process of a "good death."

Background

Substitute decision-makers are integral to the care of dying patients and these decision-makers make many healthcare decisions for patients.[1] Conflict of healthcare providers with substitute decision-makers is not uncommon.[2,3] These conflicts can involve families feeling pressured to make decisions; feeling their loved one is a burden to healthcare resources[2]; decisions to withdraw or withhold treatment[2]; management decisions[3]; and concerns over who has the right to make decisions.[3,4] Most conflict situations can be distilled down to the presence of a "Calman's gap."[5] "Calman's gap" is the inverse relationship of the discrepancy between a patient's actual functional status, and his/her expectation of what it should be.[5] The larger the gap, the poorer the quality of life; the smaller the gap, the better the quality of life.[5,6] Neuenschwander et al.[6] adapted this concept of "Calman's gap" to describe a discrepancy in the family's understanding or acceptance of the patient's condition, and their overall expectations.

A conflict between a physician and the surrogate of a dying patient can contribute to a "bad death" experience for the patient and family. A "bad death" could involve having uncontrolled symptoms or distress, a lack of acceptance of the death, the death not being in agreement with the patient's or family's wishes, or the family being burdened.[7,8] Patients and families may fear "bad dying" even more than death itself.[9]

Conflicts between physicians and surrogate decision-makers can also negatively impact the family members of the dying patient.[10,11] Surviving caregivers of patients with a poorer quality of life at death experienced a poorer quality of life, and a higher risk of developing major depression.[12] This negative ripple effect of a "bad death" may start with the lack of end-of-life preferences being discussed and/or documented.[12]

There has been little published on the strategies to prevent or manage conflict deemed useful by family physicians in their unique position as primary care physicians who have ongoing relationships with the patient and the family. The purpose of this study is to describe the conflict experiences that family physicians have with substitute decision-makers of dying patients and to identify the factors that may facilitate or hinder the end-of-life decision-making process. This will provide insight on how to best manage these complex situations and may ultimately improve the overall care of dying patients.

Methods

Design

To gain a better understanding of family physicians' experiences of conflict with substitute decision-makers and to develop an approach to address these conflicts, we used Grounded Theory methodology.[13] Grounded theory develops an understanding of a problem, and delves into the process to determine how the problem can be resolved.[14]

This study received ethical approval from the Health Research Ethics Board Panel B of the University of Alberta, Edmonton, Canada.

Study Setting and Sample

The research team consisted of two family physicians in Edmonton, Alberta. The principal investigator has a special interest in Palliative Medicine, and the other investigator has expertise with grounded theory. Both have experience managing conflict with surrogates of dying patients. The recruitment letter was sent by email to 28 potential Edmonton-based English-speaking family physicians to enlist physicians who experienced conflict with surrogates of dying patients in any clinical setting within the past 5 years. Interested physicians who met the inclusion criteria, were sent an information letter and consent form.

Purposeful sampling sought a variation in the sample for such factors as years in practice, gender, location, and clinical practice type.[15] Sample variation identifies common themes that transcends a focused sample.[15] Theoretical sampling was also used to provide further insights on the evolving understanding obtained during data analysis.[13]

The inclusion criteria included experience of conflict with substitute decision-makers to ensure that the sample was appropriate, since participants would have knowledge of the research topic.[16]

We had sought to interview 12 subjects, as the literature shows that samples of 5–20 are adequate in qualitative studies.[15] Category and theoretical saturation[13] was achieved by the eighth participant interviewed, since no new information on key themes was identified in the later interviews.

Our final sample group (Table 1) included 11 family physicians who had a variety of practice experiences. These physicians ranged from 3 to 40 years in clinical practice.

Data Collection

Individual semi-structured interviews were used in this study because of the sensitive nature of the topics being discussed,[17] and to elicit case-oriented narratives and deeper exploration of developing themes.[18]

An open-ended interview guide for the semi-structured interviews was developed to ensure key areas were explored, based on the researchers' previous clinical experiences and the introductory literature review. The draft interview guide was pilot-tested on colleagues who were not participating in the study. The initial question was: *"Could you please tell me in*

Table 1   Demographics of study participants

Study participant (RANDOM ORDER)	Gender	Type of practice	Type(s) of location	Medical school graduation year	Years in practice
1	M	Private clinic, nursing home, home	Rural & urban	1996	11
2	F	Academic clinic, hospital, home visits	Urban	2000	8
3	M	Private clinic, hospital, community clinic	Urban	2002	6
4	F	Academic clinic, hospital, hospice, home visits	Urban & rural	2002	6
5	F	Academic clinic, hospital, hospice	Urban	1998	10
6	M	Private clinic, hospice, home visits	Urban	1978	32
7	F	Private clinic, hospital, hospice, nursing home, home visits	Urban	1988	20
8	F	Private clinic, hospital	Urban	1995	13
9	M	Academic clinic, hospital, hospice, home visits	Urban & rural	1977	32
10	F	Academic clinic, private clinic, hospital, home visits	Urban	2004	3
11	M	Academic clinic, private clinic, hospital, hospice, home visits	Urban	1969	40

an anonymous manner, about the time(s) when you experienced conflict during an end-of-life decision-making discussion with a substitute decision-maker of a dying patient?"

The first author conducted each semi-structured interview in person. The interviews took 45 to 75 minutes to complete, and were audio-taped, transcribed verbatim and checked for accuracy.

Thorough field notes were taken after each interview to capture key verbal and nonverbal communications and observations.[17] A journal was kept to assist with documenting the audit trail and included memorandums about possible linkages between data; emerging or contradictory areas that needed further exploration; and the researchers' evolving perceptions/understandings and potential biases.[17]

Data Analysis

The transcripts, field notes, and journal memorandums were analyzed manually for emerging themes and key quotes.[19] Analysis was done concurrently with data collection, using an iterative analysis technique, so that future interviews were shaped by the themes identified in prior interviews. Each investigator read and coded each interview transcript separately and then met regularly to review and compare the themes and concepts generated. Differing perspectives were discussed and challenged and in some cases explored in future interviews to gather new information that developed a deeper understanding and achieved consensus that moved beyond the initial individual perspectives. Someone outside the medical field also coded transcript excerpts to confirm the initial coding of themes. An audit trail was created throughout the data collection and analysis stages to help with the constant comparison of data. Memorandums helped to analytically interpret the data, including emerging concepts and relationships as they emerged. Through sorting the memorandums into different groupings, and constantly comparing how each memorandum related to another,[13] relationships emerged between the different concepts, giving the categories dimension and position within a theoretical framework.[19,20]

The software program, NVivo 8[21] was used after the manual coding stage to aid in the management of the qualitative data.

Rigour of Study Methods

Several methods were used to ensure the rigour, validity, and reliability of this study.[22] Triangulation was achieved through field notes to capture observations not captured in the audiotapes, thereby gathering data from more than one source to ensure comprehensiveness.[17,22,23] Triangulation was also achieved through theoretical sampling.[13] An audit trail was created throughout the data collection. "Member checking," whereby the findings were verified by some of the participants, was also completed to ensure credibility of the data analysis.[17,22,23]

Results

The family physicians expressed a desire to achieve a "good death" and described their role in positively influencing that experience of death for their patients. They were concerned primarily that any conflict with substitute decision-makers would hinder their ability to help their patients achieve this.

> . . . although we can't change the ultimate end point, I think we can change the journey to the end point and I think that's very powerful and very important in Family Medicine and probably needs to be emphasized.

Finding Common Ground to Achieve a "Good Death" for the Patient, Figure 1 emerged as an approach to managing conflict, and to achieving that good death. The three key components in this process that facilitate a patient's "good death" were identified as: (1) *Building Mutual Trust and Rapport,* (2) *Understanding One Another,* and (3) *Making Informed, Shared Decisions* (Figure 1). This iterative process involves going back and forth as necessary. As each layer of the foundation is built, the process of finding *Common Ground* has fewer barriers to overcome to achieve the mutual goal of a "good death."

Facilitators and barriers to this process were identified. Barriers to *Finding Common Ground* contributed to the conflict in these end-of-life discussions. The inability to resolve an overt conflict may lead to an impasse at any stage of this process. A process for *Resolving an Impasse* is described (Figure 2).

The Process of Finding Common Ground to Achieve a "Good Death" for the Patient
Component 1: Building Mutual Trust and Rapport

Through *Building Mutual Trust and Rapport* (Figure 3), roles are clarified and key players come together as bits of information are shared in manageable quantities with multiple contacts over time. The key players include the physician, other members of the multidisciplinary team (such as nurse practitioners, nurses, social workers, chaplains, physiotherapists, respiratory therapists, and dieticians, who can be involved in both the inpatient and outpatient settings) and the key surrogates, as ideally identified by the patient. Compassionate delivery of difficult information to surrogates is essential. Normalizing and checking in on the family's emotions is especially valuable in building a trusting relationship with surrogates.

> So I think you can enable the patients and families to digest things in smaller chunks so you can basically give them more information over time, and you see them over time, and they have a trust in you . . . to come to a better understanding of things.

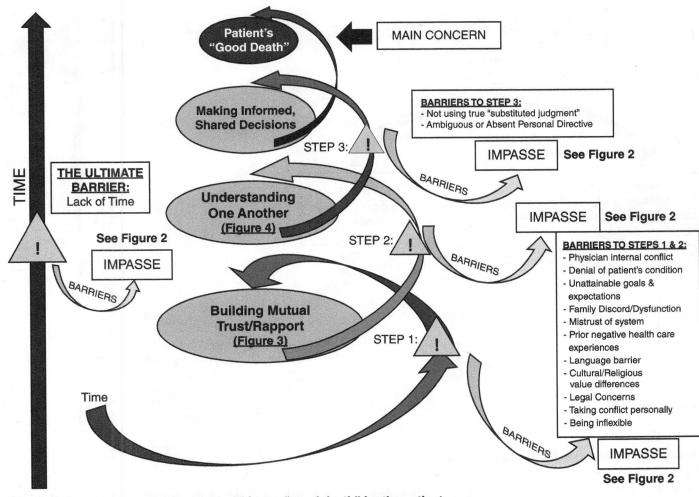

Figure 1   Finding common ground to achieve a "good death" for the patient.

Component 2: Understanding One Another

Once *Mutual Trust and Rapport* is established, the next major step is *Understanding One Another*. Once people feel understood, they are better able to listen to others, as opposed to focusing on being heard. *Understanding One Another* (Figure 4) entails each participant advocating for the patient while actively listening and educating each other about their respective opinions. Misconceptions are clarified and corrected. The physician also facilitates the surrogates' grief process and navigates the family through the dying process and the medical system.

> And, tell me a little bit about . . . what your understanding is of what's going on here and what are your sorts of thoughts about what's going to happen now? . . . then I learn kind of where we're at.

Component 3: Making Informed, Shared Decisions

With the establishment of trust and the ability to understand one another, a productive relationship is developed to make informed decisions together to best enable the patient's "good death".

After the death of their loved one, the family will be left to live with their decisions. Exploring perceptions on how decisions will affect them after the death may help inform those involved.

> And I think . . . people need to think about the dying person's wishes, but ultimately when that person's gone, you still have to go on and they would want you to go on and be happy, so how do you think this would affect you?

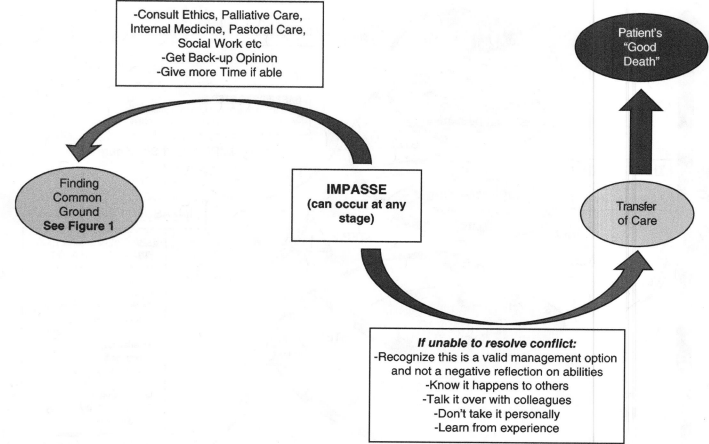

Figure 2   When common ground cannot be achieved—resolving an "impasse".

A physician's previous discussion about the patient's wishes when the patient was competent, and clear documentation of this conversation, can help the family understand the patient's wishes and take some of the pressure off of them.

> This is a very difficult situation that you're in, having to make a decision for your loved one when they're not able to tell you what they want, and that's a lot of pressure on you, but actually we have this to guide us and help us out.

Key Barriers to the Process of Finding Common Ground to Achieve a "Good Death" for the Patient

Barriers were described that could impede the process of *Finding Common Ground* (Figure 1) leading to conflict and possibly resulting in an impasse (Figure 2).

The physician's own internal conflict may impede delivering a consistent message to the family. Hence, the physician must first come to terms with understanding and accepting the patient's prognosis, illness trajectory and best medical management plan.

The family's denial of the patient's terminal illness makes it difficult for surrogates to be receptive to information about realistic management options. There may be an unrealistic expectation of what medicine can do.

> The wife wasn't really grasping it and probably in some denial . . . so she was sort of saying, "Can we do this? Can we do this? Can we do more?"

> I think a lot of it has to do with unrealistic expectations for the patients and family though . . . They expect of medicine what medicine cannot do. . . .

The lack of a prior relationship between the physician and the dying patient and family means that this relationship is beginning at a very intense and emotional time.

> . . . because I take on "orphan" palliative patients a lot of the time, you're meeting people for the first time at precisely the most emotionally stressful time of the patient and usually the family's life . . . the potential for me for conflict is greater when I'm coming in as a new physician.

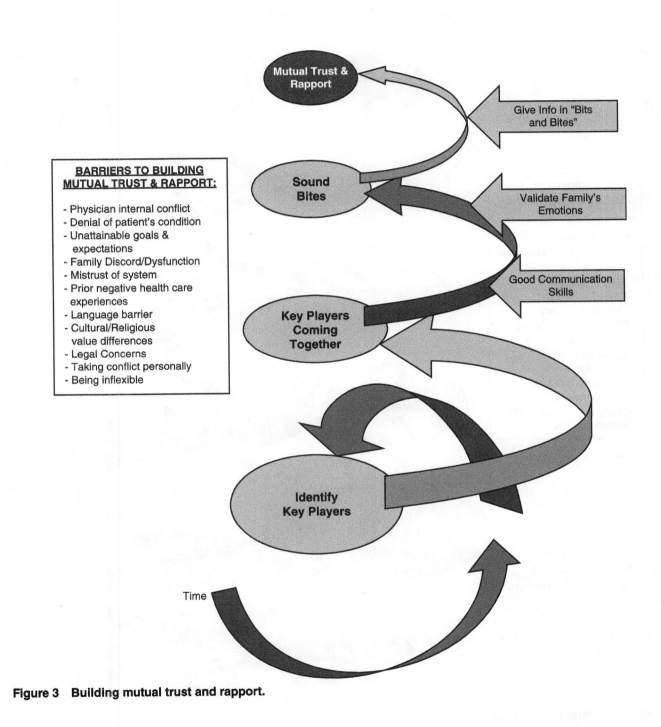

BARRIERS TO BUILDING MUTUAL TRUST & RAPPORT:

- Physician internal conflict
- Denial of patient's condition
- Unattainable goals & expectations
- Family Discord/Dysfunction
- Mistrust of system
- Prior negative health care experiences
- Language barrier
- Cultural/Religious value differences
- Legal Concerns
- Taking conflict personally
- Being inflexible

Figure 3   Building mutual trust and rapport.

Another major barrier is if there has not been any previous *effective* advance care planning by the patient and family. Family physicians are in the best position to facilitate the discussion about end-of-life care goals and wishes with patients.

So I really think it is our responsibility, first and foremost, we are the people that know them the best. We are the people that can have this discussion and we've got the continuity and the longevity. We know how to bring this up, we know when to bring it up. . .

It really has to be the family physician . . . in an ideal world, it would always be brought up by the family physician and we would have clear understandings about future wishes of patients.

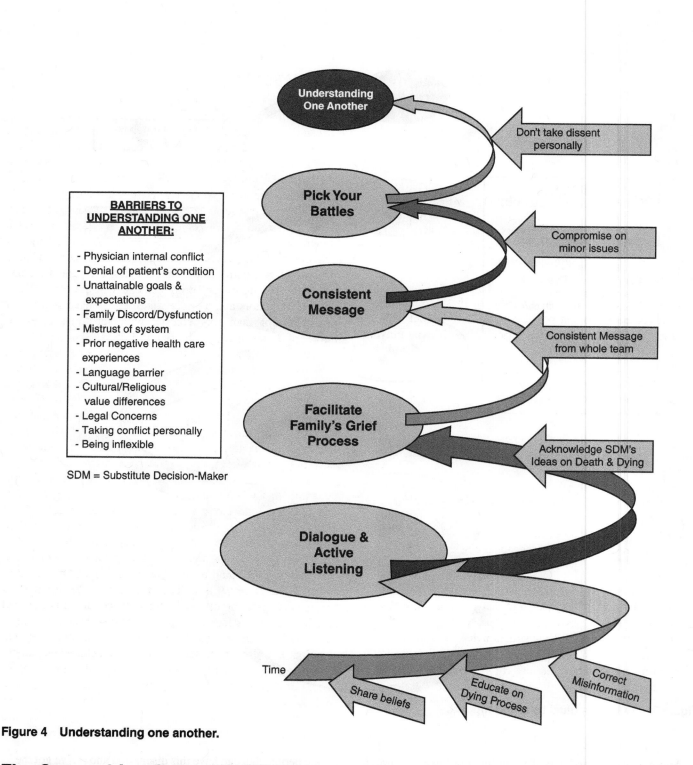

BARRIERS TO
UNDERSTANDING ONE
ANOTHER:

- Physician internal conflict
- Denial of patient's condition
- Unattainable goals &
  expectations
- Family Discord/Dysfunction
- Mistrust of system
- Prior negative health care
  experiences
- Language barrier
- Cultural/Religious
  value differences
- Legal Concerns
- Taking conflict personally
- Being inflexible

SDM = Substitute Decision-Maker

Figure 4   Understanding one another.

The Overarching Concept of Time *to the Process of* Finding Common Ground

Time is the ultimate facilitator and allows the progression through the three steps of the framework leading to *Common Ground* (Figure 1).

It takes time. I think understanding the perspective of the substitute decision-maker, or even the patient. And time. And that whole thing of finding common ground, I think is important. And it takes time to find that common ground.

Time is also the ultimate barrier since the overall time for a patient's clinical decline is ultimately out of everyone's hands.

Physicians, other healthcare team members, and surrogates need to get to *Common Ground* as efficiently as possible.

Part Two: Resolving an "Impasse"

There are times where an "impasse" may occur between the surrogates and the family physician due to unresolvable conflict (Figure 2).

Several strategies emerged as helpful to manage an impasse so as to still achieve a "good death". One strategy involves seeking a second opinion from members of the multidisciplinary healthcare team, such as nurses, social workers, and chaplains, to try to move back to the process of trying to build some *Common Ground*.

> don't think that you're by yourself in these situations . . . If you ever feel that you're coming into conflict with someone, always just ask for help and get different perspectives on situations and different ways of dealing with things . . . don't ever get angry with it. You know, just stop the conversation if you feel like you're not getting anywhere, and leave and ask for help.

There may come a point, however, where the physician may either feel that the conflict is potentially compromising the patient's care, or *Common Ground* is not achievable. In these instances, transferring the patient's care to a colleague may be the best course of action for everyone concerned, and improve the outcome towards a "good death." Changing physicians may bring a new perspective and dynamic. Family physicians who have had to transfer care because of an impasse realized this was a valid treatment option and not a negative reflection of their skills or abilities.

> knowing that one, I was able to transfer care, like I was able to kind of just let go of it at that point, and also try not to internalize it too much, and realize that a lot of the issues were a product of the situation and not something that I had failed on or I had produced or caused, and sort of learn from it rather than use it to kind of flail myself with or sort of feel like I was not doing a good enough job. But that takes a while, right?

Experience was the key to helping family physicians cope with conflict with substitute decision-makers. Experience benefits the physician trying to prevent overt conflict, resolve a conflict situation, or deal with an impasse. These incidents are valuable experiential learning opportunities.

> conflict, dealing with conflicts, I think, makes you more grounded, makes you more experienced to deal with these kind of situations in the future. That's how I feel . . . I learn a lot. We all learn a lot from conflicts.

Discussion

Family physicians can work to achieve *Common Ground* with substitute decision-makers of dying patients as a means to prevent and/or manage conflict and facilitate the mutual goal of achieving a "good death" experience for everyone involved. Through our exploration of family physicians' conflict with substitute decision-makers, we developed a cohesive, practical approach that could assist clinicians with finding *Common Ground* with surrogates when providing care to dying patients. "Common Ground" is a key element of the Patient-Centered Clinical Method in Family Medicine as conceptualized by McWhinney.[24] He describes "finding Common Ground" as a "process of clarifying issues, encouraging the patient's questions, and seeking his or her agreement with the plan."[24] The specific facilitators and barriers identified for each step in our framework for managing conflict with substitute decision-makers of dying patients was found to fit McWhinney's more general description of finding common ground within the Patient-Centered Clinical Method.[24] This further supports our framework since entering these various indicators and concepts into our framework lead to the same core variable of *Finding Common Ground*. This supports the Glaserian grounded theory concept of "inter-changeability of indicators" since other indicators can be incorporated or explained by our framework, indicating that the framework is relatively complete.[25]

Our framework emphasizes that this process of achieving *Common Ground* relies on time as the ultimate facilitator. Multiple contacts with the surrogates are required to deliver and discuss medical information in manageable quantities. Multiple contacts over time also foster the formation of a trusting relationship between the physician and the surrogates so that each can start to understand each other effectively. There is great benefit to facilitating the family and substitute decision-makers through their grief process to improve the collaborative, shared decision-making process. Not only does the physician need to help surrogates understand the reality of the patient's medical situation, but also, there needs to be time, acknowledgement, and support given for the family to *grieve* the loss of their hopes for the future with the patient, even prior to the death. As it is the family who will need to be able to live with their decisions beyond the patient's death, decisions made should not increase their risk of developing future anxiety or depression.[10,11] Thus, embarking on this process to achieve *Common Ground* should be initiated at the first contact of the healthcare team with any surrogate, ideally *before* any conflict has arisen. Each of these detailed elements provide the foundation for the physician, the healthcare team, and substitute decision-makers to work together effectively, and prevent or manage any conflicts so as to make informed decisions which will optimize the achievement of the patient's "good death."

Unfortunately, just as time is the ultimate facilitator for this process, it is also the ultimate barrier. At any point of this process, a lack of time prevents conflicts from being effectively resolved, and an impasse could occur. Further contributing factors to an impasse also emerged from our study and some of these concepts support what has already been described in the literature.

Unrealistic expectations and loved ones' denial of the patient's condition were both identified as fundamental barriers to achieving Steps 1 and 2 (Figures 1, 3, and 4). Managing these helps to close "Calman's gap" as defined earlier.[5,6] This may also be an indicator that both the physician and surrogates are *being understood*. Hence, achieving the ideal situation of matching expectations could facilitate finding *Common Ground*. Matching expectations are indicators of the concept of closing "Calman's gap"[5,6] which, to some degree, represent our concept of achieving Common Ground. This is again evidence of an inter-changeability of indicators, and supports our findings.[25]

Even when other identified barriers to Steps 1 and 2 in Figure 1, such as family discord or dysfunction, mistrust of the medical system, language barriers or cultural value differences (Figures 1, 3, and 4), can be reconciled, there may still be difficulties with decision-making due to absent, or ineffective advance care planning with the patient. A lack of preparedness for the role of a substitute decision-maker, and a lack of clear understanding of using true substituted judgement,[26,27] (whereby the surrogate is responsible for making the medical decision that the *patient* would have made), further increases the risk for irresolvable conflict to lead to an impasse. These were identified as the key barriers to achieving Step 3 in Figure 1.

The specific approach to resolving an impasse in this study has not been previously described. This approach to managing an impasse gives permission to consider transferring care as a viable management option, if multiple genuine attempts to resolve conflicts have been unsuccessful. When a physician feels that ongoing conflict may actually either affect patient care, cross a physician's personal moral boundary, or cause a loss of the affective neutrality imperative in a doctor-patient relationship, a "hand-off"[28] of the patient and the surrogates to another physician could be accepted as an appropriate method of termination of the therapeutic relationship.[28] This allows a fresh start to occur for all involved,[28] and may ultimately improve the chances of the end goal of a "good death" to still be accomplished. A large European survey showed that physicians often perceive ethical difficulties related to a patient's impaired decision-making capacity (94.8%), or disagreement with caregivers over making decisions for incompetent patients (81.2%).[29] Thus, the framework of how to approach an impasse, with the option of transferring care, may help physicians to better cope with these difficult dilemmas and foster effective relationships with surrogates of dying patients, thereby increasing job satisfaction and decreasing job stress.[30]

Our results underscore what has been recommended for the last decade about educating the general public about death, dying, and planning for this eventuality.[31] Richard Smith,[32] remarked in a *British Medical Journal* editorial that health services need to change its view of death and dying so as improve the chances for achieving good deaths. He argues: "If death is seen as a failure rather than as an important part of life then individuals are diverted from preparing for it and medicine does not give the attention it should to helping people die a good death."[32] If society as a whole was better informed about the dying process, conceivably, this would help facilitate more open discussion about end-of-life care and wishes.[33] The framework described in this study may help in educating the public on how to have these discussions effectively with healthcare providers and surrogates, and to not delay these conversations. Perhaps then, terms such as "code status" or "Personal Directives" will not be seen as "icons of death," but rather an opportunity to delineate one's definition of a "good death."

Family physicians are in an ideal position to guide patients through the advance care planning process and to encourage their potential surrogates to actively participate. In the 2004 Ipsos-Reid survey[34] on Canadian Hospice Palliative Care, 44% of Canadians had discussed their EOL wishes with family, and only 9% had discussed these with their physicians. Family physicians can take advantage of their established relationship to determine how best to broach these sensitive end-of-life issues with each patient, and positively influence death experiences for patients and their families. Since primary care physicians or family physicians are best trained to treat the whole person, and to coordinate care within the healthcare system, they are "the best prepared of all physicians to hear and implement patients' wishes regarding care."[35] Even when a patient must be transferred to a care facility where the family physician cannot continue to be the primary attending physician, the early work that the family physician may have done with the patient and substitute decision-makers in delineating his/her end-of-life wishes can still be of benefit. "Informational continuity"[36] can result through the direct transfer of this information, including the patient's values, beliefs and any specific end-of-life preferences, from the family physician to the new attending physician. With this transfer of information, the key foundational work that the family physician will have furthered can then be built upon. The next steps in any conversation regarding a patient's wishes may then be less overwhelming to the surrogates because the concepts will not be wholly foreign. Thus, *Common Ground* may be attained more efficiently for the next provider. This concept may be generalized to other primary care providers, such as general internists, and primary care nurse practitioners.

A major barrier to pre-emptive advance care planning is the amount of time required to have these conversations with patients and their surrogates. Family physicians need to be financially supported to take the time necessary for these complicated discussions. This seems even more urgent given Canada's aging population. An Ontario study found that detailed advance care planning can save health care costs in nursing home facilities.[37] This argues for the economic benefits of financially supporting Canadian family physicians to implement detailed advance care planning for all of their patients as part of their comprehensive practice.

Limitations of Study

This study involved family physicians who work only in Northern Alberta, Canada. While the participants work in a variety of clinical settings, the findings of this study may not be applicable in other clinical settings, or different healthcare systems.

Initially, the research team had preconceptions and possible selection bias which may have limited exploring the experiences of those who did not perceive having had conflict. Perhaps those who did not perceive conflict with surrogates have refined skills in preventing or handling conflict.

Ethical constraints inhibited interviews with substitute decision-makers and dying patients to provide further insight.

Future directions

Future work may include further theoretical sampling with family physicians who self-report not experiencing conflict to gain more insight from their perspectives. Theoretical sampling of intensive care specialists, nephrologists, oncologists and others who work closely with dying patients, to explore the ways in which they manage conflict with surrogates of dying patients may be beneficial. Studies with other primary care providers would further the insights gathered from this study.

Initiatives are necessary to encourage and facilitate family physicians to foster their unique relationships with their patients, and to commence these important end-of-life conversations so as to help their patients achieve "good deaths." Effective methods to improve "informational continuity"[36] of advance care planning within a healthcare system are required as well.

Conclusion

Conflict between physicians and substitute decision-makers of dying patients can occur for a multitude of reasons, and can potentially contribute to a patient's "bad death" with ramifications for everyone involved. A novel framework for developing *Common Ground* is described to help resolve these conflicts,

and may assist in achieving a "good death." These results may aid in educating physicians, learners, and the public on how to have productive collaborative relationships during end-of-life decision-making for dying patients, and ultimately improve their deaths.

References

1. Tulsky JA: Beyond advance directives: importance of communication skills at the end of life. *JAMA* 2005, 294(3):359–365.
2. Abbott KH, *et al.:* Families looking back: one year after discussion of withdrawal or withholding of life-sustaining support. *Crit Care Med* 2001, 29(1):197–201.
3. Breen CM, *et al.:* Conflict associated with decisions to limit life-sustaining treatment in intensive care units. *J Gen Intern Med* 2001, 16(5):283–289.
4. Torke AM, *et al.:* Physicians' experience with surrogate decision making for hospitalized adults. *J Gen Intern Med* 2009, 24(9):1023–1028.
5. Calman KC: Quality of life in cancer patients—an hypothesis. *J Med Ethics* 1984, 10(3):124–127.
6. Neuenschwander H, Bruera E, Cavalli F: Matching the clinical function and symptom status with the expectations of patients with advanced cancer, their families, and health care workers. *Support Care Cancer* 1997, 5(3):252–256.
7. Kehl KA: Moving toward peace: an analysis of the concept of a good death. *Am J Hosp Palliat Care* 2006, 23(4):277–286.
8. Payne SA, Langley-Evans A, Hillier R: Perceptions of a 'good' death: a comparative study of the views of hospice staff and patients. *Palliat Med* 1996, 10(4):307–312.
9. Steinhauser KE, *et al.:* In search of a good death: observations of patients, families, and providers. *Ann Intern Med* 2000, 132(10):825–832.
10. Kirchhoff KT, *et al.:* The vortex: families' experiences with death in the intensive care unit. *Am J Crit Care* 2002, 11(3):200–209.
11. Carr D: A "good death" for whom? Quality of spouse's death and psychological distress among older widowed persons. *J Health Soc Behav* 2003, 44(2):215–232.
12. Wright AA, *et al.:* Associations between end-of-life discussions, patient mental health, medical care near death, and caregiver bereavement adjustment. *JAMA* 2008, 300(14):1665–1673.
13. Glaser B: *Doing Grounded Theory: Issues and Discussions.* First edition. Mill Valley, CA: Sociology Press; 1998:254.
14. Heath H, Cowley S: Developing a grounded theory approach: a comparison of Glaser and Strauss. *Int J Nurs Stud* 2004, 41(2):141–150.
15. Kuzel AJ: Sampling in Qualitative Inquiry. In *Doing Qualtitative Research.* Edited by Crabtree BF, Miller WL. Thousand Oaks, California: Sage Publications; 1999:33–45.
16. Morse JM, Barrett M, Mayan M, Olson K, Spiers J: Verification strategies for establishing reliability and validity in qualitative research. *I J Qual Methods* 2002, 1(2):10.

17. Rowan M, Huston P: Qualitative research articles: information for authors and peer reviewers. *CMAJ* 1997, 157(10):1442–1446.

18. Miller WL, Crabtree BF: Depth Interviewing. In *Doing Qualitative Research*. Edited by Crabtree BF, Miller WF. Thousand Oaks, California: Sage Publications; 1999:5.

19. Charmaz K: *Constructing grounded theory: a practical guide through qualitative analysis*. London: Sage Publications; 2006:208. xiii.

20. Creswell JW: *Research design: qualitative, quantitative, and mixed mixed methods approaches*. 3rd edition. Los Angeles: Sage Publications; 2009:260. xxix.

21. QSRInternational: *Nvivo 8*. 2008. [cited 2010 September 18]; Available from: www.qsrinternational.com.

22. Cohen DJ, Crabtree BF: Evaluative criteria for qualitative research in health care: controversies and recommendations. *Ann Fam Med* 2008, 6(4):331–339.

23. Mays N, Pope C: Qualitative research in health care. Assessing quality in qualitative research. *BMJ* 2000, 320(7226):50–52.

24. McWhinney IR: *A textbook of family medicine*. 2nd edition. New York: Oxford University Press; 1997:448. xii.

25. Glaser BG, Strauss AL: *The discovery of grounded theory: strategies for qualitative research. Observations (Chicago, Ill.)*. Chicago: Aldine Pub. Co; 1967:271. x.

26. Lang F, Quill T: Making decisions with families at the end of life. *Am Fam Physician* 2004, 70(4):719–723.

27. Kluge EH: Incompetent patients, substitute decision making, and quality of life: some ethical considerations. *Medscape J Med* 2008, 10(10):237.

28. Stokes T, Dixon-Woods M, McKinley RK: Ending the doctor-patient relationship in general practice: a proposed model. *Fam Pract* 2004, 21(5):507–514.

29. Hurst SA, *et al.*: Ethical difficulties in clinical practice: experiences of European doctors. *J Med Ethics* 2007, 33(1):51–57.

30. Ramirez A, Addington-Hall J, Richards M: ABC of palliative care. The carers. *BMJ* 1998, 316(7126):208–211.

31. Field MJ, Cassel CK: *Approaching Death: Improving Care at the End of Life*. Washington, D.C: Institute of Medicine; 1997.

32. Smith R: A good death. An important aim for health services and for us all. *BMJ* 2000, 320(7228):129–130.

33. Vig EK, *et al.*: Beyond substituted judgment: How surrogates navigate end-of-life decision-making. *J Am Geriatr Soc* 2006, 54(11):1688–1693.

34. Ipsos-Reid: *Hospice Palliative Care Study: Final Report. The GlaxoSmithKline Foundation and the Canadian Hospice Palliative Association*. 2004, 41.

35. Perkins HS: Controlling death: the false promise of advance directives. *Ann Intern Med* 2007, 147(1):51–57.

36. Haggerty JL, *et al.*: Continuity of care: a multidisciplinary review. *BMJ* 2003, 327(7425):1219–1221.

37. Molloy DW, *et al.*: Systematic implementation of an advance directive program in nursing homes: a randomized controlled trial. *JAMA* 2000, 283(11):1437–1444.

Critical Thinking

1. Describe the kinds of situations that healthcare providers and families may face when advocating for their dying loved ones.

2. Did the article suggest what a "good death" could involve? "Bad death"?

Internet References

American Psychological Association (APA): End-of-Life Care Fact Sheet

http://www.apa.org/pi/aids/programs/eol/end-of-life-factsheet.aspx

National Institute on Aging: End of Life: Helping with Comfort and Care

http://www.nia.nih.gov/health/publication/end-life-helping-comfort-and-care/finding-care-end-life

Article

Prepared by: Elaina F. Osterbur, *Saint Louis University*

Six Steps to Help Seniors Make the CPR/DNR Decision

There's a lot of misinformation and misunderstandings when it comes to cardiopulmonary resuscitation (CPR) or a do not resuscitate (DNR) order. Here's an insider's view and six steps you can follow to help seniors have meaningful conversations to make this critical decision and feel confident it is right.

VIKI KIND

Learning Outcomes

After reading this article, you will be able to:

- Identify the traditional form of CPR and why this concept has changed over time.
- Discuss the six steps in the decision-making process.
- Identify health goals that may influence a CPR/DNR process.

A common and extremely important decision seniors face when writing their advance health-care directives or experiencing a medical crisis is whether to choose cardiopulmonary resuscitation (CPR) or to request a do not resuscitate order (DNR). There is a lot of misinformation and misunderstandings when it comes to the CPR decision. As a Certified Senior Advisor (CSA)®, you are in a position to provide relevant and accurate information to help seniors and their families make a decision that reflects the senior's values and health goals.

How CPR Has Changed

CPR used to be very simple to understand. *Cardio* stands for heart; *pulmonary* stands for lungs; and *resuscitation* means to revive from death. In the past, when a patient died, someone would push on the person's chest to try to restart the heart while giving mouth-to-mouth resuscitation to help the person breathe. But over time, CPR has become more complex as health-care professionals discover different and advanced ways to try to bring a person back to life. What seemed like an easy question,

"Does the person want CPR?" has turned into a decidedly complicated decision.

Do You Want to Be a DNR?

There are three ways to say "do not resuscitate"—DNR, DNAR, and AND; the differences are very important. The second choice, "do not *attempt* resuscitation" (DNAR), more appropriately explains that just because you attempt CPR doesn't mean it will work.

The third and newest term, "allow natural death" (AND), is a more gentle way of saying "do not resuscitate." Instead of telling you what won't be done for the senior, the doctor is offering the senior a peaceful, natural death without resuscitation efforts. Along with introducing the concept of allowing a natural death, this language creates an opportunity to discuss what the senior might envision at the end of life, as well as the benefits of hospice and palliative care.

Steps to Having the CPR/DNR Conversation

As a clinical bioethicist, my approach to the CPR/DNR conversation is threefold:

- Educate the person about CPR.
- Help the person put the medical decision into the context of his or her life.
- Have the person make the decision.

If the senior or the senior's decision maker would like your assistance, the following steps will help you guide and support the person in making a choice that represents the senior's values and health goals.

Step 1: Inform

Ask the Senior, "What Do You Know about Cardiopulmonary Resuscitation (CPR)?"

Most seniors will say, "They push on your chest, blow in your mouth, and/or shock you with paddles." You need to explain that CPR also includes *medications* to help restart your heart and *intubation,* which means they put a tube down your throat. Also, you will be put on a *breathing machine* (sometimes called a ventilator or a respirator). I have been shocked to see how many seniors are outraged when I tell them what really happens during CPR, because they never would have chosen to be put on a ventilator. They are also angry that they didn't have all the facts.

Another option that may be offered is the misleading choice of being a "chemical code only," which means medicine will be given but no chest compressions. As nurses and doctors will tell you, if the doctor gives the medicine but doesn't do the chest compressions to move the blood around, the medicine will not circulate in the body. Without circulation, the medicine cannot do its job. That said, if family members can't accept that the senior is going to die, this choice is occasionally offered, even though it very probably won't work. Some seniors, families, and physicians also find comfort in this choice because "something is being done." But as a bioethicist, I don't think people should be offered options that have no benefit. If a person wants CPR, then he or she should choose everything CPR offers to have a chance at being brought back to life.

Step 2: Explain

Help Seniors Understand the Chance of CPR Working for Them.

If you ask health-care professionals, "How many of you would like to die by CPR?" no one ever raises a hand. What they know is that the chance of CPR working is minimal—sometimes even 0 percent. On television shows such as *ER,* CPR brings the patient back to life about 75 percent of the time (Diem, Lantos, & Tulsky, 1996), but in real life it only works, at best, 17 percent of the time on healthy patients (Peberdy et al., 2003). In many situations, the chance of success is zero.

In the article "CPR Survival Rates for Older People Unchanged," by Serena Gordon (2009), William Ehlenbach, M.D., the lead author of a study on CPR in the elderly, explains that "CPR has the highest likelihood of success when the heart is the reason, as in an ongoing heart attack or a heart rhythm disturbance. If you're doing well otherwise, CPR will often be successful. But, if you're in the ICU [intensive care unit] with a serious infection and multiple organ failure, it's unlikely that CPR will save you."

Step 3: Discuss

"You May Come Back to Life in a Worse Condition Than You Were Before, Both Mentally and Physically."

Most people don't understand what can happen if CPR brings someone back to life. When the health-care team is pushing on the person's chest, there is a chance of broken ribs or a collapsed lung. The longer the patient isn't able to breathe, the greater the chance is for brain damage. There may also be damage to the windpipe if the person is placed on a ventilator.

Another way that television shows mislead you is by letting you think a person will be healthy enough to go home about 67 percent of the time (Diem, Lantos, & Tulsky, 1996). In reality, if CPR is able to bring the patient back to life, the chance of this person going home with good brain function is about 7 percent (Kaldjian et al., 2009). Some patients may survive CPR but are never able to leave the hospital. Others may remain hooked up to ventilators for the rest of their lives. The success rate will depend on the health of the patient, the patient's age, how quickly the CPR was begun, and other medical factors.

Step 4: Reflect

"The Type of Death You May Be Choosing with CPR May Not Be the Kind of Death You Want."

With CPR, the senior might not have the opportunity for a peaceful and profound death experience. When you picture the last minutes of a person's life, do you see strangers straddling the patient on a bed, pushing on the patient's chest, while the family waits outside in the waiting room? Or do you see a time with family and friends gathered around the bedside, with words of love being expressed, music being played, or prayers being said?

The CPR decision is about more than medicine. It frames the dying experience for the patient and their loved ones. I would encourage people to balance the chance of CPR working and bringing the person back in a good condition with the desire for a dignified death. This is why many health-care professionals wouldn't want to die by CPR; there is nothing peaceful or dignified about this type of death.

Step 5: Clarify

"I Want to Make Sure You Understand There May Be a Time in Your Life When You Would Want CPR and a Time When CPR Would No Longer Be an Option You Would Choose."

This is where to stop and re-emphasize the difference between choosing CPR when you are healthy and choosing CPR at the end of your life. The senior's medical instructions should clarify in what health condition the senior would choose a DNR.

5 CPR Decision-Making Tips for Seniors

1. Make sure you understand what really happens during CPR.
2. CPR doesn't work like you see on television.
3. CPR will not change the underlying cause of your condition, and it might make you worse.
4. Think about the kind of death you are choosing.
5. The decision about CPR is only one part of a good end-of-life plan.

The senior might say, "While I am still healthy and able to interact with the people I care about, I would want to receive CPR. When I near the end of my life, or when I can no longer enjoy spending time with my loved ones, I would not want to receive CPR." This decision is more than a "medical choice"; it is really a quality-of-life choice. Thus, the senior will need to define what makes his or her life worth living.

Step 6: Process
Moving the Medical Decision into the Context of the Senior's Life.

At this point in the conversation, the goal is to help the senior process what he or she has just learned. Let the senior lead the conversation and explore what CPR represents to him or her. Leave some silence for the senior to consider the significance of these issues. If the senior is hesitant, you can try asking one of these questions: "For many people, CPR just prolongs the dying process. What do you think about this?" or "Is there value in fighting until your last breath, even if this might increase your suffering?"

But don't rush the senior because you are uncomfortable in the silence. He or she may need some time to think about what you have shared. You might also encourage the senior to take his or her time with the decision by saying, "You don't need to make a decision about this today."

What Else May Affect the Decision?
Decision Maker's Emotions

As a bioethicist, I get called in to resolve conflicts when a loved one is demanding CPR for the patient and the doctor is frustrated because he or she knows CPR won't work since the person is terminal. When a family member says to me, "I won't sign the DNR," I ask the person, "Why don't you want to sign it?" Then I listen. The demand for CPR may be desperation, grief, guilt, familial obligations, religious beliefs, a fear of death, misunderstanding what CPR can do, or a reaction to a past negative experience with the health-care system.

The other day, a family was refusing to sign the DNR and the health-care team thought that they were refusing because they were very religious. It turns out that the family was not making the decision based on their religious values. They were refusing to sign the DNR because a family member had once come back to life when everyone had said there was no hope. Given their experience, they believed not only that miracles can happen, but that they do happen. Once the health-care team understood the family's perspective, it made sense to them why the family was so insistent on "doing everything."

Professional's Beliefs

As professionals, we may get caught up in thinking we always know what is best for the clients we are serving. We approach these situations with our own perspective about what would be the "right decision." But these types of choices are not about us and our agendas—they are about the senior.

It is important to educate the senior about CPR but then you have to let the individual make his or her own decision. These end-of-life conversations are a process, not a one-time event. Don't push the person to sign the DNR. Pushing the senior will erode the trust he or she has in you and will create a confrontational relationship.

When the Person Wants CPR and the Doctor's Choice

If the person chooses CPR, I would encourage the senior to find out if the hospital has a family presence policy that allows loved ones to witness any attempts at resuscitation. Being able to be in the room has been shown to help the family feel comforted by knowing that all efforts were made to help their loved one. The family will also have the opportunity to say good-bye during the CPR attempt, instead of being told after the fact that the senior has died. Of course, the hospital has the right to refuse to have the family in the room if the family is disruptive.

There are times when a patient can want CPR but the doctor can refuse. This is when CPR no longer has a chance of working and is therefore no longer a valid medical option. A patient cannot make the doctor give an ineffective or non-beneficial treatment, and sometimes CPR falls into that category because it simply won't work.

Another issue is when certain doctors won't agree to a DNR because of moral opposition. While doctors are allowed to live by their morals and to refuse to participate in acts that go against their values, they are still obligated to let patients know about valid medical options and then let the patient or the decision maker decide. If the doctor is unwilling to do this, then he or she should help the patient find a physician who will discuss and honor the DNR decision.

Lastly, make sure that the DNR request in an advance directive is transferred into the hospital chart. If the DNR is not on the chart, it doesn't exist. Encourage the senior or the decision maker to review the advance health-care directive with the health-care team in the emergency room and again when moved to an inpatient room.

Our role as CSAs in the CPR/DNR conversation is to educate, to understand the senior's perspective, and to support the person who has this difficult choice to make. Encourage the seniors and the families you work with to ask for a meaningful conversation with their health-care providers. The ultimate goal is to ensure that the senior's health goals are listened to and respected.

References & Related Reading

Diem, S. J., J. D. Lantos, and J. A. Tulsky. 1996. "Cardiopulmonary Resuscitation on Television: Miracles and Misinformation." *New England Journal of Medicine* 334: 1578–82.

Ehlenbach, W. J., A. E. Barnato, J. R. Curtis, W. Kreuter, T. D. Koepsell, R. A. Deyo, and R. D. Stapleton. 2009. "Epidemiologic Study of In-Hospital Cardiopulmonary Resuscitation in the Elderly." *New England Journal of Medicine* 361: 22–31.

Gordon, S. 2009, July 1. "CPR Survival Rates for Older People Unchanged." *HealthDay: News for Healthier Living.*

Kaldjian, L. C., Z. D. Erekson, T. H. Haberle, A. E. Curtis, L. A. Shinkunas, K. T. Cannon, and V. L. Forman-Hoffman. 2009. "Code Status Discussions and Goals of Care among Hospitalised Adults." *Journal of Medical Ethics* 35(6): 338–42.

Peberdy, M. A., W. Kaye, J. P. Ornato, G. L. Larkin, V. Nadkarni, M. E. Mancini, R. A. Berg, G. Nichol, and T. Lane-Truitt. 2003. "Cardiopulmonary Resuscitation of Adults in the Hospital: A Report of 14, 720 Cardiac Arrests from the National Registry of Cardiopulmonary Resuscitation." *Resuscitation* 58(3): 297–308.

Critical Thinking

1. How do states differ in their requirements for advance directives?
2. What is the role of the family in the CPR/DNR decision-making process?

Create Central

www.mhhe.com/createcentral

Internet References

Caring Connections
www.caringinfo.org/i4a/pages/index.cfm?pageid=32891

MedlinePlus
www.nlm.nih.gov/medlineplus/advancedirectives.html

VIKI KIND is a clinical bioethicist, professional speaker, hospice volunteer, and author of the award-winning book *The Caregiver's Path to Compassionate Decision Making: Making Choices for Those Who Can't.*

Article   Prepared by: Elaina F. Osterbur, *Saint Louis University*

"Affordable" Death in the United States: An Action Plan Based on Lessons Learned from the *Nursing Economic$* Special Issue

CHRISTINE T. KOVNER, EDWARD LUSK, AND NELLIE M. SELANDER

Learning Outcomes

After reading this article, you will be able to:

- Identify the end-of-life reforms and why they are necessary.
- Discuss the advantages and disadvantages of palliative care and hospice care.
- Discuss the proposed action plan and the impact it could potentially achieve in end-of-life care.

The preceding six articles presented in this special issue of *Nursing Economic$* illustrate with uncommon clarity the nature and scope of the end-of-life cost problems facing the U.S. health care system. They tactfully navigate the sensitive and often contentious subject of death, while acknowledging that it must be addressed by patients, by their families, and ultimately by all Americans, if we are to efficiently and expertly dodge the catastrophic effects of the "perfect cost storm" that several of the authors reference. The storm—rising health care costs, particularly at the end-of-life, and the aging baby-boomer generation—is just beginning to lap at our shores; predictably soon it will be a tsunami. Taking the necessary actions to deal with the nexus of the Cost and the Dignity of Death issues will require making difficult decisions about the extent and types of care delivered, as well as the mode of health care delivery offered in the United States. The authors of the articles that you have just read provide convincing evidence for why and how these decisions should now be made. To give a sense of the most salient points that each of the preceding authors make, we will next summarize them. Following our summaries, we will offer an eight-point action plan that policymakers and lobbyists would do well to consider to avoid the impending tsunami that inaction will surely invite.

Lessons Learned from Papers Addressing the Question, How Can We Afford to Die?

In "End of Life Care in the United States: Current Reality and Future Promise—A Policy Review," Lisa A. Giovanni, BSN, RN, details the end-of-life reforms, or lack thereof, in the 2010 Patient Protection and Affordable Care Act and the inherent potential of the 1991 Patient Self-Determination Act, specifically as it pertains to advance directives and their ability to curtail end-of-life health care costs. Stressing "that the unique needs of the terminally ill remain poorly addressed," she explains the benefits of hospice and palliative care and advance directives, and suggests their integration, bringing forward their individual benefits but also anticipating the synergy created by folding these initiatives together. Giovanni also raises an alert that must be considered—that of disparity in access and funding for these cost-controlling measures.

Marlene McHugh, DNP, DCC, FNP-BC; Joan Arnold, PhD, RN; and Penelope R. Buschman, MS, RN, PMHCNS-BC, FAAN, in their article, "Nurses Leading the Response to the Crisis of Palliative Care for Vulnerable Populations," posit that nurses are innately qualified to provide palliative care. They poetically suggest that the qualities and duties of palliative care compose the essence of nursing and that all nurses can be palliative care generalists, whereas nurses with more specialized, advance knowledge in the field can lead the implementation and expansion of palliative care. Beyond simply encouraging the expansion of palliative care, McHugh and co-authors argue palliative care must be expanded to vulnerable populations, as these populations are especially in need of palliative care and should have easy access to it. The authors go on to detail recent innovations in encouraging and expanding palliative care in the United States and recommend all nurses should be aware of these initiatives. Ultimately, the authors want patients, not settings, to dictate the quality and type of care received at end-of-life. They conclude with a hopeful vision of the future: "all nursing care is palliative care" and adopting this viewpoint "can transform health with nurses taking the lead."

In "Death Is Not an Option How You Die Is: Reflections from a Career in Oncology Nursing," Brenda M. Nevidjon, MSN, RN, FAAN, and Deborah Mayer, PhD, RN, AOCN, FAAN, describe the fears associated with dying that they have witnessed in decades of practice in oncology nursing and which they also support with evidence. Nevidjon and Mayer also address the costs associated with dying and ask the profound question, "Life at what cost?" By denying that death is an inevitable reality, we make it impossible to discuss our end-of-life care rationally. Nevidjon and Mayer provide resources and cite examples of successes in beginning this conversation, but assert that providers have not gone far enough. Ultimately, they suggest that to answer this question, providers must begin the end-of life conversation in their own homes.

Deborah Witt Sherman, PhD, CRNP, ANP-BC, ACHPN, FAAN, and Jooyoung Cheon, MS, RN, in "Palliative Care: The Paradigm of Care Responsive to the Demands for Health Care Reform in America," go beyond asserting that something must be done to curtail costs and improve the quality of end-of-life care and identify a remedy: palliative care. Sherman and Cheon offer convincing evidence that palliative care is poised to become a "universally available approach" to health care, which addresses both the quality of life needs of patients and families as well as the costs of delivering end-of-life treatment and services. Although they address the differences between hospice and palliative care, they focus quite intently on palliative care because of its broader potential (it can be coupled with curative treatments and it can be used to ease the suffering associated with long-term, not just end-of-life, diseases) and because of its proven cost-saving and quality-improving characteristics. The logical extension of their idea is that costs at the end of life, which seems to be the most contentious aspect of "controlling" health care costs in general, can be routinely subsumed in the palliative care domain and so controlled. In addition to documenting the positive aspects of palliative care, Sherman and Cheon offer convincing evidence that advance practice nurses, as a result of their educational training, proficiency in practice, and professional commitment, are and should continue to be the integral players in the rapid and continued expansion of palliative care nationally and internationally.

Virginia P. Tilden, DNSc, RN, FAAN; Sarah A. Thompson, PhD, RN, FAAN; Byron Gajewski, PhD; and Marjorie Bott, PhD, RN, provide a well-documented rendering of the escalating cost problem created by high nursing home employee turnover rates in their article, "End-of-Life Care in Nursing Homes: The High Cost of Staff Turnover." The consequence of this high turnover is further compounded by a new trend the authors cite: "By 2020, 40% of those over 65 are projected to die in nursing homes." Tilden and colleagues study of 85 Midwestern nursing homes also found that high turnover rates were significantly related to lower quality of dying for patients and their families. Similar to the end-of-life health care conundrum at large, the problem with high nursing home employee turnover is both economic and personal. They argue performance-linked reimbursement policy is the "hammer" that will, over time, put the health care delivery system back on track. To this extent, they see the active employment of incentive systems and punitive reimbursement policy as measures to reduce costs by minimizing staff turnover. This intelligent design uses both carrot and stick incentives at a time when they are needed.

Dorothy J. Wholihan, DNP, ANP-BC, GNP-BC, ACHPN, and James C. Pace, DSN, MDiv, ANPBC, FAANP, offer an exciting plan to engage Americans in conversation regarding their end-of-life care—something every human will have to confront eventually. Their article, "Community Discussions: A Proposal for Cutting the Costs of End-of-Life," proposes initiating discussions of end-of-life care earlier in life—before people are terminally ill. Although this is not a new concept, they suggest these discussions should take place in the community, not in the ICU. By opening up the topic of end-of-life care to the community, the issues and apprehensions surrounding creating and implementing advance directives are lessened. As evidence for this, the authors cite numerous studies showing early adoption and sensitive cultural creation of advance directives makes these documents more effective. Ultimately, the potency of the authors' argument is that if scripted properly, based on individual, family, and community beliefs and norms, advance directives can contribute to a dignified end-of-life strategy consistent with the community discourse an individual is engaged in over his or her lifetime. This may finally allow the health care delivery system to move away from providing heroic and ineffective end-of-life treatments and toward a more palliative approach.

These six works competently address the myriad issues warranting consideration in the development of an action plan, which addresses the question, "How can we afford to die?" These articles have many common arguments and fit together nicely; that is to say, our proposed action plan basically wrote itself.

The Action Plan

Following are the eight central points of our action plan derived from a synthesis of the research summarized in this special issue. We fully recognize the complicated systemic-dynamic change necessary to achieve our action plan will require pilot testing, redesign refinements, further pilot testing, a full-scale launch, and then periodic monitoring and evaluation. We propose this action plan because, at some point, systemic change will happen; we want these change efforts to be pro-active—driven by design rather than re-active—not spawned by panic. After outlining our proposed action plan, we will discuss its desirability, feasibility, and sustainability.

1. All individuals over 18 years old should have advance directives long before they find themselves at the "seventh age:" the end of life. Nurses, physicians, and other health care providers should be required to follow these advance directives. Many of the authors

who have contributed to this special issue suggest and demonstrate advance directives have significant cost-cutting potential, but recognize that even when patients do complete them, they are not always honored. The contributing authors posit ways to increase completion and use of advance directives. These suggestions, which we believe to be the essentials in scripting effective advance directives, are: (a) reimbursement policies should compensate health care providers for helping their patients to complete advance directives, (b) advance directives should be discussed and created in the context of an individual's community, and (c) cost sensitivity should be discussed transparently as part of the intended effect of the advance directives.

2. Hospice and palliative care (as defined in the "Introduction" to this special issue) must be available for all patients treated at hospitals or using services that are supported in part by any municipal/local, state, or federal-derived revenue. Derived revenue is any tax revenue that accrues by way of the taxing/redistribution authority following the accounting principles as laid out in Statement No. 34 of the Governmental Accounting Standards Board.

3. The decision to provide a patient with hospice and/or palliative care will be determined by the patient, his or her family, case manager, and nurses and physicians of the organization where the patient is receiving care. All the while, the patient's advance directive must be kept in mind and adhered to in accordance with the patient's wishes. This is, of course, where the cost sensitivity of the advance directive will play a major role in dealing with the nexus of the Cost and Dignity of Death issues.

4. Traditional reimbursement sources will bear the cost of providing individuals with hospice and palliative care; specifically, private insurance with no/low deductibles or co-pays and a combination of municipal, state, and federal sources. Reimbursement agreements should be as simple as possible, following the usual concept of equitable redistributions. This may sound daunting; however, simple rules such as "telescoping" where one first exhausts private insurance, then municipal, then state, and finally federal may make the funding and reimbursement processes simpler and more equitable. We also propose that an individual's personal wealth should not be exhausted before municipal, state, or federal sources are used.

5. To increase the availability of hospice and palliative care facilities, for which there will be a sharp increase in demand due to the aging baby-boomer generation as well as the fact the central feature of our action plan requires the expansion of such facilities, legislators and other elected officials should consider incentivizing or subsidizing new construction or conversions of hospice and palliative care facilities using tax abatements, payments in lieu of taxes, or issuing bonds on behalf of private firms in order to lower the cost of development. This may be particularly viable in cities experiencing high vacancy and foreclosure rates where the cost of purchasing land is already low. One such city is Cleveland, which is home to the world-renown Cleveland Clinic.

6. Social networking should be used by health care organizations and local, state, and federal governments to promote choosing hospice or palliative care over heroic, and often futile, end-of life treatments. Successfully increasing the use of hospice and palliative care is contingent upon convincing individuals and their caregivers to choose these less-expensive and quality-of-life improving options, as well as detailing them in their advance directives. As Wholihan and Pace recommend, a way to encourage individuals to include hospice care in their advance directives is through extensive and intensive community dialogue and communication. Additionally, fully using social networking in this regard may also be beneficial. This is the powerful communication tool, made famous by Mark Zuckerberg's *Facebook,* and should not to be dismissed as a fad. Although we were unable to find scholarly sources connecting social networking and improved health outcomes or increased engagement in health care decision making, some studies indicate social networking may increase civic and social engagement (Pasek, More, & Romer, 2009; Valenzuela, Park, & Kee, 2009). Make no mistake: everything is contingent upon developing sensible advance directives.

7. A greater number of nurse faculty at U.S. colleges and universities will be required to meet the increased demand by nurses who need advance training and education in hospice and palliative care. Nurses can, and traditionally, have played a major role in hospice or palliative care; expanding hospice or palliative care will necessitate an increase of the numbers of specialized nurses (American Association of Colleges of Nursing, 2005).

8. We recommend that Tilden and colleagues' list of punitive reimbursement policies (penalties for hospital re-admission, value-based and pay-for-performance plans, and other payment reforms that emphasize quality and penalize systems that deliver poor care), as well as possible incentives, be linked to documented patient outcomes and be audited by the Government Accounting Office (GAO). We recommend the GAO audit the expansion of hospice and palliative care because of the unbiased, analytical role it has played in objectively evaluating U.S. legislation and governmental actions. GAO-audited and approved services would be reimbursed. Un-audited or unnecessary/non-recommended treatments would not be reimbursed under this proposed system, *unless the treatment was in accordance with a patient's advance directive.* This "unless-caveat" regarding the advance directives needs to be considered carefully; if many patients have advance directives that make positive, cost-conscious systemic change impossible, most of the other efforts discussed as part of our action plan will go for naught.

Other Important Contextual Issues

- The GAO audit will include an assessment of the benefits of a specific treatment or service relative to its cost for a particular patient population under examination. The audit will focus on a series of questions. For example, "How was the treatment or service delivered given the alternatives?" or "What were the benefits of the treatment relative to its cost?" The answers to such questions will be considered relative to reasoned *a priori* expectations for the group within which the particular patient falls. That is to say: Context matters in assessing the effects of medical treatment plans.

- As an additional control as well as enrichment of the development of the patient treatment plan, nurses should be integrated into the treatment team decision making group on hospice and palliative care units. Nurses, as a result of their training and experience, can make significant contributions in developing hospice and palliative treatment plans. Specifically, we suggest hospice and palliative care treatment plans are signed by both a trained hospice or palliative care nurse and the patient's physician. This additional documenting voice is just a simple way of recording the opinion of another health care professional as part of the treatment plan. Over time, such dual recording will likely improve the quality of care.

- It is clear that increasing hospice and palliative care use and advance directives will require the creation of many systemic support initiatives; as a result, we recommend that our action plan be the purview of an independent decision making group that is out of the influential reach of partisan lobbying. Simply put: Lobbying is counterproductive to effective cost and quality control; the case in point is that in most countries that have more socialized health care delivery systems lobbying is illegal. We imagine this group would maintain its independence and operate within the governmental context, following the models of the Federal Reserve Board and the Public Company Accounting Oversight Board.

Features of the Eight-Point Action Plan

Let us now consider the features of this action plan. Following we discuss the desirability, feasibility, and sustainability of the action plan presented here.

Desirability. We believe expanding and incentivizing hospice and palliative care and respecting advance directives, which are central aspects of the eight-point action plan, is desirable because of their inherent effectiveness and efficiency. Specifically, effectiveness is addressed because patients' advance directives will dictate the progression of their care, thus potentially avoiding heroic, ineffective, and unwarranted end-of-life treatments. Additionally, the action plan will be efficient by curtailing costs by adhering to the GAO-audited reimbursement procedures as set forth in action plan item eight.

Feasibility. The expansion of hospice and palliative care would not be feasible, from a cost or dignity perspective, if the execution of the eight-point action plan worked against the legal, religious, moral, or financial fabric of American social and cultural norms and expectations. Engaging communities in discussions of health, recommending cost-sensitive advance directives, using discharge planning in hospitals, suggesting hospice or palliative care at the end-of-life alternatives, and financing health care through insurance and audited redistributive measures have all long been used by those trying to curtail health care costs in the United States. Expanding and incentivizing hospice and palliative care is only a modest re-organization of these aspects of the U.S. health care delivery system, the action plan of which will realign these systemic features to conserve resources and preserve individual end-of-life dignity.

Sustainability. Sustainability is the most difficult-to-predict aspect of the eight-point action plan. Expanding and incentivizing the use of hospice and palliative care with an eye to conservation of scarce resources will, by definition, move the U.S. health care delivery system in the sustainability direction. Simply put: Economies affected by cost-sensitive incentives will translate into more resources being available to cover needed services. However, the Patient Protection and Affordable Care Act of 2010 (the first health legislation in decades seeking to directly help millions of uninsured Americans) will undoubtedly put greater financial pressure on the current reimbursement system, as many more millions of citizens obtain access to health care. This increased pressure may compromise the gains made in affecting economies through the eight-point action plan. Here is where experimentation, monitoring, and redesign will be needed to maintain the hospice and palliative care initiatives as features of the U.S. health care delivery system. This of course may call into question the distribution of resources of all of the federal programs from the Department of Defense to the Department of Health and Human Services as in the Zero-Based Budget context.

Concluding Comments

A recent poll from the California Health Foundation notes there is a great disparity between what people say they want (to die a natural death at home) and what actually occurs. Eighty-two percent of respondents reported "that it was important to have end-of-life wishes in writing," and yet less than 25% had done so (Wood, 2012). Ultimately, this special issue begs the question: Given our political and economic realities of 2012, can we realistically imagine positive, cost-reducing changes in the way we deliver health care in the United States? To realize the expansion of our hospice and palliative care action plan, many details must be worked out. For example, how will the incentives listed by Tilden and co-authors be employed given the GAO audit? And how will the appointment process to the independent decision making group be organized and monitored? Of course this is normal; one should not read this special issue of *Nursing Economic$* and think, "Well, I see problems here and there," and then stop thinking. One should see this special issue as a catalyst for developing ways to deal with the difficulties of negotiating end-of-life care. In this regard we appreciate the "spirit" of Peter Neumann's (2012) editorial where he introduces the central issue that defined this special issue of *Nursing Economic$*. Neumann begins with the following "directive" taken from the American College of Physician [ACP] Ethics Manual:

> Physicians have a responsibility to practice effective and efficient health care and to use health care resources responsibly. Parsimonious care that utilizes the most efficient means to effectively diagnose a condition and treat a patient respects the need to use resources wisely and to help ensure that resources are equitably available (p. 585).

With this as the logical backdrop, Neumann systematically considers the difficulties in "doing what is needed" and keeping everyone satisfied and also controlling the resources needed to affect the needed delivery. He offers the following as guidance to begin the discussion needed to avoid the impending storm:

> The challenge is how to have a more honest conversation. A candid discussion could set expectations, inform policy debates, and help the country prioritize uses for resources within and outside the health care sector. There seems to be little evidence, however, that such a conversation will take place, at least in the public sphere. There is no political advantage in talking realistically about our problems. The election-year rhetoric will continue to emphasize prevention, quality, and health information technology. On the campaign trail, the speechifying will be about fraud and abuse, the evils of rationing, and the need to improve our way to sustainability. That is why the new ACP guidelines are so valuable. Their focus on responsibility, their direct acknowledgment of the need to consider constraints, their recognition that less care may be better care, and their call for individual physicians to use resources wisely are rare and welcome. The ACP should be applauded for its engagement of costs. Is "parsimonious" the right word? Perhaps there are better ones, but "frugal," "prudent," "thrifty," "cost-conscious," and others would also raise objections. Whatever we call this necessary quality, the conversation could use a dose of reality. Calling it parsimonious is a reasonable start (p. 586).

To close this important *Nursing Economic$* special issue, let us have the courage to be proactive, evaluate the impact of our actions, make modifications, and continue to learn and evolve the health care delivery system to produce a responsive and responsible way to address the problems that we have gotten ourselves into. As Pogo so wisely quipped: "We have met the enemy and he is us." Let's prove him wrong.

References

American Association of Colleges of Nursing. (2005). Faculty shortages in baccalaureate and graduate nursing programs: Scope of the problem and strategies for expanding the supply. Retrieved from http://www.aacn.nche.edu/publications/whitepapers/faculty-shortages

Neumann, P.J. (2012). What we talk about when we talk about health care costs. *New England Journal of Medicine, 366*(7), 585–586.

Pasek, J., More, E., & Romer, D. (2009). Realizing the social Internet? Online social networking meets offline civic engagement. *Journal of Information Technology & Politics 6*(3–4), 197–215.

Valenzuela, S., Park, N., & Kee, K.F. (2009). Is the social capital in a social network site?: Facebook use and college students' life satisfaction, trust, and participation. *Journal of Computer-Mediated Communication 14*(4), 875–901.

Wood, D. (2012). Nurses critical to fulfilling patients' end-of-life wishes. *Nurse Zone: Nursing News*. Retrieved from http://www.nursezone.com/Nursing-News-Events/morenews/Nurses-Critical-to-FulfillingPatients%E2%80%99-End-of-life-Wishes_39216.aspx

Additional Readings

Activities of Daily Living Evaluation. (2002). *Encyclopedia of nursing & allied health*. Retrieved from http://www.enotes.com/topic/Activities_of_daily_living

CBS. (2009). Why the Federal Reserve needs to be independent. *Money Watch*. Retrieved http://www.cbsnews.com/8301-505123_162-39740151/why-the-federal-reserve-needs-to-be-independent

CBS. (2011). There goes the neighborhood. *60 Minutes*. Retrieved from http://www.cbsnews.com/8301-18560_162-57344513/there-goes-the-neighborhood

Hulse, C., & Cooper, H. (2011, July 31). Obama and leaders reach debt deal. *New York Times*. Retrieved from http://www.nytimes.com/2011/08/0 1/us/politics/01FISCAL.html

Kelley, M.A., Angus, D., Chalfin, D.B., Crandall, E.D., Ingbar, D., Johanson, W., . . . Vender, J.S. (2004). The critical care crisis in the United States. *CHEST 125*(4), 1514–1517.

Krause, J.H. (2010). Following the money in health care fraud: Reflections on a modern-day yellow brick road. *American Journal of Law and Medicine 36*(2–3), 343–369.

Morris, L. (2009). Combating fraud in health care: An essential component of any cost containment strategy. *Health Affairs 28*(5), 1351–1356.

Newport, F. (2011). Congress ends 2011 with record-low 11% approval. *Gallup*. Retrieved from http://www.gallup.com/poll/151628/Congress-Ends-2011-Record-LowApproval.aspx

Poulsen, G. (2011). *Improving quality, lowering costs: The role of health care delivery system reform*. Testimony before the Senate Health, Education, Labor and Pensions Committee. Retrieved from http://help.senate.gov/imo/media/doc/Poulsen.pdf

Robert, H.M. (1915). *Robert's Rules of Order: Revised for deliberative assemblies*. Retrieved from http://www.bartleby.com/176

Social Security Advisory Board. (2009). *The unsustainable cost of health care*. Retrieved from http://www.ssab.gov/documents/TheUnsustainableCostofHealthCare_508.pd

Critical Thinking

1. The article suggests that there is an "impending tsunami that inaction will surely invite." What is this tsunami?

2. What is meant by community discussions regarding advance directives?

3. How will the cost of health care be affected by these proposed changes in its delivery?

Create Central

www.mhhe.com/createcentral

Internet References

American Association of Colleges of Nursing
www.aacn.nche.edu

AARP
www.aarp.org

CHRISTINE T. KOVNER, PhD, RN, FAAN, is a Professor, College of Nursing, and Nurse Attending, NYU Langone Medical Center, New York University, New York, NY. EDWARD LUSK, PhD, MBA, MA, CPA, is a Professor of Accounting, State University of New York—Plattsburgh, Plattsburgh, NY, and Emeritus, the Department of Statistics, the Wharton School of the University of Pennsylvania, Philadelphia, PA. NELLIE M. SELANDER, MUP, is a Research Assistant, College of Nursing, New York University, New York, NY.

Kovner et al., Christine T. From *Nursing Economic$*, May/June 2012, pp. 179–184. Copyright © 2012 by Jannetti Publications, Inc., East Holly Avenue/Box 56, Pitman, NJ 08071-0056; (856) 256-2300, FAX (856) 589-7463; for a sample copy of the journal, please contact the publisher. Used with permission. www.nursingeconomics.net

Article

Prepared by: Elaina F. Osterbur, *Saint Louis University*

Palliative Care: A Paradigm of Care Responsive to the Demands for Health Care Reform in America

DEBORAH WITT SHERMAN AND JOOYOUNG CHEON

Learning Outcomes

After reading this article, you will be able to:

- Discuss the cost savings of palliative care and its impact on quality of life.

- Discuss the health-care demands for palliative and hospice care in the United States.

- Discuss the provisions in the Affordable Care Act and how the act affects end-of-life-care decisions.

I n March 2010, the affordable Care Act was passed by Congress and signed into law by President Obama. This act expands access to health care to over 30 million Americans (Pelosi, 2010). The Act increases insurance coverage for pre-existing conditions, and increases projected national medical spending with the expansion of Medicaid to include more low-income Americans (Foster, 2009; Keehan et al., 2011), while projecting a reduction in spending on Medicare of $400 billion over a 10-year period (Pelosi, 2010). The Affordable Care Act of 2010 requires the Centers for Medicare and Medicaid Services to implement a 3-year demonstration project which allows patients to receive aggressive treatment as well as palliative/hospice care concurrently (Office of the Legislative Counsel, 2010). This will require a rethinking of hospice eligibility criteria to be less stringent than having a current prognosis of 6 months or less to live for patients with advanced illness (Casarett, 2011). This moves in the right direction as the addition of palliative-hospice care to aggressive treatment reduces health care utilization and costs (Brumley et al., 2007; Temel et al., 2010).

The project also evaluates the cost saving of palliative home health care programs and will evaluate patients' quality of life. The expectation is that the results of this 3-year project will indicate that palliative care, in addition to life-sustaining treatment, will improve patients' survival when compared to usual care (Temel et al., 2010). Palliative care has great relevance to efforts to reform the health care system, insuring quality, consistency, and effectiveness of health care delivery (Meier & Beresford, 2009).

Palliative Care as a Paradigm of Care

Palliative care is a paradigm of care, which expands the traditional disease-model of treatment to anticipate, prevent, and alleviate the suffering associated with serious, progressive, chronic, life-threatening illness at any point during the illness trajectory (National Consensus Project [NCP] for Quality Palliative Care, 2009). It is now recognized as a specialty in medicine, nursing, and social work with an inherent interdisciplinary nature (Grant, Elk, Ferrell, Morrison, & von Gunten, 2009). Palliative care addresses the physical, emotional, social, and spiritual needs of patients and their families with the goal of improving their quality of life. This occurs through the aggressive treatment of pain and other symptoms, as well as optimizing function and assisting patients and families with health care decision making (NCP, 2009). Through conversations with patients and families regarding advanced care planning, palliative care focuses on matching treatments with the patient's and family's values and preferences (Meier & Beresford, 2009). It improves communication across all care settings and results in continuous and well-coordinated care during illness transitions.

The experience of serious life-threatening illness is overwhelming for patients. Studies indicate that 53% of patients averaged across all disease stages report pain, with one-third rating pain as moderate to severe (Giese-Davis et al., 2011; Morrison, Flanagan, Fishberg, Cintron, & Siu, 2009; Morrison et al., 2003; Satin, Linden, & Phillips, 2009). Often concurrent with pain are associated symptoms of depression, delirium, or functional decline. Patients with cancer also report nonpain symptoms such as dyspnea, anxiety, and insomnia (Mitchell et al., 2011; Spiegel, 2011; van den Beuken-van Everdingen et al., 2009). These symptoms are exacerbated by the uncertainty associated with severe illness and often have an impact on spiritual and social well-being which impairs quality of life (Meier & Brawley, 2011). The ultimate outcome is impaired quality of life with spiritual and social ramifications. Palliative care focuses on addressing all aspects of suffering, which not only improves quality of life, but survival. With consideration regarding the goals of care, palliative care considers the risk and benefit ratio of tests, procedures, and treatments, which may adversely affect quality of life, create additional suffering, providing limited benefit while driving up the costs of health care (Meier & Brawley, 2011).

The impact of illness is felt not only by the patient but also by family caregivers. Wright and colleagues (2008) documented the association between patients' end-of-life care and quality of life of caregivers. The burdens of family caregiving include time and logistics, physical tasks, financial costs, emotional burdens, and other health risks (Rabow, Hauser, & Adams, 2004). The physical stress of caregiving can lead to significant physiological changes and medical illness with a greater risk of mortality. In turn, health risks and serious illness require increasing utilization of health care resources and escalated health care costs as caregivers suffer from heart disease, hypertension, and impaired immune function, placing them at greater risk for cancers, HIV/AIDS, and other infections (Family Caregiver Alliance, 2006). Emotionally, caregivers suffer from symptoms of anger, depression, and anxiety and often become demoralized and exhausted (Zarit, 2006). As a vulnerable population, many caregivers of advanced cancer patients either meet DSM-IV criteria for, or are being treated for, psychiatric problems (Vanderweker, Laff, Kadan-Lottick, McColl, & Prigerson, 2005), and demonstrate impaired cognitive functioning (McGuire et al., 2000). Caregiving demands result in lost wages or leaving the workforce entirely, both of which have severe economic implications, and personal, social, and institutional consequences. As leisure, religious, and social activities are abandoned, there is heightened marital and family stress, with long-term consequences for the health and the stability of the family (Dumont, Dumont, & Mongeau, 2008). Given that palliative care offers patient and family-centered care, it promotes a sense of safety in the health care system for both patients and their family caregivers (NCP, 2009).

The Similarities and Differences of Palliative and Hospice Care

In response to the central question of "How we can afford to die?" we contend that palliative and hospice care offer holistic and comprehensive care that is individualized to the needs of patients and families, and consistent with their goals of care. Palliative care thereby limits unwanted, inappropriate, and ineffective interventions which drive up the cost of health care significantly. Palliative care can be provided at the same time as life-prolonging treatments. In contrast, hospice care, as a form of palliative care, is the care of patients and families during the last few weeks or months of life. Both palliative and hospice care are based on the principles of patient/family-centered care and holistic care including comprehensive assessment and treatment which is offered by an interdisciplinary team of health professionals. The difference between palliative care and hospice care is essentially the timing; palliative care is offered from the time of diagnosis with life-threatening illness through the death of the patient and into the bereavement period for families, while hospice care is offered at the end of life (Jennings, Ryndes, D'Onofrio, & Baily, 2003).

The clinical models of palliative care include palliative consultation services, inpatient palliative care units, and community home-based programs in nursing homes and assisted living facilities as well as care in ambulatory outpatient clinics. Similarly, hospice care can be offered in hospice units of hospitals or nursing homes as well as in residential hospices and home hospices.

The Increasing Demand for Palliative Care

Palliative care is poised to become a universally available approach to meet the needs of the sickest and most vulnerable populations and is an important factor in improving health care in America (Meier, 2010). With the increase in life expectancy for patients with cancer, HIV/AIDS, or end-stage organ diseases, as well as the expected growth of the aging population, palliative care is in demand. Seminal data from the 1994 SUPPORT studies indicate more than 50% of caregivers of Americans hospitalized with a serious illness report less than optimal care and more than 30% of families report significant economic burden (Covinsky et al., 1994). Teno and colleagues (2004) report that 1 in 4 patients report inadequate treatment of pain and dyspnea; 1 in 3 families report inadequate emotional support; and 1 in 3 patients report they receive no education related to the treatment of their symptoms following a hospital stay nor are arrangements made for follow-up care after hospital discharge. Given these significant gaps in care, hospitals are recognizing the value of palliative care in providing relief of pain and other symptoms, continuity of the care, as well as educational and emotional support for patients and families experiencing serious illness (Teno et al., 2004). As such, palliative care is important in health care reform where the emphasis is quality health outcomes while considering the value and cost of care.

Cost Savings and Health-Related Outcomes of Palliative Care

The Federal Government estimates the U.S. population ages 85 and over will grow from 5.3 million in 2006 to nearly 21 million by 2050 (Federal Interagency Forum on Aging Related Statistics, 2008). In the United States, capita spending on health care outranks anywhere else in the world with a reported $2.4 trillion spent on health care in 2008 (Medicare Payment Advisory Commission, 2009). Furthermore, 68% of all Medicare spending will be to address the needs of Medicare patients with greater than four chronic conditions. "Five percent of Medicare enrollees with the most serious illness account for over 43% of Medicare expenditures with the top 25% of enrollees accounting for 85% of the costs" (Congressional Budget Office, 2005).

Additionally, there is a rapid growth in the eligible nursing home population which represents 6%–7% of the Medicaid population, but over half of the Medicaid expenditures (Huskamp, Stevenson, Chernew, & Newhouse, 2010; Kaiser Family Foundation, 2011; Meier, Lim, & Carlson, 2010; Mitchell et al., 2009). Hospitals are responding to the economic crisis and escalating cost of health care by cutting administration costs, reducing staffs, reducing services, divesting assets, and considering merger and other economic restraints which have significant implications related to quality of care (American Hospital Association, 2008).

Increased cost of health care does not equate with a higher quality of care. Although it is estimated the U.S. Gross National Product (GNP) will increase from 16% to 20% by 2015 for medical spending, data indicate higher medical spending does not lead to better patient's outcomes. In fact, regions of highest utilization, such as having the greatest number of specialist visits, hospital days, and ICU use, have the highest mortality rates (Fisher, Wennberg, Stukel, & Gottlieb, 2004; Fisher et al., 2003; Mitka, 2006).

Morrison and colleagues (2008) examined the cost and ICU outcomes associated with palliative care consultation in eight U.S. hospitals. For individuals with live discharges, it was reported that palliative care, when compared to usual care, reduced the total costs of admission by $2,642, lowered the cost per day by $279, as well as lowered the direct costs per admission by $1,696. Palliative care also significantly lowered the costs of direct costs per admission, laboratory costs, and ICU costs. For individuals who had a hospital death, palliative care significantly lowered the total cost of admission by $6,896, lowered the total costs per day by $549, and lowered the direct costs per admission by $4,908. For this population, significant reductions also occurred for direct costs per day, laboratory costs, and ICU costs.

Morrison and colleagues (2008) indicated that for a 400-bed hospital, the annual cost savings by palliative care is more than $1.3 million per year. Penrod and colleagues (2010) further reported patients receiving palliative care were 44% less likely to be admitted to an ICU when compared to usual care patients. Evidence clearly indicates palliative care reduces the overuse of unnecessary, marginally effective, or ineffective treatments and leads to less hospital re-admissions as a result of greater continuity of care and the development of safe transition plans upon initial discharge (Morrison et al., 2008; Penrod et al., 2010; Penrod et al., 2006; Smith et al., 2003).

Brumley and colleagues (2007) also reported the palliative care shifts care out of hospital to the home. Specifically, palliative care significantly increases home health visits while lowering physician office visits, emergency visits, hospital days, and skilled nursing facilities days. According to a report published by the Institute of Medicine, savings greater than $6 billion per year would occur if palliative care teams were fully integrated into the nation's hospitals (Morrison et al., 2011).

In addition to cost savings, data indicate palliative care is beneficial in achieving positive health-related outcomes for patients, families, and health professionals. More specifically, palliative care outcomes include:

- Improvement of quality care while lowering length of stay and cost.
- Emotional, spiritual, and social support of patients and families.
- Improvement of quality of life for patients and families.
- Improvement in patient/family satisfaction.
- Handling of time-intensive family/patient/team meetings.
- Better coordination of care.
- Specialty-level assistance to the attending physician.
- Support for attending physicians and discharge planning staff.
- Improvement in nurse and physician satisfaction (NCP, 2009).

Given that health care spending continues to increase in most countries as a percentage of the GNP, Higginson and Foley (2009) affirm there is intensive pressure to reduce health care costs, which are particularly high in the last year of life. They conclude palliative care not only results in cost savings for health care systems, but quantifiable benefits in the reduction of pain and suffering, and improvement in the quality of care and quality of life. In short, the palliative care/hospice partnership creates a common sense allocation of health care resources as patients move across the illness trajectory and approach the end of life. With palliative and hospice care, the wishes and preferences of patients and families are respected, often with a desire to withdraw life-prolonging treatments and insure their comfort and dignity as death approaches.

Palliative Care Responds to the Health Care Demands in America

The 2008 State-by-State Report Card of America's care of serious illness indicates that over the last 10 years, palliative care has been one of the fastest-growing trends in health care (National Palliative Care Research Center, 2011). The report card indicates 85% of large hospitals with 300 or more beds have a palliative care team. However, only 54% of public hospitals, 26% of for-profit hospitals, and 37% of community hospitals offer palliative care services (National Palliative Care Research Center [NPCRC], 2011). Although it is recognized that palliative care is the new paradigm for managing serious illness and 92% of people polled believe palliative services should be available at all hospitals, millions of Americans with serious illness do not have access to palliative care. Despite a 138% increase in the number of palliative care programs, the accessibility and availability of such programs vary greatly by region and by state (NPCRC, 2011).

In 2008, the nation's palliative care report card indicated an overall grade of C. The good news is the overall grade improved to a grade of B in 2011 (NPCRC, 2011), indicating that overall, states now exceed the minimal standards of quality palliative care. In fact, although more than half of the 50 states received a grade of B, seven states now report they have more than 80% of hospitals with palliative care services, thereby receiving a grade of A, indicating excellence in palliative care. Clearly, there is still improvement to be made as 12% of states received a non-passing grade of D or F. In many of these states, there are disparities given geographic availability and the shortage of trained palliative care health professionals. Furthermore, public and community provider hospitals are often the only options for Americans without health care insurance as well as for those living in geographically isolated areas. The result is greater health disparities resulting from less access to palliative care for these underserved populations. The mandates of health care reform will lead institutions to voluntary certification in palliative care as recommended by the Joint Commission on Accreditation of Healthcare Organizations and an expectation for hospitals to achieve Magnet® status.

Global Demands for Palliative Care

Palliative care is a global imperative as 56 million people die each year in resource-rich as well as resource-poor countries with associated physical and emotional suffering (Seymour et al., 2009). "At the end of the first decade of the 21st Century, the provision of palliative care is beginning to feature in the political and policy agendas of many different countries as they seek to respond to the challenges of epidemiological and socio-demographic change, particularly given aging populations" (Seymour, 2011, p. 18).

With the belief that palliative care should be regarded as a human right, Wright, Wood, Lynch, and Clark (2008) have mapped the levels of palliative care development globally. Although palliative care is now regarded as a human right, the distribution of services is generally unavailable in many countries in the world. The typology of worldwide palliative care was constructed by identifying countries with: (a) no identified hospice/palliative care activities; (b) the capacity for developing palliative care, however no palliative services available; (c) the provision of localized palliative care; (d) and countries where palliative care is being integrated with mainstream health care services. The results of this mapping determined palliative care services can be found in 115 out of 234 countries. More specifically, the results indicated there was no identified activities in 78 (33%) countries, 41 (18%) countries had capacity building, and 80 (34%) countries had localized provision of palliative care, while 35 (15%) countries approached integration.

With over half of the world's countries still without palliative care, the challenges that remain include the awareness of palliative care to improve quality of life for patients and families, increased access to opioid medications, education, and government support for palliative care. Centeno and colleagues (2007) suggested the importance of implementing different models of palliative care service delivery. They proposed not only hospice consultation support teams, but day centers which are common in the United Kingdom, as well as mobile teams. In an aging society with stretched budgets, the future will bring new challenges to sustain, expand, and optimize the 8,000 dedicated palliative care services that currently exist in the world (Gomes, Harding, Foley, & Higginson, 2009).

International Recommendations for the Advancement of Palliative Care

As a global leader in hospice and palliative care, funding and financing issues in the Australian hospice and palliative care sector is informative (Gordon, Eagar, Currow, & Green, 2009). In Australia, responsibilities for managing the health care system are shared by both levels of government—the states and territories. The delivery of palliative care services therefore is the responsibility of both states and territories. The funding of palliative care varies according to the type of care offered by specialist providers, generalist providers, and support services in nongovernment, private, and public sectors. In Australia, there is no national model for funding inpatient or community services, as these services are a states/territories responsibility. Given that palliative care is evolving at a rapid rate in Australia, it is recommended that flexible evidenced-based models of care delivery emerge along with equally flexible funding and financing models with consideration of the case mix of patient and type of providers (Gordon et al., 2009).

In directing the future of the palliative care field, Gomes and colleagues (2009) and Lynch and co-authors (2009) reported on the outcomes of an international meeting of clinicians, health economists, researchers, policymakers, and advocates. Based on this meeting, seven recommendations related to palliative care were identified: (a) the need for shared definitions of palliative care, (b) identification of the strengths and weakness of different payment systems, (c) determination of country-specific and international research priorities, (d) consideration of appropriate economic evaluation methods, (e) evaluation of the cost of palliative care, (f) the need for palliative care education and training programs for interdisciplinary health care professionals, and (g) the development of national standards to regulate and determine palliative care planning and development. Countries such as the United Kingdom, Canada, Australia, and the United States are at the forefront in providing quality palliative and hospice care and national as well as international leaders in the specialty are addressing these recommendations.

Advance Practice Nurses Play a Pivotal Role in Palliative Care

With the rapid growing increase in both the number and quality of palliative care programs in the United States and worldwide, the contribution of advance practice nurses in advancing the specialty is striking. "Advance practice nurses often embody in a single person palliative care's focus on the whole person and the medical practitioner's ability to diagnose conditions, prescribe medications and order treatment interventions while recouping salary costs through billing for consultations" (Meier & Beresford, 2006, p. 624). The importance of whole-person care is emphasized by Meier and Brawley (2011), who state that "New delivery and payment models that promote quality of care, instead of the current fee-for-service model that promotes quantity of care, may change incentives that encourage procedures and interventions over whole-person care" (p. 2751).

In many hospitals, it is the advance practice nurse who spearheads the development, implementation, and evaluation of palliative care services. Advance practice nurses have pivotal leadership roles as clinical consultants, administrators, educators, health policymakers, and researchers. With advance nursing degrees in adult primary care, geriatrics, psychiatric nursing, pediatrics, or family nursing, palliative care nurses combine their primary specialization with specialist-level knowledge in palliative care gained through concurrent master's degrees or post-master's certification in palliative care. Palliative care competencies and expertise are demonstrated by passing the Advance Practice Palliative Care Certification Examination offered by the National Board for Certification of Hospice and Palliative Nurses. Eligibility to take the examination requires documentation of an advanced practice master's degree in nursing and 500 clinical hours in palliative care within the year prior to taking the examination. Advance practice nurses can bill for their services given they have achieved advance practice nursing licensure and certification and are working within their scope of practice as defined by their certification agency.

As a leader in palliative care, advance practice nurses are often the health professionals who make the case to hospital administration to implement a palliative program. The unique missions, needs, and the constraints of the hospital must be considered when designing a successful palliative care program (Center to Advance Palliative Care, 2011). In developing a business plan, the advanced practice nurse considers interdisciplinary resources, feasibility and accessibility, cost control, revenue generation, integrating and leveraging of existing services, deciding the palliative care program structure and model, where to house the program, as well as how to coordinate patient care across settings. The business plan includes the operational plan for implementation such as space needs, staffing roles and requirements, basic policies and procedures, and projections of patient volume and program capacity. The operational plan explains the program start-up and ongoing costs, as well as the expected sources of revenue or cost avoidance.

In creating the business plan, the advance practice nurse utilizes financial and strategic planning tools. The advanced practice nurse demonstrates how the palliative program will contribute to the hospital's financial viability, with consideration of program volume, length of stay, daily census, hospital billing revenues, estimated cost savings, and potential contributions by philanthropy (Center to Advance Palliative Care, 2011). The executive summary of the plan describes the context for the proposal, the program's key features, the needs or problems identified through institutional and market analysis, and how the palliative program will meet these needs as well as the expected impact and outcomes for quality care. With advanced clinical knowledge and expertise related to health care systems, advance practice nurses are credited for the rapid advancement of the specialty and for their futuristic perspectives on addressing the demands of health care reform while providing quality care.

Health Care for the Seriously Ill and Dying: An Exemplary Action Plan in the State of Maryland

Within the context of cancer care and a focus on quality and affordable health care, the Maryland Cancer Control Plan for Palliative and Hospice Care (Sherman et al., 2011) provides a valuable action plan or "Blueprint for Success in Palliative and Hospice Care." This comes at a time when citizens of Maryland and all of the United States most need a complement to health care, including cancer care. With an aging population in the State of Maryland and nationally, an increase in the number of cancer diagnoses, and an increase in the number of survivors of cancer and other life-threatening illness who still face a number of physical and emotional symptoms, a comprehensive "all hands on deck" approach to health care is critical. Quality and affordable health care during any stage of the illness trajectory, particularly as the disease progresses and death approaches, involves collaborative efforts of patients, families, communities, health care professionals, institutions, health care policymakers, legislators, and payers (see Table 1). By active involvement and joint efforts, these key stakeholders can insure quality of care and quality of life, lower cost, increased access, coordination and continuity, and the reduction of health disparities (Sherman et al., 2011).

Maryland's Action Plan for Palliative and Hospice Care (Sherman et al., 2011, p. 4) highlights the importance of the achievement of the "4 A's"—Awareness, Acknowledgment, Access, and Action—by each of the identified stakeholder groups.

- *Awareness* implies knowledge and appreciation gained through one's perceptions or by means of information about palliative and hospice care.
- *Acknowledgment* is the recognition and acceptance of the value of palliative and hospice care.
- *Access* is the right, privilege, or ability to make use of resources and information related to palliative and hospice care.
- *Action* is the development, implementation, and evaluation of initiatives to promote palliative and hospice care, which will lead to inclusion of palliative and hospice care into the standards of care and setting of future goals.

According to Maryland's Action Plan, each of the identified stakeholder groups develops an awareness of palliative

Table 1 Identification of Key Stakeholder Groups in Palliative and Hospice Care

Patients, Families, and Communities

- *Patients:* Individuals with a diagnosis of cancer at any phase of the illness experience.
- *Family:* Any individual who provides direct or indirect support of a patient experiencing cancer.
- *Community:* A group of interacting people living in a common location and who share common values or interests.

Health Care Professionals and Associated Staff

- *Health Care Professionals:* All members of the palliative care and hospice interdisciplinary team including physicians, nurses, social workers, psychologists, chaplains, pharmacists, physical or occupational therapists, as well as patients' oncologist or primary care physician.
- *Associated Staff:* All individuals involved in the caring process who offer direct or indirect support in the care of oncology patients and their families across all health care settings.

Institutions

All health care delivery systems that provide palliative or hospice care, such as medical centers, hospitals, rehabilitation hospitals, sub-acute and long-term care facilities, assisted-living facilities, hospices (inpatient, home, or residential), or related office/outpatient clinics.

Health Care Policymakers, Legislators, and Payers

State and Congressional legislators, the state executive branch of government, two key federal agencies, the Centers for Medicare and Medicaid and the Centers for Disease Control and Prevention, insurers, philanthropists, as well as the business community, including employers and caregiver advocacy organizations.

Source: Sherman et al. (2011)

care, acknowledges its value, promotes access to quality palliative and hospice care, and takes action to implement a standard of practice in palliative and hospice care. Goals, objectives, and strategies related to palliative and hospice care (see Table 2) have been identified for each of the stakeholder groups in relation to the 4 A's, which serve as cornerstones of the blueprint for success for palliative and hospice care for patients and families experiencing cancer in the state of Maryland.

As described in Maryland's Action Plan, patients, families, and communities must become educated about palliative and hospice care, and advanced care planning. This will lead to conversations with health care providers, hospital administrators, policymakers, and insurers, which might not have occurred otherwise. Their knowledge and resulting expectations related to palliative and hospice care will drive the creation of health care environments where physical symptoms and emotional and spiritual needs are acknowledged and

Table 2 Goals, Objectives, and Strategies

A more detailed version of the Goals/Objectives/Strategies can found on the Palliative and Hospice Care page of the Maryland Cancer Plan web site: www.marylandcancerplan.org.

Goal: Implement a blueprint for success for palliative and hospice care for patients and families experiencing cancer in the state of Maryland.

Objective 1 (Awareness): By 2015, develop an awareness campaign to educate Maryland citizens about palliative and hospice care within 50% of Maryland jurisdictions.

Strategies (by stakeholder group):

1. *Patients/Families/Communities* should seek information on palliative and hospice care and advanced care planning from their health care providers, public library, national and local cancer agencies, and local health department.
2. *Health Care Professionals and Associated Staff* should increase communication related to palliative care issues in patients' conversations, health care publications, and media/marketing.
3. *Institutions* should initiate palliative care activities with the goal of obtaining buy-in from various constituencies.
4. *Health Care Legislators/Policymakers/Payers* should conduct an internal education effort on strategies to reduce barriers that Maryland residents face in regard to quality palliative and hospice care. The education effort should include widespread distribution, discussion, and the development of an action plan based on:
   - The 2009 Workgroup Report on "Hospice Care, Palliative Care and End of Life Counseling," released by the Maryland Attorney General's Counsel for Health Decisions Policy workgroup, and
   - Reports of the Maryland State Advisory Council on Quality of Care at the End of Life.

(continued)

Objective 2 (Acknowledging the Value): By 2015, increase the participation in and support of palliative and hospice care initiatives by stakeholders as outlined in the strategies.

Strategies (by stakeholder group):

1. *Patients/Families/Communities* should participate in campaigns that support/promote palliative and hospice care and advanced care planning.

2. *Health Care Professionals and Associated Staff* should actively participate in palliative education and palliative care initiatives as demonstrated by attendance at national conferences, increase in certification and credentialing rates, and referral to palliative care services and hospice care.

3. *Institutions* should develop a strategic plan that incorporates goals and related tactics to institutionalize palliative care as it relates to ongoing professional education, implementing and maintaining supportive services for patient/families, supporting research and evidence-based practice, and driving health care policy and legislative initiatives that promote palliative care.

4. *Health Care Legislators/Policymakers/Payers* should conduct outreach efforts via email, town halls, and focus groups to educate constituents about the knowledge, financial, and administrative barriers Maryland cancer patients and their families face in regard to palliative and hospice care and get their input on options to reduce them.

Objective 3 (Access): By 2015, increase access to palliative and hospice care services in Maryland.

Strategies (by stakeholder group):

1. *Patients/Families/Communities* should request access to palliative and hospice services.

2. *Health Care Professionals and Associated Staff* should develop and implement educational programs (formal and informal) related to palliative and hospice care.

3. *Institutions* should:
   - Develop a mechanism to track the percentage of palliative care consultations for hospital patients admitted with cancer, and
   - Ensure clinical support through hiring a skilled and credentialed/certified team of interdisciplinary palliative care professionals and associated support staff in order to implement a palliative care consult service or other delivery models (such as an inpatient unit, outpatient clinic, home care program, and/or establishing partnerships with community hospices).

4. *Health Care Legislators/Policymakers/Payers* should explore legislative options for expanding access to and payment for palliative and hospice care, building on best practices.

Objective 4 (Action): By 2015, stakeholders will take ownership of the Blueprint for Success and act on 70% of the strategies recommended for each stakeholder group.

Strategies (by stakeholder group):

1. *Patients/Families/Communities* should advocate for effective and compassionate palliative care across health care settings to insure that the goals of care are achieved.

2. *Health Care Professionals and Associated Staff* should incorporate the National Quality Forum Preferred Practices of Palliative Care as a standard of care within the institution.

3. *Institutions* should initiate quality improvement studies to evaluate the provision of quality palliative care by tracking:
   - Requests for palliative care consults.
   - Patient/family and community outcomes.
   - Health care professional outcomes.
   - Economic outcomes.

4. *Health Care Legislators/Policymakers/Payers* should support pilot programs that test:
   - The feasibility and impact of training lay workers to serve as palliative and hospice care counseling coaches and navigators.
   - Reimbursement models for providing end-of-life care counseling.
   - The impact of innovative clinical-financial models of palliative and hospice care for cancer patients and their families designed to reduce knowledge, financial, and administrative barriers to their use.

Source: Sherman et al. (2011)

addressed in a holistic manner throughout the illness trajectory. Increased awareness, improved communication, and the expectation to be involved in decisions regarding health care will ensure a better quality of life regardless of the quantity of life.

Health care professionals and associated personnel are being educated to staff the rapid national increase in palliative care programs. Through medical, nursing, and social work training programs; graduate programs in nursing; the integration of palliative care into nursing and medical school curricula; and interprofessional fellowship programs in palliative care, educational initiatives are well underway across the country. Such education reinforces the importance of interprofessional collaboration and teamwork. By developing palliative care and hospice competencies, health professionals develop the science and art of palliative care, educate and mentor those entering the profession and other colleagues, and inform patients and families about the value of palliative and hospice care, thus increasing referrals and promoting access to quality care (Sherman et al., 2011).

At the institutional level, administrators also are important stakeholders as they recognize national priorities and initiatives related to palliative care and acknowledge its value to quality patient care. It is critical administrators incorporate palliative care goals and tactics into the institution's strategic plan, and budget substantial resources for educational outreach to insure appropriate utilization of palliative care. This conveys the message of the value of palliative and hospice care in terms of cost savings, cost avoidance, quality care, and patient and family satisfaction. Furthermore, administrators utilize philanthropic and other contributions, which can add to a revenue base for hiring a skilled and credentialed team of interdisciplinary professionals. As in the State of Maryland, each state's attorney general's office should expect health care facilities to develop systems to utilize health professionals currently trained in palliative and hospice care. They will staff services and promote the coordination of care across health care settings, while monitoring the frequency and quality of care provided by practitioners (Sherman et al., 2011).

Maryland's Action Plan recognizes health care legislators, policymakers, and payers need to be aware of the barriers to access to quality palliative care and develop a Bill of Rights related to palliative and hospice care. These critical stakeholders can facilitate changes in health policy, quality standards, and reimbursement incentives to provide for ongoing education and training in palliative care and insure excellence in care across the illness trajectory. Change can also be affected as state governments promote the development of Centers of Excellence in palliative care, which in turn support community provider hospitals, as well as 24/7 urgent care centers and clinics which are challenged in providing continuity of care. By developing and instituting initiatives which support quality improvement studies, data can be tracked regarding the number of palliative care consults, patient and family outcomes, health care professional outcomes, and financial and economic outcomes.

In addition, policy solutions can fund career development awards in palliative care and increase the number of dollars spent on educating health professionals, as well as addressing the more complex issues of payment reform and reimbursement for palliative care services. Further consideration should also be given to the legislative agenda to address relevant health care reform initiatives such as the comparative effectiveness of palliative care and hospice with traditional hospital care, bundled payments, and funding of demonstration projects that test the integration of comprehensive palliative care in the care of patients with complex medical needs. Health care policymakers should be encouraged to implement programs that will improve the quality of care while slowing the growth of total health care spending in the nation: it is this platform that defines palliative care and its goals (Sherman et al., 2011).

Conclusion

In thinking about the metaphor of "a perfect storm" with all of the issues of quality care, affordability of care and economic constraints both nationally and internationally, the emergence of palliative care as a specialty in the United States is a means of "tackling a perfect storm" (NPCRC, 2011, p. 11). Over the last 10 years, there has been growing recognition of the importance of concurrent palliative care regardless of prognosis and of whether the goal of care is cure, life prolongation, or solely comfort (Meier & Brawley, 2011). "Palliative care ensures that the person is viewed in his or her entirety, not as a collection of organs and medical problems" (NPCRC, 2011, p. 12). Not only does palliative care reduce costs and improve quality of care, it reduces high levels of suffering and distress among patients with serious illness at any age and at any stage of disease; improves communication; addresses the needs of family caregivers; reduces unwanted, unnecessary, and painful interventions; improves patient, family, and staff's satisfaction; and improves survival (NPCRC, 2011).

Palliative care is an economic imperative in reducing the cost of health care. But, even more importantly, palliative care is a humanistic imperative to insure quality of life is promoted during all phases of the illness experience for both patients and their family caregivers. "The interface of energies and visions between patients, families, communities, healthcare professionals, institutions, healthcare policymakers, legislators, and payers is critical to create much-needed reform as well as the crafting of policies that will promote the well being of patients, families, and communities facing serious, life-threatening illness. It is this interface that provides not only an informed perspective but can achieve a 'meeting of the minds' to insure high-quality care and continuous care" (Sherman et el., 2011, p. 7). Palliative care, as a relatively new paradigm of care, responds to the demand for health care reform in America.

References

American Hospital Association. (2008). *The economic crisis: Impact on hospitals.* Retrieved from http://www.aha.org/content/00-10/08-fullsurveyresults.pdf

Brumley, R., Enguidanos, S., Jamison, P., Seitz, R., Morgenstern, N., Saito, S., . . . Gonzalez, J. (2007). Increased satisfaction with care and lower costs: Results of a randomized trial of in-home palliative care. *Journal of the American Geriatrics Society, 55*(7), 993–1000.

Casarett, D.J. (2011). Rethinking hospice eligibility criteria. *JAMA, 305*(10), 1031–1032.

Centeno, C., Clark, D., Lynch, T., Racafort, J., Praill, D., De Lima, L., . . . EAPC Task Force. (2007). Facts and indicators on palliative care development in 52 countries of the WHO European region: Results of an EAPC task force. *Palliative Medicine, 21*(6), 463–471.

Center to Advance Palliative Care. (2011). *Building a hospital-based palliative care program.* Retrieved from http://www.capc.org/building-a-hospital-based-palliative-care-program

Congressional Budget Office (2005). *High-cost Medicare beneficiaries.* Retrieved from http://www.cbo.gov/ftpdocs/63xx/doc6332/05-03-MediSpending.pdf

Covinsky, K.E., Goldman, L., Cook, E.F., Oye, R., Desbiens, N., Reding, D., . . . Phillips, R.S. (1994). The impact of serious illness on patients' families. SUPPORT investigators' study to understand prognoses and preferences for outcomes and risks of treatment. *JAMA, 272*(23), 1839–1844.

Dumont, I., Dumont, S., & Mongeau, S. (2008). End-of-life care and the grieving process: Family caregivers who have experienced the loss of a terminal-phase cancer patient. *Qualitative Health Research, 18*(8), 1049–1061.

Family Caregiver Alliance (2006). *Caregiving.* Retrieved from http://www.caregiver.org/caregiver

Federal Interagency Forum on Aging Related Statistics (2008). *Older Americans 2008: Key indicators of well-being.* Retrieved from http://www.aoa.gov/agingstatsdotnet/Main_Site/Data/2008_Documents/OA_2008.pdf

Fisher, E.S., Wennberg, D.E., Stukel, T.A., & Gottlieb, D.J. (2004). Variations in the longitudinal efficiency of academic medical centers. *Health Affairs (Project Hope) (Suppl. Variation),* VAR19–32.

Fisher, E.S., Wennberg, D.E., Stukel, T.A., Gottlieb, D.J., Lucas, F.L., & Pinder, E.L. (2003). The implications of regional variations in Medicare spending. Part 2: Health outcomes and satisfaction with care. *Annals of Internal Medicine, 138*(4), 288–298.

Foster, R.S. (2009). *Estimated financial effects of the "Patient Protection and Affordable Care Act of 2009," as Proposed by the Senate Majority Leader on November 18, 2009.* Retrieved from https://www.cms.gov/ActuarialStudies/Downloads/SPPACA_2009-12-10.pdf

Giese-Davis, J., Collie, K., Rancourt, K.M., Neri, E., Kraemer, H.C., & Spiegel, D. (2011). Decrease in depression symptoms is associated with longer survival in patients with metastatic breast cancer: A secondary analysis. *Journal of Clinical Oncology, 29*(4), 413–420.

Gomes, B., Harding, R., Foley, K.M., & Higginson, I.J. (2009). Optimal approaches to the health economics of palliative care: Report of an international think tank. *Journal of Pain and Symptom Management, 38*(1), 4–10.

Gordon, R., Eagar, K., Currow, D., & Green, J. (2009). Current funding and financing issues in the Australian hospice and palliative care sector. *Journal of Pain and Symptom Management, 38*(1), 68–74.

Grant, M., Elk, R., Ferrell, B., Morrison, R.S., & von Gunten, C.F. (2009). Current status of palliative care—clinical implementation, education, and research. *CA, 59*(5), 327–335.

Higginson, I.J., & Foley, K.M. (2009). Palliative care: No longer a luxury but a necessity? *Journal of Pain and Symptom Management, 38*(1), 1–3.

Huskamp, H.A., Stevenson, D.G., Chernew, M.E., & Newhouse, J.P. (2010). A new Medicare end-of-life benefit for nursing home residents. *Health Affairs (Project Hope), 29*(1), 130–135.

Jennings, B., Ryndes, T., D'Onofrio, C., & Baily, M.A. (2003). Access to hospice care: Expanding boundaries, overcoming barriers. *The Hastings Center Report, (Suppl.),* S3–7, S9–13, S15–21.

Kaiser Family Foundation (2011). *Medicaid's long-term care beneficiaries: An analysis of spending patterns across institutional and community-based settings.* Retrieved from http://www.kff.org/medicaid/upload/7576-02.pdf

Keehan, S.P., Sisko, A.M., Truffer, C.J., Poisal, J.A., Cuckler, G.A., Madison, A.J., . . . Smith, S.D. (2011). National health spending projections through 2020: Economic recovery and reform drive faster spending growth. *Health Affairs (Project Hope), 30*(8), 1594–1605.

Lynch, T., Clark, D., Centeno, C., Rocafort, J., Flores, L.A., Greenwood, A., . . . Wright, M. (2009). Barriers to the development of palliative care in the countries of central and eastern Europe and the commonwealth of independent states. *Journal of Pain and Symptom Management, 37*(3), 305–315.

McGuire, D.B., DeLoney, V.G., Yeager, K.A., Owen, D.C., Peterson, D.E., Lin, L., & Webster, J. (2000). Maintaining study validity in a changing clinical environment. *Nursing Research, 49*(4), 231–235.

Medicare Payment Advisory Commission. (2009). *Report to Congress: Medicare payment policy.* Retrieved from http://www.medpac.gov/documents/Mar09_March%20report%20testimony_WM%20FINAL.pdf

Meier, D.E. (2010). The development, status and future of palliative care. In D.E. Meier, S.L. Isaacs, R. Hughes (Eds.), *Palliative care: Transforming the care of serious illness.* San Francisco, CA: Jossey-Bass. Retrieved from http://www.rwjf.org/files/research/4558.pdf.

Meier, D.E., & Beresford, L. (2006). Advanced practice nurses in palliative care: A pivotal role and perspective. *Journal of Palliative Medicine, 9*(3), 624–627.

Meier, D.E., & Beresford, L. (2009). Palliative care seeks its home in national health care reform. *Journal of Palliative Medicine, 12*(7), 593–597.

Meier, D.E., & Brawley, O.W. (2011). Palliative care and the quality of life. *Journal of Clinical Oncology, 29*(20), 2750–2752.

Meier, D.E., Lim, B., & Carlson, M.D. (2010). Raising the standard: Palliative care in nursing homes. *Health Affairs (Project Hope), 29*(1), 136–140.

Mitchell, A.J., Chan, M., Bhatti, H., Halton, M., Grassi, L., Johansen, C., & Meader, N. (2011). Prevalence of depression, anxiety, and adjustment disorder in oncological, haematological, and palliative-care settings: A meta-analysis of 94 interview-based studies. *The Lancet Oncology, 12*(2), 160–174.

Mitchell, S.L., Teno, J.M., Kiely, D.K., Shaffer, M.L., Jones, R.N., Prigerson, H.G., . . . Hamel, M.B. (2009). The clinical course of advanced dementia. *The New England Journal of Medicine, 361*(16), 1529–1538.

Mitka, M. (2006). Less may be more when managing patients with severe chronic illness. *JAMA, 296*(2), 159–160.

Morrison, R.S., Dietrich, J., Ladwig, S., Quill, T., Sacco, J., Tangeman, J., & Meier, D.E. (2011). Palliative care consultation teams cut hospital costs for Medicaid beneficiaries. Health Affairs (Project Hope), 30(3), 454–463.

Morrison, R.S., Flanagan, S., Fischberg, D., Cintron, A., & Siu, A.L. (2009). A novel interdisciplinary analgesic program reduces pain and improves function in older adults after orthopedic surgery. *Journal of the American Geriatrics Society, 57*(1), 1–10.

Morrison, R.S., Magaziner, J., Gilbert, M., Koval, K.J., McLaughlin, M.A., Orosz, G., . . . Siu, A.L. (2003). Relationship between pain and opioid analgesics on the development of delirium following hip fracture. *The Journals of Gerontology. Series A, Biological Sciences and Medical Sciences, 58*(1), 76–81.

Morrison, R.S., Penrod, J.D., Cassel, J.B., Caust-Ellenbogen, M., Litke, A., Spragens, L., . . . Palliative Care Leadership Centers' Outcomes Group. (2008). Cost savings associated with US hospital palliative care consultation programs. *Archives of Internal Medicine, 168*(16), 1783–1790.

National Consensus Project for Quality Palliative Care (NCP). (2009). *Clinical practice guidelines for quality palliative care* (2nd ed.). Pittsburgh, PA: National Consensus Project for Quality Palliative Care. Retrieved from http://www.nationalconsensusproject.org/guideline.pdf

National Palliative Care Research Center (NPCRC). (2011). *America's care of serious illness: A state-by-state report card on access to palliative care in our nation's hospitals.* Retrieved from http://reportcard-live.capc.stackop.com/pdf/state-by-state-report-card.pdf

Office of the Legislative Counsel. (2010). *Compilation of Patient Protection and Affordable Care Act of 2010, S 3140, 111th Congress, 2nd Session.* Retrieved from http://docs.house. gov/energycommerce/ppacacon.pdf

Pelosi, N. (2010). *Letter to the Honorable Nancy Pelosi providing estimates of the spending and revenue effects of the reconciliation proposal.* Washington, DC: Congressional Budget Office. Retrieved from http://www.cbo.gov/ftpdocs/113xx/doc11379/AmendReconProp.pdf

Penrod, J.D., Deb, P., Dellenbaugh, C., Burgess, J.F., Jr, Zhu, C.W., Christiansen, C.L., . . . Morrison, R.S. (2010). Hospital-based palliative care consultation: Effects on hospital cost. *Journal of Palliative Medicine, 13*(8), 973–979.

Penrod, J.D., Deb, P., Luhrs, C., Dellenbaugh, C., Zhu, C.W., Hochman, T., . . . Morrison, R.S. (2006). Cost and utilization outcomes of patients receiving hospital-based palliative care consultation. *Journal of Palliative Medicine, 9*(4), 855–860.

Rabow, M.W., Hauser, J.M., & Adams, J. (2004). Supporting family caregivers at the end of life: "They don't know what they don't know." *JAMA, 291*(4), 483–491.

Satin, J.R., Linden, W., & Phillips, M.J. (2009). Depression as a predictor of disease progression and mortality in cancer patients: A meta-analysis. *Cancer, 115*(22), 5349–5361.

Seymour, J. (2011). Changing times: Preparing to meet palliative needs in the 21st century. *British Journal of Community Nursing, 16*(1), 18.

Seymour, J.E., Kennedy, S., Arthur, A., Pollock, P., Cox, K., Kumar, A., & Stanton, W. (2009). *Public attitudes to death, dying and bereavement: A systematic synthesis.* Retrieved from http://tinyurl.com/35g6lsc

Sherman, D.W., Evans, S., Halstead, L., Kelleher, C., Kenworthy, C., Olson, L., & Piet, L. (2011). In *Maryland comprehensive cancer control plan: Palliative and hospice care* (pp. 1–10). Retrieved from http://fha.maryland.gov/cancer/cancerplan

Smith, T.J., Coyne, P., Cassel, B., Penberthy, L., Hopson, A., & Hager, M.A. (2003). A high-volume specialist palliative care unit and team may reduce in-hospital end-of-life care costs. *Journal of Palliative Medicine, 6*(5), 699–705.

Spiegel, D. (2011). Mind matters in cancer survival. *JAMA, 305*(5), 502–503.

Temel, J.S., Greer, J.A., Muzikansky, A., Gallagher, E.R., Admane, S., Jackson, V.A., . . . Lynch, T.J. (2010). Early palliative care for patients with metastatic non-small-cell lung cancer. *The New England Journal of Medicine, 363*(8), 733–742.

Teno, J.M., Clarridge, B.R., Casey, V., Welch, L.C., Wetle, T., Shield, R., & Mor, V. (2004). Family perspectives on end-of-life care at the last place of care. *JAMA, 291*(1), 88–93.

van den Beuken-van Everdingen, M.H., de Rijke, J.M., Kessels, A.G., Schouten, H.C., van Kleef, M., & Patijn, J. (2009). Quality of life and non-pain symptoms in patients with cancer. *Journal of Pain and Symptom Management, 38*(2), 216–233.

Vanderwerker, L.C., Laff, R.E., Kadan-Lottick, N.S., McColl, S., & Prigerson, H.G. (2005). Psychiatric disorders and mental health service use among caregivers of advanced cancer patients. *Journal of Clinical Oncology, 23*(28), 6899–6907.

Wright, A.A., Zhang, B., Ray, A., Mack, J.W., Trice, E., Balboni, T., . . . Prigerson, H.G. (2008). Associations between end-of-life discussions, patient mental health, medical care near death, and caregiver bereavement adjustment. *JAMA, 300*(14), 1665–1673.

Wright, M., Wood, J., Lynch, T., & Clark, D. (2008). Mapping levels of palliative care development: A global view. *Journal of Pain and Symptom Management, 35*(5), 469–485.

Zarit, S. (2006). Assessment of family caregivers: A research perspective. In *Family Caregiver Alliance (Eds.), Caregiver assessment: Voices and views from the field.* Report from a National Consensus Development Conference (Vol. II) (pp. 12–37). San Francisco, CA: Family Caregiver Alliance.

Critical Thinking

1. In the face of long-term growth of older Americans, how will demand change in a decade, in a quarter-century?

2. Will the acceptance of palliative and hospice care as viable end-of-life treatment measures lead to new technologies?

Create Central

www.mhhe.com/createcentral

Internet References

Family Caregiver Alliance
www.caregiver.org/jsp/content_node.jsp?nodeid=368
Medicare Payment Policy: March 2013—Medicare Payment Advisory Commission
www.medpac.gov/documents/Mar13_entirereport.pdf

DEBORAH WITT SHERMAN, PhD, CRNP, ANP-BC, ACHPN, FAAN, is a Professor, University of Maryland, School of Nursing, Baltimore, MD. **JOOYOUNG CHEON, MS, RN,** is a Doctoral Student, University of Maryland, School of Nursing, Baltimore, MD.

Sherman, Deborah Witt and Cheon, Jooyoung. From *Nursing Economic$*, May/June 2012, pp. 153–162, 166. Copyright © 2012 by Jannetti Publications, Inc., East Holly Avenue/Box 56, Pitman, NJ 08071-0056; (856) 256-2300, FAX (856) 589-7463; for a sample copy of the journal, please contact the publisher. Used with permission. www.nursingeconomics.net

Article   Prepared by: Elaina F. Osterbur, *Saint Louis University*

Palliative Care: Impact on Quality and Cost

JESSICA D. SQUAZZO

Learning Outcomes

After reading this article, you will be able to:

- Discuss the definition of palliative care.

- Identify the role of family in the discussion of palliative care.

- Discuss the professional's role in the management of palliative care options for patients and families.

Palliative care is an emerging piece of the healthcare system that many predict will have a profound ability to improve quality of care, communication and coordination for seriously ill patients and their families and, through this process, reduce reliance on emergency departments and hospitals. Different in name and function than hospice and end-of-life care, palliative care is a unique, team-oriented approach to caring for the sickest of patients who are also, without doubt, the costliest.

Though not a new concept, it is perhaps one of the least understood service lines. It is, however, showing signs of growth, with the number of U.S. hospitals offering palliative care rising rapidly, according to the Center to Advance Palliative Care. Data from the Center and the American Hospital Association reveal that the number of programs in U.S. hospitals with 50 or more beds increased from 658 (24.5 percent) to 1,635 (66 percent) from 2000 to 2010—a 145.8 percent increase.

One person on the front lines of the emergence of palliative care programs in the U.S. healthcare system is Diane E. Meier, MD, FACP, director of the New York-based Center to Advance Palliative Care. "My mission is to improve access to palliative care across all settings," Meier told the audience at the ACHE program "Palliative Care: Impact on Quality and Cost." The program, funded in part by the Foundation of ACHE's Fund for Innovation in Healthcare Leadership, was held Sept. 11, 2012, in conjunction with ACHE's Atlanta Cluster Program.

During her keynote address, Meier, who is also vice chair of public policy and professor of geriatrics and palliative medicine and Catherine Gaisman Professor of Medical Ethics at Mount

Sinai School of Medicine in New York City, made the case for why palliative care is so important to healthcare today and how organizations can begin to develop such programs.

According to Meier, it isn't difficult to make the business case for establishing palliative care programs, especially at a time when, she said, the largest cause of bankruptcy in the U.S. is healthcare bills, and a very large portion of our population is underinsured.

"It is the costliest, very small proportion of patients that drive the vast majority of spending," she said. "Healthcare spending is highly concentrated on the sickest and most vulnerable 5 percent of patients. Palliative care models have been shown to improve quality of life for these patients and families, to prolong life in a number of studies and, as a result, to enable patients to avoid the preventable crises and emergencies that land them in the hospital. The costliest patients are palliative care patients. That's why palliative care is so critical to improving quality and reducing costs."

Defining Palliative Care

Meier said one key way to help organizations think about palliative care and distinguish it from other service lines is to remember that, "Palliative care is not what we do when there's nothing else to do." Palliative care is delivered *at the same time* as appropriate disease-related therapies, she said. "You don't move to hospice until disease-directed therapies are no longer working or their burdens begin to outweigh their benefits."

Palliative care differs from hospice or end-of-life care because the patients benefiting from palliative care programs aren't necessarily dying. Often they are patients who are very sick but have a good prognosis and are expected to live. Most people with serious and complex chronic illness in the United States are not dying, but living with significant burden of illness for many years. Meier said the fact that there are pediatric palliative care programs operating at some organizations highlights the importance of not linking palliative care to end-of-life care. In Meier's program at Mount Sinai, they are very accustomed to taking care of patients who are likely to be cured, such as bone marrow transplant patients, she said.

Meier shared the Center to Advance Palliative Care's definition of palliative care with the audience. The definition was crafted using language that was most highly rated among the public, according to a public opinion survey conducted by the Center, so as to use language that is meaningful and important to patients and families:

"Palliative care is specialized medical care for people with serious illnesses. This type of care is focused on providing patients with relief from the symptoms, pain and stress of a serious illness—whatever the diagnosis. The goal is to improve quality of life for both the patient and the family. Palliative care is provided by a team of doctors, nurses and other specialists who work with a patient's other doctors to provide an extra layer of support. Palliative care is appropriate at any age and at any stage in a serious illness, and can be provided together with curative treatment."

As described in the above definition, palliative care is delivered by a care "team." The team consists of key players such as physicians, nurses and advance practice nurses, social workers, chaplains or spiritual advisors, pain management specialists and others. The emphasis is on treating the patient's medical condition but also helping him or her through the difficult practical challenges and emotional and spiritual distress that accompany a serious illness.

Patients' family members and other loved ones also play a key part in palliative care. In a successful palliative care program, they are part of the conversation at the moment treatment begins. Palliative care programs also provide the proper counseling and support, including bereavement programs, if necessary, to patients' loved ones.

Meier said the impact of serious illness on patients' family members—including increased mortality and morbidity and post-traumatic stress disorder—cannot be ignored. "The cost to society from this is incalculable . . . [resulting in] people who can't function as mothers, who can't go to work, who can't return to their role in society," she said. "That is a fault in the system we don't think about much."

Palliative care addresses three domains, said Meier. By addressing these domains, quality of care is improved and because patients feel better and remain in control, costs are reduced:

- Physical, emotional and spiritual distress
- Patient-family-professional communication about achievable goals for care and the decision making that follows
- Coordinated, communicated continuity of care and support for practical needs of both patients and families across settings

Evidence showcasing these and other benefits of palliative care programs is mounting, with hundreds of studies showing how palliative care can improve care quality, Meier said. A Harvard Medical School/Massachusetts General Hospital study published by the *New England Journal of Medicine* in 2010 found that in a randomized trial of patients receiving standard cancer care with palliative care co-management from the time of diagnosis versus a control group receiving standard cancer care

only, the group receiving palliative care co-management experienced improved quality of life, reduced major depression, reduced "aggressiveness" in treatment (e.g., less chemotherapy before death, less likely to be hospitalized during the last month of care, etc.), *and improved survival rates* (11.6 months versus 8.9 months). Other studies have pointed to cost savings including reductions in use of costly imaging and pharmaceuticals and reductions in ED visits and time spent in the ICU.

Making Palliative Care Work

Meier provided attendees with an overview of what it takes in a healthcare organization to make palliative care succeed. At the top of the list is medical staff engagement. "If you don't have respectful and strong relationships with front-line medical staff working with the patients and families, it won't work," Meier said. "A social worker alone can't do it. Palliative care teams without a doctor are not going to work well." Meier says having medical staff on the palliative care team provides added credibility to the information presented to patients and their families.

Other strategies for convincing physicians and others in the organization to get on board with palliative care include identifying opinion leaders in the organization and getting their interest and investment to help you sell the idea to others; interviewing others in the organization about what problems/issues they perceive and how they feel they should be addressed (this aids in relationship building); gathering quality data; focusing on quality; and, finally, seeking senior leadership's support for a universal, systemwide palliative care screening checklist. "Palliative care should be part of the admission process," said Meier. "They should be screening for unmanaged illness just as they screen for pressure ulcer or fall risk."

Palliative care is sure to gain more ground in the future, as it is already on the radar of several national healthcare groups such as the National Quality Forum, which has listed it as one of six of its National Priorities for action; The Joint Commission, which in September 2011 released its Palliative Care Advanced Certification Program; MedPAC; and the Institute for Healthcare Improvement.

"Palliative care is key to survival under a capitated, global budget," said Meier. "When fee-for-service goes away and you're not managing the sickest 5 percent in the best way possible, they will bankrupt your budget."

After her keynote address, Meier introduced the program's three panelists, who each discussed their organization's experiences with palliative care.

Advance Care Planning

Bernard "Bud" Hammes, PhD, director, medical humanities, and director, Respecting Choices, at Gunderson Lutheran Health System in La Crosse, Wis., discussed advance care planning (ACP) as a complement to palliative care. He said the health system, which serves approximately 560,000 people in 19 counties in western Wisconsin, has invested heavily in the quality of the planning process—the process of knowing and honoring a patient's informed plans.

Hammes outlined the three key desired outcomes of advance care planning:

- Creating an effective plan, including selecting a well-prepared healthcare agent or proxy when possible and creating specific instructions that reflect informed decisions geared toward a person's state of health
- Having advance care plans available to the treating physician
- Incorporating the plans into medical decisions when and wherever needed

"Planning isn't enough," said Hammes. "We have to make sure these plans are available to the treating physicians, and they incorporate them correctly into decisions."

Hammes discussed the relationship of ACP to advance directives. According to Hammes, the successful implementation of an advance directive is directly tied to the quality of the planning process or advance care planning. "If the process of planning has a poor quality to it, the plan will not work," said Hammes. "Quality of communication with the patient and the family predicts the quality of the outcome."

There are four key elements in designing an effective ACP program, according to Hammes. They are:

1. **Systems design**—build an infrastructure that assists in hardwiring excellence, including effective, standardized documentation, reliable medical records storage and retrieval, and an ACP team and referral mechanism. According to Hammes, advance care planning must be made routine among staff members and a part of the care process. "It has to be hardwired into how we relate to our patients," he said. "No matter where patients are being treated, the written care plan must be available to the treating physicians."

2. **Advance care plan facilitation skills training**—build confidence among staff and create an effective ACP team. Hammes said Gunderson Lutheran Health has experienced success with teams featuring "facilitators" who on behalf of doctors talk with patients about their values and goals in order to develop their care plans. Facilitators help take some of the burden off already-busy physicians.

    Once the team is in place, staff training and use of a standardized curriculum are paramount. This ensures delivery of a consistent, reliable ACP service, according to Hammes.

3. **Community education and engagement**—reach out to communities with consistent messages about advance care planning. Because care in the La Crosse region involves two integrated health systems, all ACP-related materials distributed throughout the community have the names of both systems on them so patients know they can contact both systems related to their advance care plans, according to Hammes. This makes it possible to work effectively with all community groups and institutions.

4. **Continuous quality improvement**—measure and improve. Hammes noted the importance of continuously measuring your organization's ACP program—and constantly looking for ways to improve it.

"We didn't create a successful system because we were smart—we created a successful system because we were persistent," said Hammes. "We redesigned it and redesigned it until it worked."

Making the Case for Palliative Care

Stacie T. Pinderhughes, MD, director of palliative medicine at Banner Good Samaritan Medical Center in Phoenix, told the audience about her experience with setting up a palliative care program at the system, which comprises 23 acute-care hospitals, when she began her job at the organization in 2010. She shared several important lessons learned.

One key lesson was to know your organization s culture before you jump in. For Pinderhughes, she was fortunate to be at a hospital where "the doctors were very receptive and open to the whole concept of palliative care," she said.

That buy-in from physicians is critical to the success of a palliative care program, according to Pinderhughes. But there was some education of physicians that had to be done, especially among the specialty groups such as hospitalists, primary care doctors and the hospital's two large intensivist groups.

She recalled how it was helpful at Good Samaritan to have physicians round with the palliative care team to gain a better understanding of how a palliative care program works and see the variety of services it offers. According to Pinderhughes, it also helped clinicians understand that palliative care is different from hospice care. "We made a deliberate decision at Banner Health System to debrand palliative care from hospice," she said.

During year one of the palliative care program, the team consisted of Pinderhughes, a nurse practitioner and one social worker. Pinderhughes said bringing a social worker on board helped make connections in the community, an important aspect of palliative care.

Another key lesson Pinderhughes and her colleagues learned was the importance of getting C-suite buy-in. Showing senior leaders the cost benefit of a palliative care program is key.

"We found significant cost avoidance among these patients, which got the attention of the C-suite early," recalled Pinderhughes. In the first year of its program, Good Samaritan's palliative care team had seen approximately 500 patients. Since the program's start, Pinderhughes said, the total cost avoidance attributed to Good Samaritan's palliative care program is approximately $1.5 million.

At the end of the program's first year, a Palliative Care System Developmental Initiative was convened and charged with developing a stable platform for the delivery of palliative care across the healthcare continuum. This group called together stakeholders across the system, including providers, risk management staff and administrators. The group began the process of defining palliative care for the system and developed a business plan, a plan for educating others about the program and an IT infrastructure for documentation. The palliative care team also defined the program's mission and vision (and alignment with Banner Health's overall mission and vision) and defined its patient population.

Pinderhughes recalled how crucial it was to have the CFO's support with developing the business plan. Good Samaritan's CFO was involved from the beginning, even accompanying the palliative care team on walk rounds. "Now he is an effective ally in the C-suite," said Pinderhughes.

Pinderhughes said the team created tools to ensure palliative care at Good Samaritan was standardized. The team created an information card, which they distributed to physicians, residents, nurses, social workers and case managers. The organization's EHR now includes a Palliative Care Rounding Tool in which palliative care team members document information. Palliative care information is also captured on the Palliative Medicine H&P (history and physical) Template the team developed.

Banner Health is now looking at developing palliative care programs in several of its hospitals and plans to work with its ACO to develop palliative care further across other settings. "We've laid the infrastructure, now we're moving to the design phase," Pinderhughes said.

Buy-In from the C-Suite

When John M. Haupert, FACHE, became CEO of Grady Health System in Atlanta in 2011, one of his priorities was improving the way the system was managing the significant number of patients in need of hospice and palliative care. At least one-third of those patients were being improperly placed in the ICU.

As a safety net provider for Atlanta and one of the nation's largest public hospitals with 625 acute-care beds, Grady's payor mix is 30-30-20-20 (charity, Medicaid, Medicare, commercial). "To make this work economically takes a lot of work," Haupert told the audience.

The development of Grady's palliative care program is one major solution developed to help more efficiently and economically manage the most vulnerable among Grady's patient population. Haupert and his staff established a vision statement for palliative care at the system, which "has become our calling card for everything we do, every action we take and every action we put our energy behind," he said. The vision is: "The program assists patients and their families by providing relief from the symptoms, pain, and stress of a serious illness with the goal of improving their quality of life. The program affirms life and recognizes death as a normal process; helps people live as actively as possible and, in the event of terminal illness, neither postpones nor hastens death but helps them experience the end of their life with dignity and comfort."

Haupert said the vision is inclusive and looks at the full continuum of palliative and hospice services. "We wanted to avoid a model consisting of just life-prolonging care," Haupert said. An ideal model, he said, is a palliative care team working *with* hospice care staff and supportive services including after-care support.

The palliative care program at Grady is constantly evolving and improving as the organization learns what works best to serve its patient population. The focus is always on doing what's best for patients and their families in difficult times. "We have a lot of work to do to treat people with the dignity they deserve," Haupert said.

Grady's palliative care program has been developed in three levels. The organization is currently working to get from level two to level three, and Haupert says they have identified the following factors that must be in place to make that happen:

- **Enhanced leadership**—including identifying clinical leaders
- **Established operational infrastructure**—including implementation of a palliative care service scorecard and deployment of resources to meet demand for services
- **Enhanced system integration**—including clinical partnerships with other service lines such as oncology and internal medicine

Haupert knows firsthand the importance of having C-suite buy-in for a palliative care initiative. "With my commitment, we will get there and make this happen," he said.

Attendee Tammie Quest, MD, associate professor of emergency medicine and director, Emory Center for Palliative Care, which has a close working relationship with Grady Health, emphasized Haupert's sentiment. It makes a difference in the success of a palliative care program when you work with senior leaders who are "incredibly motivated and enthusiastic," she said.

"When you don't have that from the C-suite, it's really hard to take these programs to the next level."

Critical Thinking

1. What are the considerations that need to be discussed between professionals and patients in order to ensure that patients are making informed decisions?

2. What is the role of advance directives in the palliative care treatment option?

Create Central

www.mhhe.com/createcentral

Internet References

National Hospice and Palliative Care Organization
   www.nhpco.org
Open Society Foundations: Health: Palliative Care
   www.opensocietyfoundations.org/topics/palliative-care

JESSICA D. SQUAZZO is senior writer with *Healthcare Executive*.

Squazzo, Jessica D. From *Healthcare Executive Magazine*, January/February 2013, pp. 27–28, 30, 32, 34, 36, 38. Copyright © 2013 by American College of Healthcare Executives—ACHE. Used with permission.

Unit 7

UNIT

Prepared by: Elaina Osterbur, *Saint Louis University*

Living Environment in Later Life

Old age is often a period of shrinking life space. This concept is crucial to an understanding of the living environments of older Americans. When older people retire, they may find that they travel less frequently and over shorter distances because they no longer work. As the retirement years roll by, older people may feel less in control of their environment due to a decline in their hearing and vision as well as other health problems. As the aging process continues, elderly people are likely to restrict their mobility to the areas where they feel most secure. This usually means that an increasing amount of time is spent at home. Estimates show that individuals aged 65 and above spend 80 to 90 percent of their lives in their home environments. The house, neighborhood, and community environments are, therefore, more crucial to elderly individuals than to any other adult age group. The interaction with others that they experience within their homes and neighborhoods can either be stimulating or foreboding, pleasant or threatening. Across the country, older Americans live in a variety of circumstances, ranging from desirable to undesirable.

According to the Administration on Aging, *A Profile of Older Americans, 2012,* 57 percent of older adults (noninstitutionalized)) live with their spouses, and 28 percent of older adults live alone. Some older adults live with their grown children, and a relatively small number of older adults live in institutional settings such as nursing homes. With the growing number of older adults, the readings included in this section illustrate the wide range of stereotypical attitudes toward older Americans. With longer life expectancy and more years in retirement, older adults are demanding a variety of retirement living options that allow for greater quality of life.

The articles in this unit focus on technologies, aging-in-place options, and alternative housing models.

Article

Prepared by: Elaina Osterbur, *Saint Louis University*

Creating Communities That Support Healthy Aging

Nancy LeaMond

Learning Outcomes

After reading this article, you will be able to:

- Identify key components of the adaptations necessary to create a community that supports healthy aging.

- Explain why communities need to consider an aging population.

The dramatic aging of our population will be one of America's greatest challenges of the 21st century. For some of us *Policy & Practice* readers, the aging of America already is part of our everyday world of thought and planning, and has been for some time. For others, it may have, so far, played only an incidental, or peripheral, role in your daily responsibilities.

But—please believe me—the aging of our population is a phenomenon that will profoundly affect all sectors of our society. Everyone who is privileged to be in a position to make a difference will be tasked with an important role in dealing with it. And when historians years from now look back at our time and at what we did, one of their primary points of measurement will be how we met this great challenge.

A key component of meeting the challenge will be our nation's communities successfully adapting to accommodate their aging residents by making changes in infrastructure and services that will benefit all age groups. If community leaders have a range of information, tools, successful strategies, and best practices available to assist them at the outset, the task will be easier and less costly. AARP is committed to being a primary go-to resource. Here are some key points everyone needs to know.

Point 1: There is no escape! The aging of America is happening everywhere

By 2030, just 17 years from now, when the last of the baby boomers turns 65, the 65 and older population will have doubled from what it is today—to more than 70 million. Today, the nation's "oldest" city is Scottsdale, Arizona, where one of every five residents is 65 or older. In 2030, one of every five residents of the entire United States will be 65 or older.

All 50 states will see a rapid acceleration in the growth of their 65 and older populations. By 2030, 10 states will actually have more 65 and older residents than school-age children. That's never happened before in our nation's history—in even one state. Utah is projected to be our "youngest" state in 2030, yet their 65 and older population will still have nearly doubled.

Point 2: Too many of our communities are just not prepared for their aging populations

A report several years ago by the International City/County Management Association documented that less than half of our country's jurisdictions were prepared for the aging of their residents. Clearly, there have been pockets of encouraging innovation and experimentation. The approach to date in too many communities and states has been one of "let's wait and see." We just can't afford any longer to play the "wait and see" game.

Point 3: Forget about the old myths concerning aging in America

Supporting "wait and see" has been a pervasive string of myths. Let's start with the myth that suggests the cherished dream of most Americans nearing retirement is to pack up and retire in Florida, or Arizona, or some other place with palm trees. The fact is, this may be true for some, but not for the vast majority.

Since 1990, roughly 90 percent of older Americans have stayed in the same county they've lived in during their working years—most in the very same home. And we expect this to continue. AARP's research on the topic has found repeatedly that more than eight of every 10 boomers want to remain in their current home or community during retirement. The number one reason is the desire to stay close to their families.

Another myth suggests that preparing a community to retain older residents will make it less attractive to younger residents. Not true! I can't stress this enough: This isn't an "old versus young" issue. Livable communities benefit residents of *all* ages and we must consider *all* ages at every stage in the planning process.

Residents of all ages benefit from safer, barrier-free buildings and streets; as well as from better access to local businesses and more green spaces. A curb-cut designed for a wheelchair user also benefits a parent pushing a baby stroller. A crosswalk safe for a senior is a crosswalk safe for a child. A community that is friendly for an 80 year old can be friendly for an 8 year old—and everyone else in between.

Then, there's the myth that creating livable communities will cost too much and will never yield a decent return on the investment. Cost too much? Well, certainly there is cost, but creating livable communities doesn't mean tearing down our communities and starting over. It means, primarily, adapting and building upon existing programs, services, and infrastructure to make them accessible and safe for residents with varying needs and capacities.

How about the cost of not making our communities livable? The cost to our communities and our families—and to our nation—of not having age-friendly housing, streets and sidewalks is enormous—well into the tens of billions of dollars.

Here's a prime example. The biggest cause of hospitalization for Americans 65 and older today isn't cancer, or heart-related episodes. It is falls. Each year, one of every three Americans 65 and older falls, and a third of those require medical treatment. The Centers for Disease Control and Prevention project that annual direct treatment costs from older Americans falling will escalate from just under $20 billion today to nearly $44 billion by 2020. That's more than the current annual budget of the federal Department of Homeland Security.

Point 4: People want solutions, and creativity is the key to finding them

We can't just look to the federal government for solutions anymore. It will require working across unique coalitions involving nonprofits, state and local governments, foundations, businesses, and engaged citizens. Finding the best ways to create successful communities for all ages will require input from just about everyone. Some solutions will emerge naturally. Others will be developed through plans of action, driven by robust research and focused commitment.

Finding the best ways to create successful communities for all ages will require input from just about everyone. Some solutions will emerge naturally. Others will be developed through plans of action, driven by robust research and focused commitment.

Communities and state and local public service administrators need to be thinking of livable communities in terms of the enormous potential for more efficient and less costly delivery of health and other human services. This will require those responsible for transportation planning, human services, and care coordination to work across department and agency lines to solve the challenges related to ensuring that seniors get access to the care they need.

Here are a couple of already successful models for building on existing community structures.

Programs in *"Naturally Occurring Retirement Communities,"* known as NORCs, are now being developed across the nation. NORCs are geographic areas or building developments that feature multigenerational populations, but which already include a significant number of residents that are 60 and older.

Eldercare agencies are creating community-based interventions that build on these "natural" concentrations of elders called NORC-Supportive Service Programs. They connect elders to a variety of health care and home care services that allow them to remain healthy and independent. By serving relatively large numbers of elders in small areas, this model benefits from economies of scale in the organization and delivery of services, and creates related cost savings. We know of more than 100 of these programs moving forward nationwide.

Preserving existing affordable housing near accessible transit is essential, especially for lower-income older adults who desire to age in their homes. Mixed-use neighborhoods with safer, denser, walkable streets engender more physical activity. Public transit users are more likely than nontransit users to meet federally recommended physical activity goals by walking. Nationally, 29 percent of those who use transit are physically active for 30 minutes or more each day, solely by walking to and from public transit stops.

AARP is playing a proactive role, as well through the work of our state offices located in the 53 states and territories. We're excited about the AARP Network of Age-Friendly Communities we launched last year in affiliation with the World Health Organization's *Age-Friendly Cities and Communities Program.* To be selected for the network, a city or community must commit to undertake a 3-year process of continually assessing and improving its age-friendliness, and involve its older residents in a meaningful way. The AARP Age-Friendly Communities Network launched with eight pilot programs in the District of Columbia, and in Georgia, Iowa, Kansas, Michigan, New York, Oregon, and Pennsylvania.

Another example is the AARP HomeFit workshops that have been held by AARP State Offices. The workshop teaches people about inexpensive modifications they can make to their homes so they can stay in their own homes and communities and remain independent as long as possible.

And, with all of the innovation underway in the states to reform their Medicaid long-term care system, human service administrators should use this opportunity to shift resources away from costly institutional nursing home care to less expensive more desirable quality home-and community-based services and supports.

Communities and state and local administrators should also recognize the contribution of caregivers who provide an estimated $450 billion dollars a year in uncompensated support to family members that allows them to remain in their homes. Caregivers can be supported by increasing access to information; connecting them to community-based respite services, and protecting them from losing their jobs because of time spent caring for loved ones.

The late author, Peter Drucker, used to say, "The best way to predict the future is to create it."

I believe strongly that we have an obligation to work together, to identify and share solutions, and to celebrate the opportunities and challenges of Americans living longer and healthier lives, and communities opening their arms to all generations.

I encourage *Policy & Practice* readers to visit our new AARP Livable Communities: Great Places for All Ages web site (*www.aarp.org/livable*). This new site is a go-to resource for the latest information, best practices, research, policy analysis, advocacy resources, including model acts that address both complete streets and universal design, and funding sources that support livable communities. It is the first time that resources from a wide-range of sources have been compiled in one place and organized with the needs of local officials in mind.

Creating Livable Communities for all ages will be a key component in creating brighter and economically stronger futures for our nation's communities. The challenges are formidable, to be sure. But for those communities that succeed, the rewards will be much greater.

Critical Thinking

1. Do you think that aging myths will cloud the views of community leaders when making change to accomodate this population?
2. Discuss current programs, innovations, and accommodations that are being made by communities and agencies.

Internet References

AARP: Livable Communities
http://www.aarp.org/livable-communities
American Public Human Services Association
http://www.aphsa.org/content/APHSA/en/home.html

Article   Prepared by: Elaina F. Osterbur, *Saint Louis University*

Happy Together

Villages are helping people age in place.

SALLY ABRAHMS

Learning Outcomes

After reading this article, you will be able to:

- Describe the variety of niche communities that exist for older adults today.
- Identify the fastest-growing niche communities in the country at the present time.

For years, boomers have denied they are going to get old. Now, with knees that need scoping and birthday cakes with way too many candles, the defiant generation is finally thinking about the future—especially where and how to live.

Visits to their parents in sterile, regimented assisted living or nursing homes are leaving boomers dismayed. They want better choices for Mom—and for themselves. While they may be a decade or more away from needing care, they're overhauling or honing traditional models and inventing new ones.

In choosing how they want to age, and where, boomers are helping shape the future of housing. "They have changed expectations every decade they've gone through; I don't think it will stop now," says John McIlwain, senior fellow for housing at the Urban Land Institute. Down the road, he says, "there won't be one single trend. People will be doing a lot of different things." They already are. The common denominator in existing and still-to-be-created models, say experts, is the desire to be part of a community that shares common interests, values or resources. People want to live where neighbors know and care about one another and will help one another as they age. That doesn't mean they'll become primary caretakers; if it gets to that point, outside professionals may need to help.

They also won't necessarily retire from their jobs if they live in a "retirement" community. Today's housing options reflect the attitude of older Americans: Stay active, keep learning, develop relationships and have fun for as long as possible.

Niche Communities

The concept: Live with others who share similar lifestyles, backgrounds or interests. **The numbers:** Around 100 across the country. **The price:** Depends on community type.

Prices can range from $800 a month for a rental at an RV park or $1,700 at an artists' community, up to several hundred thousand dollars to buy a unit at a university community, with monthly addons of $2,000 or more that include some meals, housekeeping, social activities and medical care.

"With 78 million baby boomers, housing options are virtually unlimited," says Andrew Carle, founding director of the Program in Assisted Living/Senior Housing Administration at George Mason University in Virginia. In the next 20 years, he says, name an interest group and there'll be a community for it. "Will there be assisted living for vegetarians or a community for Grateful Dead fans? Residential cruise ships with long-term care? Absolutely."

Today's niche communities are already varied. They're geared to healthy adults but often have an assisted care component. They include places like Rainbow's End RV Park in Livingston, Texas, which offers assisted living, Alzheimer's day care, respite for caregivers and short-term care for the sick or frail. The Charter House in Rochester, Minn., provides a home for former Mayo Clinic staffers, among others. The Burbank Senior Arts Colony in Los Angeles attracts retired or aspiring artists, musicians, actors and writers. Aegis Gardens in Fremont, Calif., caters to older Asians.

The swanky Rainbow Vision in Santa Fe, N.M., is primarily—but not exclusively—for gay, lesbian, bisexual and transgender (GLBT) clients. While it has assisted living, there's also a cabaret, an award-winning restaurant and a topnotch spa. With 3 million GLBT older Americans—a figure projected to nearly double by 2030—and typically no adult children to care for them, such communities are expected to multiply.

Hands down, the fastest-growing niche community sector is university-based retirement communities (UBRCs). So far there are 50 or more on or near such college campuses as Dartmouth, Cornell, Penn State and Denison University. While residents are usually in their 70s, 80s and up—besides independent living, there is assisted living and nursing care—UBRCs will appeal to boomers, the most highly educated demographic, when they grow older, says Carle. Residents can take classes and attend athletic or cultural events at the nearby college campus, professors lecture at the UBRC, and young students can complete internships.

Five years ago, Harvey Culbert, 75, a former medical physicist from Chicago, and his wife moved to Kendal at Oberlin, which is affiliated with the Ohio college. He has audited, for free, a course in neuroscience, sings in a college group, and is taking voice lessons from a retired Kendal music teacher. "I'm always interested in improving what I do," he says.

Cohousing

The concept: A group, usually composed of strangers at the start, creates a communal-type housing arrangement that is intergenerational or all older people, with separate units but some shared common space. The group may buy the property, help design it, make all rules by consensus and manage it independently. Residents eat some dinners together and often form deep relationships. **The numbers:** 112 intergenerational cohousing communities, with another 40 to 50 planned; four elder cohousing projects, with 20 or so in the works. More than half are in California. **The price:** $100,000 to $750,000, monthly fees $100 to $300; 10 percent of projects offer rentals for $600 to $2,000 a month.

Intergenerational cohousing is geared to families with younger children but also draws boomer couples and singles. The youngest elder cohousing residents are in their 60s. Members live in separate, fully equipped attached or clustered units, and share outdoor space and a common house where communal meals take place. The common house also contains a living room and guest (or caretaker's) quarters. What's in the rest of the space depends on the members; it could be a media or crafts room, or a studio for exercise and meditation.

"I think cohousing is a marvelous way to live," says Bernice Turoff, an 85-year-old widow and member of the intergenerational Nevada City Co-housing community in California. "It's a close community where people really care about one another. If you get sick, 14 people say, 'How can I help you?' "

Charles Durrett, her neighbor and an architect who, along with his wife, Kathryn McCamant, brought the concept of cohousing to the United States from Denmark in the 1980s, says older members act as surrogate grandparents. Last year, when one of the older residents was dying, all ages pitched in to help or visit.

Today, older boomers live in both intergenerational and elder cohousing. "I'd be surprised if cohousing doesn't double every couple of years in the next 20 years," says Durrett. Getting popular: cohousing in cities.

Green House

The concept: A new style of nursing home created by gerontologist William Thomas that looks, feels and operates more like a cozy house than an institution. Ten or so residents live together and get ultra-individualized care from nursing staff that knows them well and cooks their meals in an open country-style kitchen. **The numbers:** 87 Green House projects serving 1,000 residents; 120 projects in development. **The price:** The same Medicaid and Medicare coverage offered to traditional nursing homes; the minority paying out of pocket are charged the going rate in the area for a more conventional nursing home.

Residents' private bedrooms and bathrooms surround a living and dining room that looks like it could be in a single-family home; a screened-in porch or a backyard offers outdoor access. As much as possible, residents make their own decisions, such as when they'll wake up.

Proponents point to studies showing a Green House can improve an older person's quality of life, provide at least comparable, if not better, care than a traditional nursing home, and reduce staff turnover. "The good news and the bad news is that you get to spend the rest of your life with 10 people," says Victor Regnier, a professor of architecture and gerontology at the University of Southern California.

Stanley Radzyminski, 90, might not be able to communicate with a few dementia residents in his Green House at Eddy Village Green in Cohoes, N.Y., but says, "I really like it here. I have my own room and privacy, and if I need help, the staff is outstanding. We all want to think we can take care of ourselves, but it's not always possible."

The Village Model

The concept: Live in your own home or apartment and receive discounted, vetted services and social engagement opportunities. **The numbers:** 56, with 17 in the Washington, D.C., area alone, and 120 in development around the country. **The price:** $100- to $1,000-a-year membership fee, with an average of $500 for a single member, $650 or so for a household.

Growing quickly in popularity, this model will become even more popular in the coming years, say housing experts. That's because studies show most older people want to age in place. The first village was established in 2002 at Beacon Hill Village in Boston; in the last four years alone, 90 percent of the villages have formed.

Village members call a central number for help of any kind. That might be transportation to the grocery store or the doctor, or the name of a plumber, acupuncturist, computer tutor, caregiving agency, home modifications specialist, babysitter for visiting grandkids, dog walker or home delivery company. Because the village may have up to 400 members (although new groups may have fewer than 100), vendors find it an attractive market. The group buys theater tickets in bulk, for example, or contracts with a service provider; consolidated services save everyone money.

Villages offer plenty of opportunities to socialize, whether it's taking yoga down the street with neighbors, attending outings to museums or movies, or participating in a book club, walking group or supper gathering.

Rita Kostiuk, national coordinator for the Village to Village Network, which helps communities establish and manage their own villages, has noticed something about the new people calling for information: "The majority are boomers."

On the horizon: Already, demographers are seeing more older Americans moving, or contemplating moving, into cities and suburban town centers. Rather than being saddled with a house requiring nonstop upkeep or feeling isolated in the burbs, they're within walking distance of shops, entertainment and public transportation. So their ability or desire to drive is not a big deal.

Another trend: divorced, widowed or never-married older women living together. Some who don't know one another are keeping such agencies as nonprofit Golden Girls Housing in Minneapolis busy. Golden Girls offers networking events for women who want to live together, lists requests for women looking, and steers them to services that can help. They don't match women, though; women do that themselves. Others opting for this setup are already friends.

David Levy, a gerontologist and lawyer by training, runs seven groups a week for caregivers. Inevitably, the conversation turns from the parents they care for to themselves. "These boomer women may be estranged from, or never had, kids, have diminished funds, and not a significant other on the horizon. They want to know, 'What's going to happen to me? Who will be there for me?'" he says.

It looks like they'll have choices.

Critical Thinking

1. What will the effect of the Green House concept be on nursing homes in the future?

2. What is the advantage that the villages offer to older people in terms of their preferred living choices?

3. What attracts older persons to moving to downtown cities and suburban town centers?

Create Central

www.mhhe.com/createcentral

Internet References

American Association of Homes and Services for the Aging
www.aahsa.org
Center for Demographic Studies
http://cds.duke.edu
Guide to Retirement Living
www.retirement-living.com
The United States Department of Housing and Urban Development
www.hud.gov

SALLY ABRAHMS writes about aging, boomer health, and workplace issues. She lives in Boston.

City Governments and Aging in Place: Community Design, Transportation, and Housing Innovation Adoption by Amanda J. Lehning

155

Article

Prepared by: Elaina F. Osterbur, *Saint Louis University*

City Governments and Aging in Place: Community Design, Transportation, and Housing Innovation Adoption

AMANDA J. LEHNING

Learning Outcomes

After reading this article, you will be able to:

- Cite the most effective strategy to get cities to adopt innovations that benefit older adults.

- Discuss what should be included in the successful advocacy to the local government for changes that would benefit older adults.

The physical environment of many cities in the United States presents barriers to elder health, well-being, and the ability to age in place. These include community design that separates residential and commercial areas (Handy, 2005), the absence of adequate alternative transportation services (Rosenbloom & Herbel, 2009), and limited accessible housing (Maisel, Smith, & Steinfeld, 2008). Recent studies (e.g., AARP Public Policy Institute, 2005) suggest an emerging consensus regarding the innovative policies and programs needed to address these physical barriers, including the following: (a) zoning and infrastructure changes that could allow older adults to remain connected to their community, (b) developing a range of transportation services and mobility options, and (c) creating a wide variety of housing supports and choices. City governments often provide services that may help older adults age in place, including senior centers, recreation programs, and social services. However, there are no previous studies that have explored city government adoption of policies that address the impact of the physical environment on older adults. Informed by an internal determinants and diffusion framework, there are two aims of this mixed-methods study. The first is to examine the characteristics associated with city government adoption of community design, housing, and transportation innovations that affect older adults. The second is to use qualitative interviews to explain the quantitative findings and provide additional findings around the process of adopting these innovations.

A growing interest in adapting the physical environment of communities to better meet the needs of older adults is a reaction to a confluence of factors, including the aging of the U.S. population, a projected increase in disability and chronic disease in future cohorts of older adults, and an inadequate long-term care system. Due to the aging of the Baby Boomer generation and increased longevity, by the middle of the 21st century, a projected 88.5 million Americans will be aged 65 and older (U.S. Census Bureau, 2009). Although the percentage of older adults with a disability decreased in recent years (Crimmins, 2004), the 85 and older population, whose members experience a greater incidence of functional and cognitive impairment, is expected to triple over the next 40 years (U.S. Census Bureau, 2008). In addition, research indicates an increase in chronic illness among Baby Boomers compared with the previous cohort (Martin, Freedman, Schoeni, & Andreski, 2009), suggesting that improvements in morbidity and disability rates will reverse in the near future. The growing number of older adults who require assistance with functioning will rely on a U.S. long-term care system characterized by high costs (Komisar & Thompson, 2007), unmet need (Zarit, Shea, Berg, & Sundstrom, 1998), and poor quality (U.S. Government Accountability Office, 2005). Further, even as 93% of older adults want to remain in their own homes (Feldman, Oberlink, Simantov, & Gursen, 2004) and governments attempt to reduce long-term care costs and increase the supply of community-based services, public reimbursement continues to favor institutional care (Harrington, Ng, Kaye, & Newcomer, 2009).

Physical Environments and Elder Health and Well-being

Community Design

In recent decades, the percentage of older adults living outside of cities has steadily increased, and a majority of elders today are suburbanites (Frey, 1999). Thus, many older adults live in communities characterized by the separation of commercial and residential areas, creating a situation in which access is severely restricted for those who no longer operate their own vehicle. The distances between residential and commercial areas, combined with the absence of sidewalks in many suburban neighborhoods, discourages walking as a mode of transportation or physical activity.

Research suggests that zoning and infrastructure changes can positively affect the health and well-being of community residents. First, mixed-use and walkable neighborhoods can help individuals maintain or increase their life space (Beard, Blaney, Cerda, Frye, Lovasi, Ompad, Rundle, & Vlahov, 2009), thereby improving access to goods and services. Second, residents of neighborhoods with a variety of walking destinations score higher on measures of social capital (Leyden, 2003). Third, mixed-use and walkable neighborhoods are related to increased physical activity (Berke, Koepsell, Moudon, Hoskins, & Larson, 2007) and decreased limitations of instrumental activities of daily living (IADL; Freedman, Grafova, Schoeni, & Rogowski, 2008).

Transportation

The majority of older adults get around their communities in a car, with 75% as the driver and 18% as a passenger (Feldman et al., 2004). Impairments such as reduced cognitive functioning, however, hamper the ability of many older adults to drive safely (Lynott et al., 2009). Older nondrivers make 15% fewer trips for medical appointments and 65% fewer trips for religious, social, or community activities compared with their driving counterparts (U.S. Government Accountability Office, 2004). Policies and programs that help older adults continue to safely operate their own vehicle, such as improving the visibility of street signs and simplifying intersections, could positively affect elder health and well-being. Approximately 33% of older adults do not have public transportation in their communities (Rosenbloom & Herbel, 2009), and many that do experience inadequate service that is viewed as unsafe, unresponsive, and inconvenient (Adler & Rottunda, 2006). Complementary paratransit services mandated by the Americans with Disabilities Act of 1990 address the mobility needs of some elders (Koffman, Raphael, & Weiner, 2004), although eligibility criteria mean that approximately 40% of older adults with a disability do not qualify for these services (Rosenbloom, 2009). A recent study found that the negative impact of driving cessation on elder well-being can be avoided if transportation needs are met through other modes of travel (Cvitkovich & Wister, 2003), suggesting that alternative transportation services, such as senior vans, can benefit elders.

Housing

The cost of maintaining a home presents a significant barrier to aging in place, and in a recent survey more than 50% of older respondents reported spending more than 30% of their income on housing (Feldman et al., 2004). Further, the majority of housing in the United States includes design features that make it inaccessible to individuals with disabilities (Maisel et al., 2008). Federal laws such as the Fair Housing Amendments of 1988 mandate the inclusion of accessible features (i.e., wide entrances and interior doors, accessible light

switches) in new multifamily housing (Kochera, 2002), but do not address accessibility in single-family homes or small multifamily buildings (American Planning Association, 2006). In addition, regulatory barriers such as restrictions for converting a garage into a dwelling unit not only keep densities low but also limit the housing options of older adults (Rosenthal, 2009). For example, in many communities zoning ordinances prevent the development of accessory dwelling units (ADUs; Pollack, 1994), an attached or detached permanent structure located on the same lot as a single-family home that includes a private kitchen and bathroom. For older adults who need to downsize because of financial or physical functioning reasons (e.g., difficulty climbing stairs), ADUs serve as an alternative form of housing, whereas for older adults who can remain in their own home but require some financial or personal care support, adding their own ADU creates a rental unit or a living space for a caregiver (Pynoos, Nishita, Cicero, & Caraviello, 2008).

Changing the home environment is associated with improved outcomes for individuals with a disability (Wahl, Fange, Oswald, Gitlin, & Iwarsson, 2009). Incorporating accessibility features is associated with a lower risk of health problems (Liu & Lapane, 2009), slower decline in IADL independence (Gitlin, Corcoran, Winter, Boyce, & Hauck, 2001), and reduced health care expenses (Stearns et al., 2000).

Purpose of the Study

As described earlier, there is growing evidence that community design, transportation, and housing innovations can have a positive impact on elder health, well-being, and the ability to age in place. However, there is little evidence as to why city governments may institute these policies and programs. To begin to address this gap in the literature, this study examined city government adoption of 11 innovations by testing 3 hypotheses informed by an internal determinants and diffusion framework. In addition, this study used qualitative interviews to explain the quantitative findings and provide additional findings around the process of adopting these innovations.

A combined internal determinants and diffusion framework is often used to guide investigations into the process of adopting an innovation, defined as a program or policy that is new to the adopting unit (Berry & Berry, 1999; Walker, 1969). Diffusion models propose that governments adopt innovations because they are influenced by other governments; policymakers often must devise solutions to problems quickly within the context of limited resources and therefore look to others as they determine the appropriate policy response (Colvin, 2006). Internal determinants models propose that factors within a government jurisdiction, such as community characteristics, determine whether the government will adopt innovations (Berry & Berry). The author selected this framework because it has been applied to previous investigations of the adoption of policy agendas rather than only one specific policy (e.g., Walker), has been used in research on local government innovations (e.g., Shipan & Volden, 2005), and allows flexibility in terms of the specific internal characteristics influencing policy adoption.

This study tested three hypotheses informed by previous studies using an internal determinants and diffusion framework.

City Governments and Aging in Place: Community Design, Transportation, and Housing Innovation Adoption by Amanda J. Lehning

157

The first hypothesis, based on the ideas of Berry and Berry (1999), is three diffusion factors will be positively associated with the adoption of these innovations. First, because uncertainty regarding the potential impact of an innovation can be overcome by observing its effects in nearby jurisdictions, governments will adopt innovations that are perceived as being beneficial elsewhere. Second, governments want to gain a competitive advantage to, for example, attract high-income households to increase their tax base, and therefore adopt policies that have popular support in other jurisdictions. Third, governments are more likely to adopt innovations when citizens advocate for these changes.

The second hypothesis is five community characteristics will be positively associated with the adoption of these innovations. In previous studies, larger total population and higher socioeconomic status of the population have positively influenced innovation adoption (Shipan & Volden, 2005; Walker, 1969). In the United States, recognition of older adults as a distinct social group that deserves special consideration in matters of public policy dates back to the passage of the Social Security Act of 1935 (Elder & Cobb, 1984). Therefore, the percent of older adults living in the community could be associated with the adoption of these innovations. Further, many of these innovations are designed for those who have a physical disability, suggesting the inclusion of the percent of the adult population with a disability.

The third hypothesis is two government characteristics will be positively associated with innovation adoption. First, higher per capita government spending may be a proxy for fiscal health, and local governments that are in poor fiscal health may be more conservative than innovative, particularly in terms of innovations that require a commitment of financial resources (Wolman, 1986). Second, policy entrepreneurs, or those who work within government to promote and advocate for policy innovations (e.g., elected officials), may be particularly influential in terms of increasing awareness and consideration of innovations (Mintrom, 1997).

Methods

This study used a sequential explanatory mixed-methods design, which involves a larger quantitative study followed by a smaller qualitative study (Creswell & Plano Clark, 2007). As this is the first study to examine the factors that influence the adoption of these specific innovations, the use of both quantitative and qualitative methods provided a more in-depth understanding of this topic. Qualitative interviews also allowed the author to expand beyond the quantitative findings to collect information that would be difficult to capture using a more structured online survey, including the process of innovation adoption.

The University of California Berkeley Committee for the Protection of Human Subjects classified this study as exempt from Institutional Review Board approval.

Quantitative Phase
Sample and Data Collection Procedures
The sample for this study included all 101 cities located in the San Francisco Bay Area. City governments were selected because they have jurisdiction over the use of land, including aspects of community design, housing, and transportation (Feldstein, 2007). Primary data were collected via online surveys developed by the author. Following a small pilot of the survey, the author sent an invitation to participate via electronic mail to the director of city planning in each city. Survey data collection took place between March and August of 2009. A total of 62 of 101 (61.4%) city planners returned completed surveys, and these data were combined with secondary data from the 2000 U.S. Census and the California 2000 *Cities Annual Report*.

Measures
Table 1 describes the measures and distribution of the dependent and independent variables. For the dependent variables, the survey asked respondents if their city had adopted the 11

Table 1 Description of Measures and Sample (*N* = 62)

Variables	Description	Frequency (%)
Dependent variables		
Community design	0: Zero or one innovation adopted	22 (35.5)
• Incentives to encourage mixed-use neighborhoods	1: Both innovations adopted	40 (64.5)
• Changes in infrastructure to improve walkability		
Transportation (range: 0–5)	0	13 (21.0)
• Education programs for older drivers	1	18 (29.0)
• Assessment programs for older drivers	2	25 (40.3)
• Infrastructure changes to improve older driver safety	3	5 (8.1)
• Alternative transportation	4	1 (1.6)
• Slower-moving vehicle ordinance	5	0

(continued)

Table 1 Description of Measures and Sample ($N = 62$)

Variables	Description	Frequency (%)
Housing (range: 0–4)	0	0
• Accessory dwelling unit ordinance	1	15 (24.2)
• Developer incentives to guarantee housing units for seniors	2	19 (30.6)
• Incentives to make housing accessible	3	15 (24.2)
• Home modification assistance	4	13 (21.0)
Total number of innovations (range: 0–11)	0	0
	1	2 (3.2)
	2	4 (6.5)
	3	4 (6.5)
	4	5 (8.0)
	5	17 (27.4)
	6	12 (19.4)
	7	11 (17.7)
	8	5 (8.1)
	9	2 (3.2)
	10	0
	11	0
Independent variables		
Diffusion factors		
Benefits	0: No knowledge of benefits in other jurisdictions	7 (11.3)
	1: Knowledge of benefits in other jurisdictions	55 (88.7)
Advantage	0: Does not believe other cities gained an advantage by adopting innovations	15 (24.2)
	1: Does believe other cities gained an advantage by adopting innovations	47 (75.8)
Public advocacy	0: Has not experienced public advocacy from residents to adopt innovations	18 (29.0)
	1: Has experienced public advocacy from residents to adopt innovations	44 (71.0)
Community characteristics		
Size (range: 2,125–776,733)	0: Population size < 50,000	42 (67.7)
	1: Population size ≥ 50,000	20 (32.3)
Education (range: 48.2%–98.8%)	0: Percent of the population with a high school diploma ≤ 89	31 (50.0)
	1: Percent of the population with a high school diploma >89	31 (50.0)
Income (range: 37,184–200,001)	0: Household median income ≤ 67,352	31 (50.0)
	1: Household median income >67,352	31 (50.0)
65 + (range: 5.1%–45.1%)	0: Percent of the population aged 65 and older ≤ 11.1	31 (50.0)
	1: Percent of the population aged 65 and older >11.1	31 (50.0)
Disability (range: 8.5%–25.5%)	0: Percent of the adult population with a disability ≤ 15.2	31 (50.0)
	1: Percent of the adult population with a disability >15.2	31 (50.0)
Government characteristics		
Spending (range: 294–6,550)	0: City per capita government spending ≤ 1,013	31 (50.0)
	1: City per capita government spending >1,013	31 (50.0)
Policy entrepreneur	0: No individual within government has advocated for innovation adoption	28 (45.2)
	1: An individual within government has advocated for innovation adoption	34 (54.8)

community design, transportation, and housing innovations shown in the table. Due to the distribution of frequencies, the community design outcome was dichotomized to compare cities with both innovations to those with one or none. Transportation, housing, and total number of innovations were measured as count variables.

For the independent variables, the survey asked respondents whether they had knowledge of benefits of these innovations in other jurisdictions, believed other cities gained an advantage by adopting these innovations, experienced public advocacy to adopt these innovations, and if there was an individual within government advocating for adoption. Data on community characteristics were obtained from the 2000 U.S. Census (the most recent year that included all necessary data for cities in the sample), and the California 2000 *Cities Annual Report* provided information on per capita government spending. Population size was coded into categories of less than 50,000 versus 50,000 or more, a demarcation of small and large cities used by federal agencies (e.g., the Office of Management and Budget) and professional organizations (e.g., National League of Cities). Due to problems with functional form, the author transformed continuous variables for community characteristics into dichotomous variables using median splits.

Statistical Analysis

The author calculated four different regression equations to examine the association between internal determinants and diffusion factors and innovation adoption. Tolerance and variance inflation factor results indicated that multicollinearity is not a concern with independent variables. Logistic regression was used to estimate odds ratios for the dichotomous outcome variable of community design innovations. Poisson regression was used to analyze the other three outcome variables (i.e., transportation, housing, and total number of innovations) as these measured counts of the number of innovations adopted. As recommended by Cameron and Trivedi (2009), robust standard errors for the parameter estimates were obtained to adjust for minor underdispersion.

Qualitative Phase
Sample and Data Collection Procedures

After completing the survey, 28 city planners indicated their willingness to participate in a follow-up interview. Ten interview participants were selected using maximum variation sampling, which allows the researcher to explore phenomena using cases that vary by characteristics (Sandelowski, 2000). The author selected interview participants representative of community characteristics (e.g., high and low education, high and low income, high and low percent of the population 65 and older, high and low percent of the population with a disability) and a range in the total number of innovations adopted. The researcher conducted, recorded, and transcribed the interviews in November and December of 2009. Interviewees were asked about the decision process involved in adopting innovations, including how the idea developed and facilitators of and barriers to adoption.

Data Analysis

Following the recommendation of Miles and Huberman (1984), qualitative data analysis consisted of three concurrent activities: data reduction, data display, and conclusion drawing/verification. Analysis of interview data was informed by previous research but was also inductive in nature, with data reduction starting at the basic level of line-by-line coding (Padgett, 1998). Following the first review of all interview transcripts, the researcher developed initial codes, which were refined after multiple iterations through the data. During data display, the researcher created spreadsheets for each code that included direct quotes as well as data from the online surveys (i.e., community characteristics and specific innovations adopted by the local government of the interview participant). This visual display allowed the researcher to further refine codes, establish a set of themes expressed by multiple interview participants, and draw conclusions about the data. The researcher then verified conclusions by a final review of the interview transcripts, a procedure that has been used by other qualitative researchers to determine the validity of qualitative data analysis (Miles & Huberman).

Results
Quantitative

Table 2 presents the results of the regression of internal determinants and diffusion factors on innovation adoption. Model 1 presents the logistic regression for the adoption of community design innovations. Cities that experienced public advocacy or had a higher percent of the population with a disability had an increased odds of adopting both community design innovations. However, these results should be interpreted with caution as wide confidence intervals indicate problems with the precision of the model.

Model 2 presents the regression of the number of transportation innovations, and public advocacy was significantly associated with innovation adoption. As shown in Model 3, cities with a higher percent of the population aged 65 and older adopted fewer housing innovations and those with a higher percent of the population with a disability adopted more housing innovations. In Model 4, which presents the regression of the total number of innovations, the relationship between percent of the population with a disability and innovation adoption was also significant. In addition, higher per capita government spending was negatively associated with innovation adoption, whereas the existence of a policy entrepreneur was positively associated with innovation adoption.

Qualitative

Qualitative interviews uncovered potential explanations for the quantitative findings and also additional findings. Three concepts were identified through analysis of the qualitative interviews: advocacy and public resistance, disability and age, and city and resident economic resources.

Advocacy and Public Resistance

Advocacy by city residents was described as a facilitator of the adoption process. According to one city planner, "Every large

Table 2 Regression Results for the Adoption of Community Design, Transportation, and Housing Innovations (N = 62)

Internal determinants and diffusion variable	Model 1[a]: community design, OR (95% CI)	Model 2[b]: transportation, B (95% CI)	Model 3[b]: housing, B (95% CI)	Model 4[b]: total number of innovations, B (95% CI)
Diffusion factors				
Benefits	1.46 (0.29–7.40)	.09 (−.29 to .46)	.02 (−.19 to .23)	−.01 (−.34 to .33)
Advantage	2.26 (0.40–12.81)	−.03 (−.43 to .37)	−.07 (−.29 to .16)	.08 (−.16 to .31)
Public advocacy	4.28* (0.88–20.73)	.35** (.02 to .68)	.11 (−.13 to .35)	.17 (−.04 to .38)
Community characteristics				
Size	3.39 (0.55–20.70)	−.03 (−.41 to .34)	.12 (−.07 to .32)	.11 (−.06 to .27)
Education	1.34 (0.23–7.77)	−.02 (−.39 to .35)	−.10 (−.34 to .14)	−.06 (−.22 to .10)
Income	2.00 (0.17–22.81)	−.15 (−.62 to .33)	.17 (−.058 to .39)	.05 (−.10 to .20)
65+	0.70 (0.16–3.08)	.04 (−.33 to .42)	−.26** (−.51 to .02)	−.11 (−.26 to .03)
Disability	8.79* (0.69–112.14)	.19 (−.33 to .72)	.28** (.03 to .54)	.22** (.05 to .40)
Government characteristics				
Spending	0.28 (0.06–1.28)	−.15 (−.49 to .18)	−.08 (−.267 to .11)	−.12* (−.26 to .01)
Policy entrepreneur	0.85 (0.18–3.91)	.21 (−.12 to .53)	.07 (−.16 to .30)	.15* (−.02 to .32)

Note: OR = odds ratio; CI = confidence interval.
[a] Logistic regression.
[b] Poisson regression.
*$p < .10$. **$p < .05$.

project had its genesis with some sort of citizens' group that came to the city with a concept and got that to move forward." Another said, "We respond to things we're pushed to do." A third city government respondent reported that "Activists come to public meetings and they share info about their needs. It is clear what they want: they call me and they definitely call their council people."

Public resistance, often discussed as concerns about mixed-use neighborhoods and higher-density development, is perceived by city planners as a barrier to adopting these innovations. One city planner referred to "the traditional NIMBY [not in my backyard] people." Another interviewee noted "There are parts of town where people don't want more dense neighborhoods . . . People prefer single-family homeownership." Another planner recalled resistance to an accessible apartment building: "The concerns raised were about how it would affect parking in the neighborhood and wanting to make sure it would be well managed and well designed."

Disability and Age

Several interviewees mentioned advocacy by and on behalf of younger individuals with disabilities. One planner explained, "When we built more accessible housing, it wasn't seniors per se, but a disability group pushed the city. The basic idea was 'why are you spending all this money to keep people in institutions when you could keep people in their homes?'." Another interview participant noted the increased visibility of

individuals with disabilities in this region compared with other parts of the United States: "There are probably not more people here with disabilities, but they are more out in the community." A third interviewee said, "I think, anecdotally, this area is a magnet for people with disabilities because we have such great services."

City and Resident Economic Resources

Interviewees indicated that they viewed some of these innovations as a way to improve the fiscal health of their city. The following quote is from a city with relatively low spending that adopted a high number of innovations: "We see all these policies and provisions coming into place to make downtown more vital, more interesting, and more economically competitive. The thought process is getting more people into downtown." Similarly, another city planner explained that a recent push by a city to create more walkable mixed-use neighborhoods was motivated in part because "people want more lively places, more lively streets, and they want more of a 24-hr presence."

In terms of resident economic resources, some cities do not see any need for public supports for their more economically advantaged aging residents. For example, as one city planner explained: "This is an affluent community, so it doesn't require as much public assistance. I think the seniors do need household assistance and sometimes medical assistance . . . We are going to promote increased density near the commercial district, and also second units so you can have your nurse living nearby, but most of these services are private in this community." According to another, "there is a sense that we have addressed a good chunk of part of the need, and I mean by income levels. I tend to focus on below market housing, but there are other niches outside of my scope. There could be a need for empty nester housing but that is not part of our focus."

Discussion

This mixed-methods study is the first attempt to explore local government adoption of community design, transportation, and housing innovations that could improve elder health, well-being, and the ability to age in place. The quantitative phase tested three hypotheses informed by an internal determinants and diffusion framework using data collected via online surveys with city planners. The qualitative phase used data collected through telephone interviews designed to explain and supplement the quantitative results.

The first hypothesis proposed that three diffusion factors would be positively associated with the adoption of community design, transportation, and housing innovations that could benefit older adults: knowledge of benefits in other jurisdictions, a belief that cities gain an advantage from adopting innovations, and public advocacy. Only public advocacy was significant, and only for community design and transportation innovations. In qualitative interviews, a number of participants reported that resident advocacy influences policy decisions. However, interviews also suggest that public resistance can present a barrier to innovation adoption. Similar to a recent study examining barriers to the adoption of ADU ordinances (Liebig et al., 2006), public resistance came up in discussions about mixed-use and higher-density development, ranging from NIMBY sentiments to residential concerns about parking problems.

The second hypothesis proposed that five community characteristics would be positively associated with innovation adoption: population size, population education, household median income, percentage of the population aged 65 and older, and percent of the adult population with a disability. This hypothesis was partially supported as the percent of the population with a disability was associated with the adoption of community design, housing, and total number of innovations. The percent of the population aged 65 and older was not significant in three of the models and was negatively associated with the adoption of housing innovations. Interview participants mentioned disability advocates more often than older adults or groups representing their interests. Historically, due to their high voter turnout and the organizational power of groups such as AARP, older adults have successfully pushed policymakers at the federal level to adopt policies (e.g., Medicare) targeted to meet their needs (Elder & Cobb, 1984). At the local level, however, interviews suggest that public advocacy for changes to the physical environment comes from residents with disabilities rather than older adults. Previous research has found that advocacy can lead to the adoption of innovations that are particularly salient to residents, such as those around sex education and gambling (Mooney & Lee, 2000), but plays a smaller role in innovations more removed from people's everyday lives, such

as hazardous waste policies (Daley & Garand, 2005). Some of the innovations examined in this study (e.g., incentives to develop accessible housing) address difficulties associated with functional status rather than age. Disability groups may be more active because individuals who have a disability are more aware of the physical barriers in their communities than older adults who face the possibility of disability in the future. Alternatively, younger individuals with disabilities may be more effective advocates for the adoption of these innovations because the general response to disability varies across age populations. It has been suggested that for younger individuals, disability is more often viewed as a result of problems in the social and physical environment, whereas for older adults disability is more typically attributed to disease (Kane, Priester, & Neumann, 2007). City governments may therefore perceive these innovations as more appropriate for younger adults with disabilities.

The implication is that service providers and advocates should facilitate the involvement of older adults through education and community-building activities. This has proved a successful strategy by the Elder Friendly Communities Project in Calgary, Canada, which has successfully brought about changes, including infrastructure improvements, by training and supporting older adults to plan and carry out actions to change their community (Austin, Des Camp, Flux, McClelland, & Sieppert, 2005). In addition, aging service providers and advocates may also need education about the ways in which the physical environment can affect older adults. Councils on Aging, for example, could broaden their service and advocacy efforts to address community design, transportation, and housing.

Contrary to the second hypothesis and previous research (Berry & Berry, 1999; Shipan & Volden, 2005), there was no significant association with population education or income in any of the four regression models. As discussed in interviews, city government perceptions of the need for many of these innovations may depend on the residents' private economic resources, and city planners in wealthier communities may assume that older residents are wealthy and do not require public assistance. It is possible that older adults with higher education and incomes are less likely to require the public provision of environmental adaptations because of their reduced risk for physical limitations (Freedman & Martin, 1999), lower rates of impairments, and slower deterioration of physical functioning (Mirowsky & Ross, 2000). Higher levels of education have been linked with improved access to care, higher quality of care, and better health behaviors (Goldman & Smith, 2002), and these elders may be able to delay or avoid disability because they can obtain personal care, assistive devices, medical care, healthy foods, and exercise equipment (Schoeni, Freedman, & Martin, 2008). Cities whose residents have a lower socioeconomic status, and are therefore more vulnerable to disease and disability, may be more receptive to advocacy efforts to put these innovations in place.

For the third hypothesis, the positive significant association between the existence of a policy entrepreneur and the total number of innovations indicates that enlisting the support of individuals with a formal role in city government may be an effective strategy to innovation adoption. This is consistent with the proposition of Walker (1973) that "the presence of a single aide on a legislative staff who is enthusiastic about a new program, or the chance reading of an article by a political leader can cause [governments] to adopt new programs more rapidly" (p. 1190). Per capita government spending had an inverse relationship with the total number of innovations. Similar to previous studies (e.g., Boyne & Gould-Williams, 2005), this finding combined with qualitative data suggests that the need for economic revitalization could inspire innovation adoption because it creates a greater need for innovative solutions. For example, because city governments receive much of their revenue from sales taxes, property taxes, and user fees (Warner, 2010), incentives for mixed-use development and the construction of residential buildings that dedicate units for seniors could improve city finances. Another implication of this research is that advocates and residents pushing for these innovations should emphasize the potential economic benefits associated with some of these changes.

Findings from the current study should be interpreted in light of its limitations, and future research should examine whether the results are applicable to other cities. First, this study achieved fairly good response rates but may still have some nonresponse error. Second, future research should address the limitation of self-report data by, for example, soliciting participation from multiple employees in each city. Third, because the nonlinear relationship between the continuous variables and outcome variables indicated problems with functional form, the author used median splits, which in turn affects model precision and could lead to overestimation or underestimation of significant statistical relationships (Maxwell & Delaney, 1993). The small sample size also affects the validity of the quantitative results. For example, the logistic regression model for community design innovations may be overestimating the odds ratios (Nemes, Jonasson, Genell, & Steineck, 2009). Fifth, results may not be generalizable outside of the San Francisco Bay Area because of its unique characteristics, including higher population income and education and rapid population growth at the end of the 20th century (Kawabata & Shen, 2007). Furthermore, the region has a reputation for embracing innovative land use and transportation policies and is often the subject of case studies of these types of innovations (e.g., Bhatia, 2007; Kawabata & Shen).

Additionally, the use of cross-sectional data does not allow for an understanding of the diffusion of innovations over time (Berry & Berry, 1990). Future research should employ techniques such as event history analysis to ascertain which innovations have been in place for years and which have been only recently adopted, uncover if there are particularly influential cities affecting the diffusion process, and further clarify the factors associated with the adoption of these innovations. Other policy researchers (e.g., Downs & Mohr, 1976) have criticized an internal determinants and diffusion framework for the variation in results reported across studies. It is not unusual for factors that are positively associated with one type of policy innovation to be negatively associated, or not associated at all, with other innovations (Downs & Mohr). The researcher selected this framework in part because of its flexibility in the specific characteristics associated with policy adoption, and therefore it is not surprising

that results differed from previous research on, for example, local antismoking policies (see Shipan & Volden, 2005).

The findings and limitations of this study suggest the need for additional research into local government adoption of community design, transportation, and housing innovations that could benefit older adults. Future research should explore modifications to an internal determinants and diffusion framework as it relates to these policies and programs. For example, although per capita government spending has been used as a proxy measure for government resources in earlier research on local government policy adoption (e.g., Shipan & Volden, 2005), other measures (e.g., city revenues) could be used in future studies. Future studies should also explore whether younger individuals with disabilities are more active in advocating for these innovations than older adults. It is possible that this finding reflects the Bay Area, which, as mentioned by interview participants, has a history of supporting disability rights and the independent living movement. It is also possible that older adults are not as engaged in public policy at the local level, and therefore more research is needed to understand how to promote their community involvement. Third, although there is emerging evidence that these innovations can improve elder health, well-being, and ability to age in place, more research is needed to explore the impact of the environment on older adults. Establishing an empirical evidence base for aging in place will ensure that local governments devote their often scarce resources toward effective policies, programs, and infrastructure changes.

Conclusion

This mixed-methods study explored city-level adoption of community design, transportation, and housing innovations that have the potential to improve elder health, well-being, and the ability to age in community. Quantitative and qualitative results indicate that advocacy is an effective strategy to encourage city adoption of innovations that affect the mobility and quality of life of older adults. Successful advocacy efforts should facilitate the involvement of older residents, target key decision makers within government, emphasize potential financial benefits to the city, and focus on cities whose aging residents are particularly vulnerable to disease and disability.

References

AARP Public Policy Institute. (2005). Livable communities: An evaluation guide. Washington, DC: AARP. Retrieved July 8, 2009, from http://assets.aarp.org/rgcenter/il/d18311_communities.pdf

Adler, G., & Rottunda, S. (2006). Older adults' perspectives on driving cessation. *Journal of Aging Studies, 20,* 227–235. doi: 10.1016/j.jaging. 2005.09.003

American Planning Association. (2006). Policy guide on housing. Policy adopted by American Planning Association (APA) Board of Directors. Retrieved January 4, 2010, from http://www.planning.org/policy/guides/pdf/housing.pdf

Austin, C. D., Des Camp, E., Flux, D., McClelland, R. W., & Sieppert, J. (2005). Community development with older adults in their neighborhoods: The Elder Friendly Communities Program. *Families in Society, 86,* 401–409.

City Governments and Aging in Place: Community Design, Transportation, and Housing Innovation Adoption by Amanda J. Lehning

163

Beard, J. R., Cerda, M., Blaney, S., Ahern, J., Vlahov, D., & Galea, S. (2009). Neighborhood characteristics and change in depressive symptoms among older residents of New York City. *American Journal of Public Health, 99,* 1308–1314. doi:10.2105/AJPH.2007. 125104.

Berke, E. M., Koepsell, T. D., Moudon, A. V., Hoskins, R. E., & Larson, E. B. (2007). Association of the built environment with physical activity and obesity in older persons. *American Journal of Public Health, 97,* 486–492. doi: 10.2105/AJPH.2006.085837

Berry, F. S., & Berry, W. (1999). Innovation and diffusion models in policy research. In P. A. Sabatier (Ed.), *Theories of the policy process* (pp. 169–200). Boulder, CO: Westview Press.

Berry, F. S., & Berry, W. D. (1990). State lottery adoptions as policy innovations: An event history analysis. *The American Political Science Review, 84,* 395–415.

Bhatia, R. (2007). Protecting health using an environmental impact assessment: A case study of San Francisco land use decisionmaking. *American Journal of Public Health, 97,* 406–413. doi:l0.2105/AJPH.2005. 073817

Boyne, G. A., & Gould-Williams, J. S. (2005). Explaining the adoption of innovation: An empirical analysis of public management reform. *Environment and Planning* C: *Government and Policy, 23,* 419–435. doi:10.1068./c40m

Cameron, A. C, & Trivedi, P. K. (2009). *Microeconometrics using Stata.* College Station, TX: Stata Press.

Colvin, R. A. (2006). Innovation of state-level gay rights laws: The role of Fortune 500 corporations. *Business and Society Review, 111,* 363–386. doi:10.1111/j. 1467–8594.2006.00277.x

Creswell, J. W., & Piano Clark, V. L. (2007). Designing and conducting mixed methods research Thousand Oaks, CA: Sage Publications.

Crimmins, E. M. (2004). Trends in the health of the elderly. *Annual Review Public Health, 25,* 79–98. doi: 10.1146/annurev. publhealth. 25.102802.124401

Cvitkovich, Y., & Wister, A. (2003). Bringing in the life course: A modification to Lawton's ecological model of aging. *Hallym International Journal of Aging, 4,* 15–29.

Daley, D. M., & Garand, J. C. (2005). Horizontal diffusion, vertical diffusion, and internal pressure in state environmental policymaking, 1989–1998. *American Politics Research, 33,* 615–644. doi:l 177/1 532673X04273416

Downs, G.W., & Mohr, L.B. (1976). Conceptual issues in the study of innovation. *Administrative Science Quarterly, 21,* 700–714.

Elder, C. D., & Cobb, R. W. (1984). Agenda-building and the politics of aging. *Policy Studies Journal, 13,* 115–129.

Feldman, P. H., Oberlink, M. R., Simantov, E., & Gursen, M. D. (2004). A tale of two older Americas: Community opportunities and challenges. New York: Center for Home Care Policy and Research.

Feldstein, L.M. (2007). General Plans and Zoning: A Toolkit on Land Use and Health. Sacramento, CA: California Department of Health Services. Retrieved February 26, 2010, from http://www.phlpnet.org/ healthy-planning/products/general-plans-and-zoning

Freedman, V., & Martin, L. (1999). The role of education in explaining and forecasting trends in functional limitations among older Americans. *Demography, 36,* 461–173. doi: 10.2307/2648084

Freedman, V. A., Grafova, I. B., Schoeni, R. F., & Rogowski, J. (2008). Neighborhoods and disability in later life. *Social Science & Medicine, 66,* 2253–2267. doi:10.1016/j. socscimed.2008.01.013

Frey, W. H. (1999). Beyond social security: The local aspects of an aging America Washington, DC: The Brookings Institution.

Gitlin, L. N., Corcoran, M. A., Winter, L., Boyce, A., & Hauck, W. W. (2001). A randomized controlled trial of a home environmental intervention to enhance self-efficacy and reduce upset in family caregivers of persons with dementia. *The Gerontologist, 41,* 15–30. doi:10.1093/geront/41.1.4

Goldman, D., & Smith, J. P. (2002). Can patient self-management help explain the SES health gradient? *Proceedings of the National Academy of Sciences, 99,* 10929–10934. doi:10.1073/pnas.l62086599

Handy, S. (2005). Smart growth and the transportation-land use connection: What does the research tell us? *International Regional Science Review, 28,* 146–167. doi:10.1177/0160017604273626

Harrington, C., Ng, T., Kaye, S. H., & Newcomer, R. (2009). Home and community-based services: Public policies to improve access, costs and quality. San Francisco: UCSF Center for Personal Assistance Services.

Kane, R. L., Priester, R., & Neumann, D. (2007). Does disparity in the way disabled older adults are treated imply ageism? *The Gerontologist, 47,* 271–279. doi:10.1093/geront/47.3.271.

Kawabata, M., & Shen, Q. (2007). Commuting inequality between cars and public transit: The case of the San Francisco Bay Area, 1990–2000. *Urban Studies, 44,* 1759–1780.

Kochera, A. (2002). Accessibility and visitability features in single-family homes: A review of state and local activity. Washington, DC: AARP Public Policy Institute.

Koffman, D., Raphael, D., & Weiner, R. (2004). The impact of federal programs in transportation for older adults. Washington, DC: AARP Public Policy Institute.

Komisar, H. L., & Thompson, L. S. (2007). National spending for long-term care. Washington, DC: Georgetown University. Retrieved July 7, 2009, from http://ltc.georgetown.edu/pdfs/whopays2006.pdf

Leyden, K. M. (2003). Social capital and the built environment: The importance of walkable neighborhoods. *American Journal of Public Health, 93,* 1546–1551.

Liebig, P. S., Koenig, T., & Pynoos, J. (2006). Zoning, accessory dwelling units, and family caregiving: Issues, trends, and recommendations.

Liu, S. Y., & Lapane, K. L. (2009). Residential modifications and decline in physical function among community-dwelling older adults. *The Gerontologist, 49,* 344–354. doi:10.1093/geront/gnp033

Lynott, J., Haase, J., Nelson, K., Taylor, A., Twaddell, H., Ulmer, J., et al. (2009). Planning complete streets for an aging America. Washington, DC: AARP Public Policy Institute.

Maisel, J. L., Smith, E., & Steinfeld, E. (2008). Increasing home access: Designing for visitability. Washington, DC: AARP Public Policy Institute.

Martin, L. G., Freedman, V. A., Schoeni, R. F., & Andreski, P. M. (2009). Health and functioning among Baby Boomers approaching 60. *The journal of Gerontology, 64B,* 369–377. doi: 10.1093/geronb/gbn040

Maxwell, S. E., & Delaney, H. D. (1993). Bivariate median splits and spurious statistical significance. *Psychological Bulletin, 113,* 181–190. doi:10.1037/0033-2909.113.1.181

Miles, M. B., & Huberman, M. A. (1984). Qualitative data analysis: An expanded sourcebook. Thousand Oaks, CA: Sage.

Mintrom, M. (1997). Policy entrepreneurs and the diffusion of innovation. *American Journal of Political Science, 41,* 738–770.

Mirowsky, J., & Ross, C. (2000). Socioeconomic status and subjective life expectancy. *Social Psychology Quarterly, 63,* 133–151.

Mooney, C, & Lee, M. H. (2000). The influence of values on consensus and contentious morality policy: US death penalty reform, 1956–82. *The Journal of Politics, 62,* 223–239.

Nemes, S., Jonasson, J. M., Genell, A., &: Steineck, G. (2009). Bias in odds ratios by logistic regression modeling and sample size. *BMC Medical Research Methodology, 9,* 56–60. doi: 10.1186/1471-2288-9-56

Padgett, D. K. (1998). Qualitative methods in social work research: Challenges and rewards. Thousand Oaks, CA: Sage Publications.

Pollack, P. B. (1994). Rethinking zoning to accommodate the elderly in single family housing. *Journal of the American Planning Association, 60,* 521–531. doi:10.1080/01944369408975608

Pynoos, J., Nishita, C., Cicero, C., & Caraviello, R. (2008). Aging in place, housing, and the law. *University of Illinois Elder Law Journal, 16,* 77–107.

Rosenbloom, S. (2009). Meeting transportation needs in an aging-friendly community. *Generations, 33,* 33–43.

Rosenbloom, S., & Herbel, S. (2009). The safety and mobility patterns of older women: Do current patterns foretell the future? *Public Works Management & Policy, 13,* 338–353. doi:10.1177/1087724X09334496

Rosenthal, L. A. (2009). The role of local government: Land use controls and aging-friendliness. *Generations, 33,* 18–23.

Sandelowski, M. (2000). Whatever happened to qualitative description? *Research in Nursing & Health, 23,* 334–340.

Schoeni, R. F., Fteedman, V. A., & Martin, L. G. (2008). Why is late-life disability declining? *The Milbank Quarterly, 86,* 47–89. doi:10.1111/j.1468-0009.2007.00513.x

Shipan, C.R., & Volden, C. (2005). The diffusion of local antismoking policies. Retrieved August 12, 2011, from: http://psweb.sbs.ohio-state.edu/intranet/rap/volden.pdf.

Stearns, S. C., Bernard, S. L., Fasick, S. B., Schwartz, R., Konrad, R., Ory, M. G., et al. (2000). The economic implications of self-care: The effect of lifestyle, functional adaptations, and medical self-care among a national sample of Medicare beneficiaries. *American Journal of Public Health, 90,* 1608–1612.

U.S. Census Bureau. (2008). An older and more diverse nation by midcentury. Retrieved June 19, 2009, from http://www.census.gov/Press-Release/www/releases/archives/population/012496.html

U.S. Census Bureau. (2009). Facts for features: Older Americans month: 2009. Retrieved June 1, 2009, from http://www.census.gov/Press-Release/www/releases/archives/facts_for_features_special_editions/013384.html

U.S. Government Accountability Office. (2004). Transportation-disadvantaged seniors: Efforts to enhance senior mobility could benefit from additional guidance and information. Washington, DC: GAO.

U.S. Government Accountability Office. (2005). Nursing homes: Despite increased oversight, challenges remain in ensuring high-quality care and resident safety. Retrieved June 2, 2009, from http://www.gao.gov/new.items/d06117.pdf

Wahl, H., Fange, A., Oswald, F., Gitlin, L. N., & Iwarsson, S. (2009). The home environment and disability-related outcomes in aging individuals: What is the empirical evidence? *The Gerontologist, 49,* 355–367. doi: 10.1093/geront/gnp056

Walker, J. L. (1969). The diffusion of innovations among the American states. *The American Political Science Revieiv, 63,* 880–899.

Walker, J. L. (1973). Comment: Problems in research on the diffusion of policy innovations. *The American Political Science Review, 67,* 1186–1191.

Warner, M. E. (2010). The future of local government: Twenty-first century challenges. *Public Administration Review,* s1, s145–s147.

Wolman, H. (1986). Innovation in local government and fiscal austerity. *Journal of Public Policy, 6,* 159–180.

Zarit, S. H., Shea, D. G., Berg, S., & Sundstrom, G. (1998). Patterns of formal and informal long term care in the United States and Sweden. AARP Andrus Foundation Final Report. State College, PA: Pennsylvania State University.

Critical Thinking

1. What effect did the percent of the population aged 65 and older have on city governments' willingness to make beneficial community changes for older persons?

2. What effect did the percent of a community's population with disabilities have on city government's willingness to make beneficial changes for older persons?

3. The growing interest in adapting the physical environment of communities to better meet the needs of older adults is a reaction to what factors?

Create Central

www.mhhe.com/createcentral

Internet References

American Association of Homes and Services for the Aging
www.aahsa.org
Center for Demographic Studies
http://cds.duke.edu
Guide to Retirement Living
www.retirement-living.com
The United States Department of Housing and Urban Development
www.hud.gov

Acknowledgments—The author would like to thank Andrew Scharlach, Michael Austin, Fred Collignon, Ruth Dunkle, Letha Chadiha, and two anonymous reviewers for valuable feedback on earlier drafts of this article.

Funding—U.S. Department of Housing and Urban Development's Doctoral Dissertation Research Grant; Society for Social Work Research; Hartford Doctoral Fellows Program; National Institute on Aging (T32-AG000117).

From *The Gerontologist*, June 2012, pp. 345–356. Copyright © 2012 by Gerontological Society of America. Reprinted by permission of Oxford University Press via Rightslink.

Article   Prepared by: Elaina F. Osterbur, *Saint Louis University*

The Real Social Network

More than a neighborhood, a village gives older people a better chance to stay in their own home longer.

MARTHA THOMAS

Learning Outcomes

After reading this article, you will be able to:

- Discuss the various services people living in a village can receive from other village members or as part of their village services provided routinely and paid for by service fees.

- Explain how Keystone's health services are better able to coordinate the services for their village patients.

On a bitterly cold morning a few years ago, Eleanor McQueen awoke to what sounded like artillery fire: the ice-covered branches of trees cracking in the wind. A winter storm had knocked out the power in the rural New Hampshire home that Eleanor shared with her husband, Jim. "No heat, no water. Nada," Eleanor recalls.

The outage lasted for nine days; the couple, both 82 at the time, weathered the ordeal in isolation with the help of a camp stove. Their three grown kids were spread out in three different states, and the McQueens weren't very close to their immediate neighbors. "We needed someone to see if we were dead or alive," Eleanor says.

But the McQueens were alone, and it scared them. Maybe, they admitted, it was time to think about leaving their home of 40 years.

Luckily, last year the McQueens found a way to stay. They joined Monadnock at Home, a membership organization for older residents of several small towns near Mount Monadnock, New Hampshire. The group is part of the so-called village movement, which links neighbors together to help one another remain in the homes they love as they grow older.

The concept began in Boston's Beacon Hill neighborhood in 2001, when a group of residents founded a nonprofit called Beacon Hill Village to ease access to the services that often force older Americans to give up their homes and move to a retirement community. More than 56 villages now exist in the United States, with another 120 or so in development, according to the Village to Village (VtV) Network, a group launched in 2010 that provides assistance to new villages and tracks their growth nationwide.

It works like this: Members pay an annual fee (the average is about $600) in return for services such as transportation, yard work, and bookkeeping. The village itself usually has only one or two paid employees, and most do not provide services directly. Instead, the village serves as a liaison—some even use the word concierge. The help comes from other able-bodied village members, younger neighbors, or youth groups doing community service. Villages also provide lists of approved home-maintenance contractors, many of whom offer discounts to members. By relying on this mix of paid and volunteer help, members hope to cobble together a menu of assistance similar to what they would receive at a retirement community, but without uprooting their household.

The earliest villages, like Beacon Hill, were founded in relatively affluent urban areas, though new villages are now sprouting in suburbs and smaller rural communities, and organizers are adapting Beacon Hill's model to fit economically and ethnically diverse communities. Each is united by a common goal: a determination to age in place. A recent AARP survey found 86 percent of respondents 45 and older plan to stay in their current residence as long as possible. "And as people get older, that percentage increases," says Elinor Ginzler, AARP expert on livable communities.

In its own quiet way, the village movement represents a radical rejection of the postwar American ideal of aging, in which retirees discard homes and careers for lives of leisure amid people their own age. That's the life Eleanor and Jim McQueen turned their backs on when they joined Monadnock at Home.

"To dump 40 years of building a home to move into a condominium doesn't appeal to me at all," Jim says. "The idea of Monadnock at Home is, I won't have to."

You could call it the lightbulb moment—literally: A bulb burns out in that hard-to-reach spot at the top of the stairs, and that's when you realize you're dependent on others for the simplest of household chores. "It's horrible," says Candace Baldwin, codirector of the VtV Network. "I've heard so many stories

What a Village Takes

Want to organize a village of your own? The Village to Village (VtV) Network offers information on helping villages get started. Membership benefits include tools and resources developed by other villages, a peer-to-peer mentoring program, and monthly webinars and discussion forums.

- To find out if a village exists in your region, the VtV website has a searchable online map of all U.S. villages now open or in development.
- The creators of Boston's Beacon Hill Village have written a book on starting a village: *The Village Concept: A Founder's Manual* is a how-to guide that provides tips on fund-raising, marketing, and organizational strategies.
- Existing resources can make your neighborhood more "villagelike," says Candace Baldwin, codirector of the VtV Network. The best place to start is your local agency on aging. The U.S. Department of Health and Human Services offers a searchable index of these services.—M.T.

from people who say they can't get on a ladder and change a lightbulb, so they have to move to a nursing home. A lightbulb can be a disaster."

Especially when the homeowner won't ask for help. Joining a village can ease the resistance, says Christabel Cheung, director of the San Francisco Village. Many members are drawn by the opportunity to give aid as well as receive it. "A lot of people initially get involved because they're active and want to do something," she says. "Then they feel better about asking for help when they need it."

Last winter Blanche and Rudy Hirsch needed that help. The couple, 80 and 82, live in a three-story brick town house in Washington, D.C.; they pay $800 per year in dues to Capitol Hill Village (CHV). During the blizzard-filled February of 2010, Rudy was in the hospital for hip surgery and Blanche stayed with nearby friends as the snow piled up. On the day Rudy came home, Blanche recalls, the driver warned that if their walkways weren't clear "he'd turn around and go back to the hospital." She called CHV executive director Gail Kohn, who summoned the village's volunteer snow brigade. A pair of young architects who lived nearby were quickly dispatched with shovels.

The Hirsches have discussed moving; they've postponed the decision by installing lifts so Rudy can get up and down the stairs. Remembering her visits to a family member who lived in a retirement home, Blanche shudders: "Everyone was so old. It's depressing."

Avoiding "old-age ghettos," says Kohn, is a major draw for villagers. She touts the intergenerational quality of Capitol Hill, full of "people in their 20s and people in their 80s," and CHV organizes a handful of events geared toward people of different ages. One program brings high school freshmen and village members together in the neighborhood's public library, where the kids offer informal computer tutoring to the older folks.

Such social-network building is a natural outgrowth of village life. Indeed, Beacon Hill Village was founded on the idea of forging stronger bonds among members. "There was a program committee in existence before the village even opened its doors," says Stephen Roop, president of the Beacon Hill Village board. "Most of my friends on Beacon Hill I know through the village."

One fall evening in Chicago, Lincoln Park Village members gathered at a neighborhood church for a potluck supper. A group of about 80—village members and college students who volunteer as community service—nibbled sushi and sipped Malbec wine as they chatted with Robert Falls, artistic director of Chicago's Goodman Theatre.

Lincoln Park Village's executive director, Dianne Campbell, 61, doesn't have a background in social work or gerontology; her experience is in fund-raising for charter schools and museums, and she lives in Lincoln Park. To village member Warner Saunders, 76, that's a big plus. "She doesn't see us as elderly clients who need her help," says Saunders, a longtime news anchor for Chicago's NBC affiliate, WMAQ-TV. "I see Dianne as a friend. If she were a social worker, and I viewed my relationship with her as that of a patient, I would probably resent that."

For Saunders, Lincoln Park Village makes his quality of life a lot better. He recently had knee and hip surgeries, and his family—he lives with his wife and sister-in-law—relies on the village for transportation and help in finding contractors. "I'd call the village the best bargain in town," he says.

Others, however, might balk at annual dues that can approach $1,000 for services that might not be needed yet. To expand membership, many villages offer discounts for low-income households.

At 93, Elvina Moen is Lincoln Park Village's oldest, as well as its first "member-plus," or subsidized, resident. She lives in a one-room apartment in an 11-story Chicago Housing Authority building within Lincoln Park. The handful of member-plus residents pay annual dues of $100 and in return receive $200 in credit each year for discounted services from the village's list of vetted providers. Since joining, Moen has enlisted the village to help paint her apartment and install ceiling fans.

But beyond home improvements, Moen doesn't ask a lot from the village yet—she's already created her own village, of a sort. When she cracked her pelvis three years ago, members of her church brought her meals until she got back on her feet; she pays a neighbor to help clean her apartment. Her community-aided self-reliance proves that intergenerational ties and strong social networks help everyone, not just the privileged, age with dignity.

Social scientists call this social capital, and many argue that we don't have enough of it. What the village movement offers is a new way to engineer an old-fashioned kind of connection. "As recently as 100 years ago most everyone lived in a village setting," says Jay Walljasper, author of *All That We Share: A Field Guide to the Commons*, a book about how cooperative movements foster a more livable society. "If you take a few steps back and ask what a village is, you'll realize it's a place where you have face-to-face encounters." He compares the village movement to the local-food movement, which also started with affluent urbanites. Think of a village as a kind of "artisanal retirement," a modern reinterpretation of an older, more enlightened way of life. And just as there's nothing quite like homegrown tomatoes, "there's no replacement for the direct connection with people who live near you," Walljasper says.

Strong, intergenerational communities—just like healthy meals—are good for everyone. Bernice Hutchinson is director of Dupont Circle Village in Washington, D.C., which serves a diverse neighborhood. Many members are well-off; some are getting by on Medicaid. "But at the end of the day," says Hutchinson, "what everyone wants is connectedness."

Connectedness alone, of course, can't ensure healthy aging. What happens next—when villagers' needs grow beyond help with grocery shopping or the name of a reliable plumber?

To meet the growing health demands of members, villages boast a range of wellness services, and many have affiliations with health care institutions. Capitol Hill Village, for example, has a partnership with Washington Hospital Center's Medical House Call Program, which provides at-home primary care visits for elderly patients.

A new village—Pennsylvania's Crozer-Keystone Village—flips the grassroots Beacon Hill model: It's the first village to originate in a health care institution. Barbara Alexis Looby, who oversees the village, works for Keystone, which has five hospitals in the southeastern part of the state. A monthly fee gives members access to a "village navigator," who schedules medical appointments and day-to-day logistics like errands. Members also get discounts on Keystone's health services. Because the village and the hospital system are aligned, says Looby, "the boundaries are flexible. You care for people when they come to the hospital, and you are in a position to coordinate their care when they leave." Keystone hopes this integration will lead to fewer ER visits and hospital readmissions.

How long can a village keep you safe at home? It depends. But Candace Baldwin, of VtV, says that the trust factor between members and the village can help family members and caregivers make choices and find services.

Michal Brown lives about 30 miles outside Chicago, where her 89-year-old mother, Mary Haughey, has lived in a Lincoln Park apartment for more than 20 years. She worries about her mom, who has symptoms of dementia. Brown saw a flyer about Lincoln Park Village in a pharmacy and immediately signed her mother up. Through the village, Brown enrolled her mom in tai chi classes and asked a village member to accompany her as a buddy.

Just before Christmas, Haughey became dizzy at her tai chi class. With her buddy's help, she made it to the hospital, where doctors discovered a blood clot in her lung. Without the village, Brown is convinced, her mother might not have survived.

Through the village, Brown has also learned about counseling services at a local hospital to help plan her mother's next steps. "We can add services bit by bit, whether it's medication management or home health care. The village knows how to get those services."

Nobody knows what Mary Haughey's future holds, but the village has given her options. And it has given her daughter hope that she can delay moving her mother to a nursing home. For now, it helps knowing that her mother is safe, and still in her own apartment, in her own neighborhood.

Critical Thinking

1. In terms of services needed by older persons, what are the advantages of joining and living in a village neighborhood?

2. How does the village movement hope to provide residents a menu of assistance similar to what they would receive in a retirement community?

3. What is the common goal of each village community?

Create Central

www.mhhe.com/createcentral

Internet References

American Association of Homes and Services for the Aging
www.aahsa.org

Center for Demographic Studies
http://cds.duke.edu

Guide to Retirement Living
www.retirement-living.com

The United States Department of Housing and Urban Development
www.hud.gov

MARTHA THOMAS is a Baltimore-based freelance writer.

Article Prepared by: Elaina Osterbur, *Saint Louis University*

AARP Network of Age-Friendly Communities

As our population ages and people stay healthy and active longer, communities need to adapt.

AARP®

Learning Outcomes

After reading this article, you will be able to:

- Identify the elements necessary for an age-friendly community.
- Discuss the agreement between the World Health Organization and AARP.
- Explain the eight broad domains that WHO maintains.

The AARP Network of Age-Friendly Communities helps participating communities become great places by adopting such features as walkable streets, better housing and transportation options, access to key services and opportunities for residents to participate in community activities.

Well-designed, livable communities help sustain economic growth and make for happier, healthier residents—of all ages.

The AARP Network of Age-Friendly Communities is an affiliate of the World Health Organization's Global Network of Age-Friendly Cities and Communities, an international effort launched in 2006 to help cities prepare for their own and the world's growing population of older adults and the parallel trend of urbanization.

AARP's Role

AARP's participation in the age-friendly network advances the Association's efforts to help people live easily and comfortably in their homes and communities as they age. AARP encourages older adults to take an active role in their communities' plans and ensures that their voices are heard. Related initiatives focus on areas such as housing, caregiving, community engagement, volunteering, social inclusion and combating isolation among older people.

As a non-profit, non-partisan organization, AARP works with local officials and partner organizations around the United States to identify communities for membership in the AARP Network of Age-Friendly Communities. AARP facilitates the community's enrollment and guides it through the implementation and assessment process.

Within a year of the AARP program's April 2012 launch, 17 communities had enrolled. We've been steadily growing ever since. (To see the current member list visit **aarp.org/agefriendly**.)

Our goal: Increase the number of communities that support healthy aging, which will thereby improve the well-being, satisfaction and quality of life for older Americans.

The Eight Domains of Livability

The AARP Network of Age-Friendly Communities targets improvements in eight domains that influence the health and quality of life of older adults. The livability domains, and what they represent, are as follows:

1. **Outdoor Spaces and Buildings:** Availability of safe and accessible recreational facilities.
2. **Transportation:** Safe and affordable modes of private and public transportation.

3. **Housing:** Availability of home modification programs for aging in place as well as a range of age-friendly housing options.
4. **Social Participation:** Access to leisure and cultural activities, including opportunities for older residents to socialize and engage with their peers as well as with younger people.
5. **Respect and Social Inclusion:** Programs that promote ethnic and cultural diversity, as well as multigenerational interaction and dialogue.
6. **Civic Participation and Employment:** Paid work and volunteer activities for older residents and opportunities to engage in the formulation of policies relevant to their lives.
7. **Communication and Information:** Access to communications technology and other resources so older residents can connect with their community, friends and family.
8. **Community Support and Health Services:** Access to home-based care services, health clinics and programs that promote wellness and active aging.

Criteria & Process

Communities participating in the AARP Network of Age-Friendly Communities commit to improving their age-friendliness and submit to a rigorous assessment cycle. How this happens:

9. An AARP state office identifies cities, towns and counties it believes can commit to a continual cycle of improvement in the eight livability domains. AARP then informs municipal officials of the program and ascertains the community's interest.
10. The mayor or municipal administrator writes a letter to the AARP state office indicating the community's commitment. AARP then advises the World Health Organization of the municipality's intent and facilitates its enrollment in the AARP and global age-friendly networks.
11. Upon entry into the age-friendly network, the community moves through the following phases:

Phase 1: Planning (Years 1–2)
- Establish mechanisms to involve older people in all stages of the age-friendly cities and communities process.
- Conduct a comprehensive and inclusive baseline assessment of the age-friendliness of the community.

- Develop a 3-year community-wide action plan based on assessment findings.
- Identify indicators to monitor progress against the plan.

Phase 2: Implementation (Years 3–5)
- Commit to implementing the approved action plan.
- Submit a progress report at the end of the 5 years that outlines progress against the baseline using the indicators developed in the action plan.

Phase 3: Continual Improvements (Year 5 and Beyond)
- Make continual improvements.
- Membership is automatically renewed following a positive assessment and the submission of a revised action plan.

Benefits of Membership

Members of the AARP Network of Age-Friendly Communities become part of a global network of communities committed to providing older adults with the opportunity to live rewarding, productive and safe lives. Benefits of membership include:

- Organizational guidance from national experts
- Streamlined admission into the World Health Organization's age-friendly network
- Resources for identifying and developing assessment and survey tools
- Information about identifying and developing community-success criteria
- Strategies for identifying and developing ways to monitor progress
- Access to a network of communities and best practices
- Access to a volunteer network of support
- Access to evaluation tools
- Invitations to organized trainings and networking events

Resources at **aarp.org/livable**

- Support and guidance from AARP
- Public recognition by AARP and others of the community's commitment to become more age-friendly

AARP and the World Health Organization: A Shared Vision

Well-designed, livable communities promote well-being and sustain economic growth, and they make for happier, healthier residents—of all ages.

The World Health Organization's age-friendly communities concept closely aligns with AARP policies and initiatives.

AARP Livable Communities supports the efforts of neighborhoods, towns, cities, counties and even states to become great places for all ages. AARP believes that communities should provide walkable streets, suitable housing and transportation options, access to key services and opportunities for residents to participate in community activities.

To empower communities across the country to better respond to the needs of their residents, AARP targets local officials, policymakers, citizen activists and people age 50-plus in its advocacy efforts, policy work and educational programs in the issue areas of housing, transportation, mobility, community design and land use and planning. Key initiatives include Complete Streets advocacy, community engagement workshops and programs to promote universal design.

Critical Thinking

1. Discuss the benefits of communities that are admitted to the WHO network.
2. Discuss the features of an age-friendly community.

Internet References

AARP's Network of Age-Friendly Communities: An Introduction
http://www.aarp.org/livable-communities/network-age-friendly-communities/info-2014/an-introduction.html

World Health Organization: Global Age-friendly Cities: A Guide
http://www.who.int/ageing/publications/Global_age_friendly_cities_Guide_English.pdf

Unit 8

UNIT

Prepared by: Elaina Osterbur, *Saint Louis University*

Social Policies, Programs, and Services for Older Americans

It is a political reality that older Americans will be able to obtain needed assistance from governmental programs only if they are perceived as politically powerful. Political involvement can range from holding and expressing political opinions, voting in elections, participating in voluntary associations to help elect a candidate or party, and holding political office.

Research indicates that older people are just as likely as any other age group to hold political opinions, are more likely than younger people to vote in an election, are about equally divided between Democrats and Republicans, and are more likely than young people to hold political office. Older people, however, have shown little inclination to vote as a bloc on issues affecting their welfare despite encouragement to do so by senior activists, such as Maggie Kuhn and the leaders of the Gray Panthers. Gerontologists have observed that a major factor contributing to the increased push for government services for elderly individuals has been the publicity about their plight generated by such groups as the National Council of Senior Citizens and the American Association of Retired Persons (AARP). The desire of adult children to shift the financial burden of aged parents from themselves onto the government has further contributed to the demand for services for people who are elderly. The resulting widespread support for such programs has almost guaranteed their passage in Congress.

Now, for the first time, groups that oppose increases in spending for services for older Americans are emerging.

Requesting generational equity, some politically active groups argue that the federal government is spending so much on older Americans that it is depriving younger age groups of needed services.

The articles in this section focus on end-of-life policy issues, Medicare, and Social Security.

Article   Prepared by: Elaina F. Osterbur, *Saint Louis University*

End-of-Life Care in the United States: Current Reality and Future Promise: A Policy Review

"Improving end-of-life care should be a national priority, not just from a cost perspective, but from a quality perspective, because we can do much better" (Carlson, 2010, p.17).

LISA A. GIOVANNI

Learning Outcomes

After reading this article, you will be able to:

- Identify solutions to end-of-life care as outlined in the article.

- Discuss how these solutions affect the quality of life of patients.

- Discuss the impact of these solutions on the provisions set forth in the Patient Protection and Affordable Care Act.

Caring for individuals at the end of their life has been a topic of conversation for decades, from political, health policy, and quality perspectives. Issues exist in multiple well-defined areas that include access to and disparities in provision of end-of-life care, problems and confusion with financing the care, inadequacies when it comes to professionals' educational preparation related to end-of-life conversations, and the quality of end-of-life care. Additionally, conversations about end-of-life care would not be complete without acknowledging the ethical and legal issues and debate that surround this topic. The purpose of this article is to examine the current reality of end-of-life care and determine what portions of current health care reform will affect end-of-life care practices and policy in the United States. Additionally, hospice, palliative care, and nursing's involvement in end-of-life care and reform are discussed. Research of current literature was conducted and concludes with a discussion of findings to support the author's personal viewpoint that current health care policy fails to recognize and endorse effective reform for end-of-life care.

Hospice and Palliative Care

One solution to end-of-life care, the hospice movement, has seen incredible growth in the United States over the past several decades. It has been over 40 years since hospice care began in the United States. Since that time, "hospice has grown into a business that served over 1 million Medicare beneficiaries, from more than 3,300 providers in 2008, according to the Medicare Payment Advisory Commission" (Zigmond, 2010, p. 6). The history of hospice in the United States dates back to 1963, when Florence Wald, then the dean of the school of nursing at Yale University, invited Dr. Cicely Saunders from London to give a series of lectures on hospice care. "Dr. Cicely Saunders, the matriarch of the worldwide hospice movement, clearly had an impact as shortly after her visit and lecture series, the first hospice in the United States opened in Branford, Connecticut, in 1973" (Connor, 2007, p. 90). Today, hospice focuses on, "caring, not curing and, in most cases: care is provided in a patient's home. Care can also be provided in freestanding hospice centers, hospitals, and nursing homes or other long-term care facilities. Hospice services, which include care management for all aspects of the patient, include family support as well" (National Hospice and Palliative Care Organization [NHPCO], 2011a, ¶ 2)

Palliative care is defined by the World Health Organization (WHO) as, "an approach that improves quality of life for patients and their families facing the problems associated with life-threatening illness, through the prevention and relief of suffering by means of early identification and impeccable assessment and treatment of problems, including physical, psychosocial, and spiritual" (WHO, 2011). NHPCO (2011a) also adds, "palliative care extends the principles of hospice care to a broader population that could benefit from receiving this type of care earlier in their disease process. Palliative care, ideally, would segue into hospice care as the illness progressed" (¶ 3). Certainly both palliative care and hospice have a rightful place and play extremely important roles in end-of-life care. Hospice and palliative care programs exist across the United States, both in for-profit and not-for-profit sectors, as well as in stand-alone organizations or as components of larger health care models. "Palliative care programs are rapidly becoming the norm in American hospitals, with more than 70% of large (more than 200 bed) hospitals reporting the presence of a program in the American Hospital Association's 2006 annual hospital survey" (Weissman, Meier, & Spragens, 2008, p. 1294).

A policy discussion would not be complete or fair without mention of the ways that the hospice and palliative care movements have improved end-of-life care for patients and their families. There is a growing understanding of hospice and palliative care among most people in society, as the realization that hospice is not a place but rather a concept gains momentum, and patients opt for palliative care services earlier in their illness. We must not fail to acknowledge the great work accomplished by hospice and palliative care professionals. This effort must continue to expand in order to reduce access disparities across the nation. "The challenge for hospice and palliative care providers can be boiled down to achieving unfettered access to quality palliative care for all who need it" (Connor, 2007, p. 98).

Problems

While use and advantages of palliative care and hospice are gaining momentum at unprecedented speed, there remains disparity in access geographically. In addition to general access disparities, the type of care patients receive at the end of their life varies according to where they live and what acute care facility they happen to be a patient in. In 2001, Raphael, Ahrens, and Fowler discussed the likelihood of dying in a hospital in the United States as depending on, not patient preference, but rather on number of hospital beds, and physician per patient statistics, which varied greatly across the nation. Medicare beneficiaries in some western and northwestern states had a less than a 20% chance of dying in a hospital, while chances for those in southern and eastern states could be greater than 50% (Raphael et al., 2001).

Research supports the fact this issue is still apparent; geography continues to play a role in end-of-life care today. McKinney (2010) points out that for patients with advanced cancer, the likelihood they will spend their last days in a hospital intensive care unit depends largely on where they live, and which hospital they seek care in. Unfortunately, Goodman and colleagues (2010) found little evidence that treatments are aligned with patient wishes. The report, which examined 235,821 Medicare patients with advanced cancer who died between the years of 2003–2007, found significant variations in end-of-life care from region to region. "Roughly 29% of patients died in a hospital, and that number reached as high as 46.7% in the borough of Manhattan in New York, to as low as 17.8% in Cincinnati, Ohio and 7% in Mason City, Iowa" (McKinney, 2010, p. 6).

Not only is there disparity in whether patients go to and utilize acute care services, but also, once there, there is disparity in what types of care they receive in those acute care organizations. Extensive variation was found in length of stay, number of physician visits, percentage of patients with 10 or more physicians, and transfers to hospice services. Wennberg and associates (2004) found striking variation in all categories.

Medicare, the largest health plan in the United States, is highly influential in end-of-life care because of the large number of beneficiaries who die each year. Numbers vary depending on the source, but according to the Medicare Payment Advisory Commission (MedPAC), "about a quarter of the total Medicare budget is spent on services for beneficiaries in their last year of life, and 40% of that is in the last 30 days of their life" (Raphael, 2001, p. 458). Multiple studies declare that of the total outlay for all Medicare costs, 30%–40% occur in the last year of life for beneficiaries (Hogan, Lunney, Gabel, & Lynn, 2001; Raphael et al., 2001). One key factor involving end-of-life care and financing includes increased numbers of older Americans, which by 2050 is predicted to reach 72.2 million (Raphael et al., 2001). By that time it is also estimated that some 27 million people, most of whom will have multiple chronic diseases, will also need some type of long-term care services (Caffrey, Sengupta, Moss, Harris-Kojetin, & Valverde, 2011).

Chronic disease is an important item to review when discussing end-of-life care, because hospice patients are no longer predominately cancer patients, but also now have diagnoses that include multiple chronic conditions. According to the National Health Statistics Report, in recent years, hospice has become increasingly used by people with noncancerous diagnosis, the rate of which has increased from 25.3% in 2000 to 57.2% in 2007 (Caffrey et al., 2011). Another factor that cannot be overlooked is that many of these future older Americans will originate from ethnic and racial minority groups; therefore, end-of-life care and reform efforts must include an assessment and understanding of the care needs for these culturally diverse groups. Since a large payer of hospice services is Medicare, there is no doubt that political debate exists when discussions about payment for this care are undertaken. However, one thing is certain, discussions regarding quality of care, health policy, and disparity must begin to occur and cannot be dismissed due to the fact these conversations are difficult to have from an ethical and legal perspective. Components of these conversations must include the cost of end-of-life care in acute settings and possible hospice and palliative care contributions as solutions to decrease those costs.

Additional problems exist related to ill-defined quality standards, and decreased numbers of professionals working in hospice or palliative care across geographical pockets, especially in rural areas of the United States. End-of-life care issues remain unsolved as a result of an inability of a nation and its people, including political leaders, to discuss what is inevitable for all—mortality. End-of-life ethical and political policy conversations are difficult and, at times, avoided. There is unwillingness or uneasiness at best, to approach this subject head on.

The Patient Protection and Affordable Care Act

This national avoidance became blatantly evident when misconceptions from a portion of the 2010 Patient Protection and Affordable Care Act (PPACA) that would have enabled physicians to be reimbursed for having advanced care planning discussions with patients, was publicized as something that would result in a "death panel" that would "ration healthcare care in the United States" (Brody, 2011). As a result, the portion of the PPACA dealing with advanced planning conversations was deleted from the final version of the policy. Unfortunately, the true intent of this portion of the proposed act was not realized by the public or policymakers, since it was dismissed too rapidly for consideration. In the end, as with multiple other facets of end-of-life care, the fallout for not addressing this issue results in financial impact to the nation, as well as a quality of life impact for the individuals and families who require end-of-life care for advanced illness in the United States.

Ironically virtually no portion of the PPACA deals with reform, reimbursement, or policy changes related to end-of-life care. There are minor sections of the PPACA that can have an effect on end-of-life care, but no portion relates directly to this vital and hugely important aspect of American health care. Unfortunately, the result is the unique needs of the terminally ill remain poorly addressed in the United States health care system. Perhaps one of the most concerning concepts when it comes to end-of-life care is the fact that so often the care provided is not necessarily the care the patient and family have elected, wanted, or even understood.

Advance Directives

The SUPPORT study, which was funded by the Robert Wood Johnson Foundation and enrolled patients over a 5-year period, was conducted to analyze decision making in patients near the end of life. Other goals of the study included gaining an understanding of communication about end-of-life interactions between patients, their families, nurses, and physicians. Results indicated that a significant number of critically ill patients did not want aggressive life-prolonging care (Celso, & Meenrajan, 2010; Fitzsimmons, Shively, & Verderber, 1995; Smith et al., 2003). Unfortunately, due to multiple reasons, including delayed timeliness in executing advance care planning until patients are terminal and out-of-date or unavailable documents (Tilden et al., 2010), issues remain involving patients advocating for themselves, families advocating for their loved ones, and health care professionals providing care that may or may not be consistent with patient preference. Perhaps the best reason for meaningful discussion and policy reform to occur is a genuine concern for a better patient experience when it comes to end-of-life care. We cannot dismiss the Triple Aim of the Institute for Health Care Improvement, which dictates the pursuit of an improved patient experience, improved health of the population at large, and reduced per capita costs (Berwick, Nolan, & Whittington, 2008). To that end, the United States simply cannot overlook all that hospice, palliative care, and advance directives

have to offer to individuals and families who face serious, life-threatening advanced illness issues.

Expert Opinion

According to NHPCO, a non-profit organization representing over 2,900 hospices in the United States, none of the PPACA that deals with accountable care organizations (ACO) mentions hospice or palliative care programs. ACOs are organizations that will have local accountability for managing populations of people throughout a continuum of lifetime care. ACOs will need to share reimbursement and determine cost-sharing strategies for all providers involved. They will also be required to care for a minimum of 5,000 enrollees and will be paid on a pre-defined outcomes measure basis. NHPCO was so dismayed that there was no mention of end-of-life care in the final ACO regulations that they communicated this fact to the Center for Medicare & Medicaid Services (CMS). In a letter dated June 6, 2011 to Dr. Donald Berwick, CMS administrator, NHPCO President and CEO J. Donald Schumacher stated, "many dying patients in institutions have unmet needs for symptom management, emotional support and being treated with respect." He went on to say, that "it is essential that hospice and palliative care organizations be partners in ACO's in order to contribute to the success of these new care models, and care for patients across the continuum of their life-time" (NHPCO, 2011b).

The American Hospital Association (AHA) recommends multiple items that should be a focus of national quality efforts; one of those recommendations is for greater self-determination related to end-of-life care (Carlson, 2010). The AHA endorses personal tools that allow patients and families to record written advance health care directives, name legally binding health care powers of attorney, and craft physician orders for life sustaining treatment. Providing the right care to the right patient at the right time defines quality. The AHA explains that the right care includes what science suggests would have the best outcomes for the patient, but also considers the patient's wishes about what's important to them (Carlson, 2010).

The Critical Role of Nursing

The Institute of Medicine (2010) in *The Future of Nursing* report calls for the need to transform nursing education, stating that nurses are critical to the success of health care reform, and that nurses need to take their rightful place in leadership endeavors, achieve higher levels of education, practice to the fullest of their ability, and be full partners with other health care professionals.

Multiple studies discuss educational deficiencies and lack of comfort levels that nurses have when it comes to conducting follow up or clarification discussions with patients about end-of-life care or treatment options (Malloy, Virani, Kelly, & Munvevar, 2010; Reinke, et al., 2010; Wittenburg-Lyles, Goldsmith, & Ragan, 2011). Changes in nursing education must occur in order to prepare professional nurses to become advocates and experts in end-of-life care. When assessing the adequacy of skill of health care professionals to initiate and conduct end-of-life conversations there are noted voids and problems.

Reinke and colleagues (2010) identified several skill sets that nurses felt were important but underutilized in end-of-life care conversations. They concluded end-of-life care interventions should address not only system and policy changes, but also improvements in individual nurse's communication skills regarding end-of-life conversations (Reinke et al., 2010). "Nurses can play a pivotal role in patient and family illness and care awareness by facilitating palliative care communication and supporting the conceptual shift to early palliative care" (Wittenberg-Lyles et al., 2011, p. 305). The communication problem exists for physicians as well. Part of this problem originates from poor preparation of professionals in their primary and early health care education programs. While many programs are adapting methods to include didactic training programs, the real experience comes from actual conversations, which of course, is not something a text or video can accomplish. Programs like the End of Life Nursing Education Consortium and continued efforts in physician mentoring and role modeling in end-of-life care conversations will prove very beneficial (Wittenberg-Lyles et al., 2011).

The development and spread of palliative care efforts and hospice education for professionals and the general public will continue to have an impact on growth and acceptance of end-of-life conversations. It is also important for individual professionals, as well as the organizations they work within, to continue to foster and participate in opportunities and experiences that will enhance ability and comfort levels regarding end-of-life conversations. This effort will be of utmost importance for not only physicians, but also for nurses.

"Communication is the cornerstone of basic nursing practice and a fundamental skill across all settings of care is to identify the patient's goals of care. As patients and families continue to face serious illness, transition to palliative care, and make difficult decisions, nurses will play a critical role and remain as the predominant professional at the bedside" (Malloy et al., 2010, p. 172). Physicians most often will champion the initial conversation with patients and families, but nurses have a responsibility and professional ethic to be present for the patient and family after initial conversations takes place. "Nurses accompany patients on their journeys; through such ongoing and intimate encounters, they support patients in confronting the weariness of living and dying" (Ferrell & Coyle, 2008, p. 247). Health care professionals, including nurses, must be vigilant about understanding their communication style and engaging in educational opportunities that enhance their ability to conduct effective end-of-life conversations with patients and families.

Future Promise and Possible Obstacles

The Patient Self-Determination Act of 1991 required all Medicare participating organizations notify patients of their rights to complete an advance directive for health treatments (American Nurses Association, 1991). The overall goal of advance directives is to allow patients to retain control over the life-prolonging treatments they receive. Current health policy sometimes fails patients in this respect, as families can argue patient's choices may change over time, or there can be delays in producing existing documents, or failures in executing the documents all together. While the intent of the federal mandate was well intentioned, it resulted in continued confusion and sporadic compliance by patients and families in completion of advance directives.

At approximately the same time as the passage of the federal Patient Self-Determination Act, another paradigm in advance care planning was initiated that had a goal of turning patient treatment preferences and advance directives into medical orders. The Oregon state legislature introduced a new program to improve adherence to patients' wishes for end-of-life care. The Patient Order for Life Sustaining Care (POLST) paradigm was created to provide a mechanism to communicate patient preference for end-of-life care treatment across care settings. The POLST document turns patient treatment preferences into medical orders, with an overall goal of ensuring that wishes for treatment are honored. "The National Quality Forum and other experts have recommended nationwide implementation of the POLST paradigm" (Hickman, Sabatino, Moss, & Nester, 2008, p. 120).

Some barriers to POLST use do exist. "The most potentially problematic barriers are detailed statutory specifications for out of hospital do-not-resuscitate orders in some states. Other potential barriers include limitations on the authority to forgo life-sustaining treatments in 23 states, medical conditions in 15 states, and witnessing requirements for out of hospital do not resuscitate orders in 12 states" (Hickman et al., 2008, p. 119). Multiple studies regarding use of POLST across care settings have been conducted to determine usefulness in understanding and following patient wishes. Results of studies yield a strong tie between use of POLST forms and adherence to patients' self-determined wishes across care settings (Hickman et al., 2010; Hickman et al., 2009; Meyers, 2004; Schmidt, Hickman, Tolle, & Brooks, 2004). Studies also revealed that patients with POLST medical orders were less likely to receive unwanted care (Hickman et al., 2010; Tilden, Nelson, Dunn, Donius, & Tolle, 2000). Multiple research studies confirm that POLST can have a positive impact on the ability of an individual to self-determine his or her end-of-life preferences.

Access to end-of-life care services is another problem. Access includes awareness of palliative and hospice services, payment and financial coverage for those benefits, and acceptance of benefits from a cultural or religious perspective. Goldsmith, Dietrich, Qingling, and Morrison (2008) concluded that significant disparities in public and educational access to hospital palliative care services exist. "Hospice care is a beneficial, yet underutilized service in advanced dementia. Hospice professionals cite prognostication as the main hindrance to enrolling patients with dementia into hospice" (Mitchell et al., 2012, p. 45).

Current reform and health policy have affected hospice organizations in several ways, the largest of which is decreases in reimbursement related to cuts from Medicare, the largest payer of hospice services. There is also increased scrutiny and regulatory efforts in the form of an additional recertification requirement of face-to-face meetings between patient and physician or nurse practitioner at time of recertification of care, which became effective January 1, 2010 (Morrow, 2010). In an industry with narrow profit margins, reimbursement reductions could worsen the already existing access problems.

Other items involving end-of-life care are present in the historic Patient Protection and Affordable Care Act. Hidden deep and not well publicized are at least two provisions that may have an impact on end-of-life care. They both relate to hospice. One section of the PPACA amends current law to eliminate the requirement for children to elect curative versus hospice care through Medicaid and CHIP programs. A second area deals with adults, "in section 3140, the PPACA authorizes a three year long Medicare Hospice Concurrent Care demonstration project involving a study to determine whether patients benefit when Medicare authorizes payment for receipt of concurrent curative treatment and hospice care" (Cerminara, 2011). The project, which does not have a start date, will begin as soon as the Secretary of Health and Human Services establishes parameters and outcome measurements, and will involve 15 hospice programs nationwide. Astonishingly, other than the previously mentioned items, there are no other portions of the PPACA that directly relate to end of life care. Once more people understand what hospice and palliative care can provide related to quality of life and a peaceful dying process, a major culture shift can begin to occur. The result would be an environment where end-of-life conversations occur prior to a patient's actual end of life. Sometimes awareness occurs because we either experience it ourselves or know someone who has experienced caring for a loved one at the end of his or her life. Despite explosive political debate, the answer really does involve a conversation.

The American Academy of Hospice and Palliative Medicine has multiple recommendations for health care reform. One of those recommendations refers to advance directives and specifically the POLST. The recommendation includes an endorsement to provide reimbursement for physician consultations that would determine goals for medical care. Nothing makes more sense, and seems farther away from death panels than prudent, frank, and transparent conversations about an individual's wishes.

The experience or wishes of the patients cannot be overlooked, especially in end-of-life care when a cure cannot be offered to patients for whatever they are suffering from. From an ethical perspective, shouldn't that be required to be conveyed? Should end-of-life care be recognized as an ethical obligation of health care providers and organizations, and what exactly does that mean? Patients must have a say in what is important to them and ultimately decide their personal wishes. Patients need to determine what defines high-quality dying for them, and decide on how they want to manage their end of life, as it relates to death (Cramer, 2010; Howell & Brazil, 2005).

Conclusion

Paying attention to health care policy, or lack thereof, or the conflicted policy Catch-22s, when it comes to end of life care is a critical responsibility of all health care professionals. In discussing the type and magnitude of changes necessary to implement cost-effective, ethically considerate, culturally acceptable changes in end-of-life care, there will no doubt continue to be difficult and painful conversations, both on individual and political fronts. But, the conversations must occur, and cannot be ignored simply because they are difficult to have. Perhaps, most importantly, the political community, who are often those who write the policy that needs to be executed, must recognize that local, organizational, and state efforts cannot be delayed related to lack of movement on a federal front. There are many examples of great work being done with regard to end-of-life care across America that have nothing to with policy or federal government intervention, and these efforts must increase and continue.

All health care professionals must realize the power they have on two levels, as individuals and as a profession, when it comes to end-of-life reform and improvement efforts. Health care professionals have an ethical responsibility to assist patients to achieve the care and life they want for their last days, and in many cases that may involve assisting them to die with dignity in a surrounding of their choice, and embraced by those they have loved for a lifetime. Hopefully, this article has created a heightened sense of awareness for health care professionals, especially nurses, to pay attention to reform efforts in the United States. Nurses, physicians, and other health care professionals have the ability, knowledge, and power to help shape new regulations and laws when it comes to end-of-life care. Although it is 2012, the insight of Ira Byock, a leading palliative care physician and long-time public advocate for improving end-of-life care, still holds true today. He summarized the current state of end-of-life care and points the way to where we must go by saying:

> A tidal wave of social change is headed our way. For the first time in human history, in the third millennium, there will be more old people than young people on the planet. In addition to the graying of the population, there will be more physical distance between families, smaller families, fewer caregivers, more chronic illness, and increased technological advances. These trends are all converging to create the perfect storm; a social tsunami of care giving that threatens to overwhelm our children's generation and us. We must rise to the challenges and build a model of healthcare that will determine the quality of care we receive tomorrow (2004, pp. 214–215).

Plan for Action

Unless we take personal, professional, and political action today, we will not be able to afford to die with dignity in the future. For multiple reasons that include an aging population, escalating health care spending, and an approach to end-of-life care that often does not conform to the wishes of patients, we cannot delay action. We need to have honest and transparent advance care planning conversations with our families and our physicians. We need to become comfortable talking about dying with those we love and interact with the most, in order to become comfortable talking about end-of-life care publically. All health care professionals should strive to create an environment for patients where the philosophy of palliative care and hospice is understood. Goals of this environment would include increased knowledge about hospice and palliative care, greater symptom control for patients with end-stage diseases, improved advance care planning, better quality of life, and ultimately less money spent on achieving better outcomes for patients facing end-of-life illness and disease.

Interactions between politicians and health care professionals, especially those involved in hospice and palliative care, must accelerate. Professionals in these fields must continue strong advocacy efforts to let the political world know what they do, and what promise their care offers related to improved quality of life and decreased overall spending. Such interactions should include tours of facilities, visits with patients and families, and letters and phone calls to politicians on specific issues that are important to the hospice and palliative care industry. These action items would cost very little, and perhaps only result in an investment of time for those involved.

Opportunities to develop advance care directives are often missed. To that end, we must revisit Medicare reimbursement for physicians participating in voluntary advanced care planning consultations, and end discussions surrounding "death panels" for good. Physicians often have a clear understanding of what defines quality of life for their patients, and this clear understanding, which takes time to develop, involves multiple discussions and explanations that physicians need and want to participate in with their patients. The positive end result would be assurance patients' wishes are understood, documented, and ultimately attainable. While health care professionals can lead the effort aimed at better advanced care planning, politicians play a vital role in assuring that policy makes sense and is not confusing to those who need it. It is simply not prudent of such a smart nation to refuse to pay physicians for this extremely important part of health care planning.

POLST legislation must continue to accelerate and expand to assure acceptance of medical orders that are understood clearly and cross all care continuums in every state. It seems possible that if several states can achieve success in overcoming legal barriers related to POLST implementation, all states can achieve it. The important and expanding work of the POLST paradigm must continue. It is incumbent upon lawmakers to create global policies that enable POLST to be available to those who critically needed it in order to enhance smoother care transitions between providers, and decrease unwanted treatment by clarifying patient's wishes into actual medical orders. The public needs to understand POLST and for whom it is intended. National television and radio commercials addressing POLST and advance care planning could have positive promotional effects, especially if hosted by the next President of the United States of America. It's too important not to consider.

The Medicare Hospice Concurrent Care Demonstration Project (as defined in the PPACA) needs to begin in order to analyze the effects of concurrent care with relation to quality of life and financial outcomes for both rural and urban demographics in the United States. This concurrent approach will address current hospice and palliative care access issues that relate to patients needing to make curative versus palliative decisions independently. A concurrent approach would also address a second population of patients who need end-of-life care but do not have a terminal cancer diagnosis, such as dementia or congestive heart disease. Demonstration results will need to be analyzed by an authoritative body such as CMS or MedPAC for final determinations as to whether quality of life was enhanced and cost savings were realized. If results are positive, then the Medicare hospice regulations that define eligibility will need to be revised. From a nursing perspective, perhaps less money would be spent treating patients who are guided into hospice care through a strong palliative care effort where symptoms are controlled and care is gradually transferred, rather than in a hurry, with short lengths of stay, as exists today for many hospice patients.

Educational voids related to end-of-life care curriculums for both medical and nursing schools should be addressed. It is important curriculums include practice and mentoring in the area of end-of-life conversations since proficiency in this type of communication will not be realized through didactic teaching alone. Conversations are critical to understanding what each patient wishes for end-of-life care.

Efforts focused on medical fraud, waste, and abuse must continue. Monies recovered for these reasons could be used for end-of-life care initiatives and start-up processes for education and advocacy efforts. While most providers are well intentioned and follow all federal and state regulations, those that do not should continue to be identified and removed from the health care service arena.

Hospice and palliative care professionals must ensure their voice is heard when it comes to creation of policy. Local, state, and grassroots end-of-life programs should continue to be developed, financed, and evaluated. While some financing may come from grants or private sources, states should actively assess what they can do to assist financing any initiative that promotes or enhances end-of-life care.

Simply put, we can begin to control the cost of end-of-life care and afford to die with dignity if we act today. We all have a role to play in securing a better means to our end, and creating a nation where quality of life and personal choice are not only a priority but also a responsibility.

References

American Nurses Association. (1991). *ANA position statement: Nursing and the patient self-determination acts.* Washington, DC: Author.

Berwick, D., Nolan, T., & Whittington, J. (2008). The triple aim: Care, health, and cost. *Health Affairs, 27*(3), 759–769.

Brody, J. (2011, January 17). Keep your voice, even at the end of life. *The New York Times.* Retrieved from www.nytimes.com/2011/01/18/health/18brody.html

Byock, I. (2004). *The four things that matter most.* New York, NY. Free Press.

Caffrey, C., Sengupta, M., Moss, A., Harris-Kojetin, L., & Valverde, R. (2011). Home health care discharged and hospice care patients: United States, 2000–2007. *National Health Statistics Report,* 38.

Carlson, J. (2010). Not finished yet: Coalition wants end of life care to be a priority. *Modern Healthcare, 40*(43), 17–18.

Celso, B., & Meenrajan, S. (2010). The triad that matters: Palliative medicine, code status, and health care costs. *American Journal of Hospice & Palliative Medicine, 27*(6), 398–401.

Cerminara, K. (2011). *Health care reform at the end of life: Giving with one hand but taking with the other.* Retrieved from www.aslme.org/print_article.php?aid=460404&bt=ss

Connor, S. (2007). Development of hospice and palliative care in the United States. *Journal of Death & Dying, 56*(1), 89–99.

Cramer, C. (2010). To live until you die. *Clinical Journal of Oncology Nursing, 14*(1), 53–56.

Ferrell, B., & Coyle, N. (2008). The nature of suffering and the goals of nursing. *Oncology Nursing Forum, 35*(2), 241–247.

Fitzsimmons, L., Shively, M., & Verderber, V. (1995). The nurse's role in end of life treatment discussions: Preliminary report from the SUPPORT project. *Journal of Cardiovascular Nursing, 9*(3), 68–77.

Goldsmith, B., Dietrich, J., Qingling, D., & Morrison, S. (2008). Variability in access to hospital palliative care in the United States. *Journal of Palliative Medicine, 11*(8), 1094–1102.

Goodman, D., Fisher, E., Chang, C., Morden, N., Jacobson, J., Murray, K., & Miesfeldt, S. (2010). Quality of end-of-life cancer care for Medicare beneficiaries, regional and hospital-specific analyses. Retrieved from www.dartmouthatlas.org/downloads/reports/Cancer_report_11_16_10.pdf

Hickman, S.E., Nelson, C.A., Perrin, N.A., Moss, A., Hammes, B.J., & Tolle, S. (2010). A comparison of methods to communicate treatment preferences in nursing facilities: Traditional practices versus the physician orders for life sustaining treatment program. *Journal of American Geriatric Society, 58*(7), 1241–1248.

Hickman, S.E., Nelson, C.A., Moss, A., Hammes, B.J., Terwilliger, A., Jackson, A., & Tolle, S. (2009). Use of the physician orders for life sustaining treatment (POLST) paradigm program in the hospice setting. *Journal of Palliative Medicine, 12*(2), 133–140.

Hickman, S., Sabatino, C., Moss, A., & Nester, J. (2008). The POLST paradigm to improve end of life care: Potential state legal barriers to implementation. *Journal of Law, Medicine and Ethics, 36*(1), 119–124.

Hogan, C., Lunney, J., Gabel, J., & Lynn, J. (2001). Medicare beneficiaries' costs in the last years of life. *Health Affairs, 20*(4), 188–195.

Howell, D., & Brazil, K. (2005). Reaching common ground: A patient-family based conceptual framework of quality end of life care. *Journal of Palliative Care, 21*(1), 19–26.

Institute of Medicine (IOM). (2010.) *IOM report brief: The future of nursing—leading change, advancing health.* Retrieved from www.iom.edu/~/media/Files/Report%20Files/2010The-Future-of-Nursing/Future%20of%20Nursing%202010%20Report%20Brief.pdf

Malloy, P., Virani, R., Kelly, K., & Munvevar, C. (2010). Beyond bad news. *Journal of Hospice and Palliative Care, 12*(3), 166–174.

McKinney, M. (2010). Where you live = how you die. *Modern Healthcare, 40*(47), 6–8.

Meyers, J. (2004). Physician orders for life sustaining treatment form. *Journal of Gerontological Nursing, 30*(9), 37–46.

Mitchell, S., Black, B.S., Ersek, M., Hanson, L.C., Miller, S.C., Sachs, G.A., . . . Morrison, R.S. (2012). Advanced dementia: State of the art and priorities for the next decade. *Annals of Internal Medicine, 156*(1), 45–51.

Morrow, A. (2010). *Obama signs health care reform bill— What's next for hospice?* Retrieved from http://dying.about.com/b/2010/03/23/obama-signs-healthcare-reform-bill-whats-next-forhospice.htm

National Hospice and Palliative Care Organization (NHPCO). (2011a). *Definition of hospice.* Retrieved from www.nhpco.org/i4a/pages/index.cfm?pageid$=$4648

National Hospice and Palliative Care Organization (NHPCO). (2011b). *Letter to CMS administrator, Donald Berwick, MD, CMS administrator.* Retrieved from www.nhpco.org/files/public/regulatory/NHPCO_Comments_on_ACO_Proposed_Rule.pdf

Raphael, C., Ahrens, J., & Fowler, N. (2001). Financing end of life care in the USA. *Journal of The Royal Society of Medicine, 94*(9), 458–461.

Reinke, L.F., Shannon, S.E., Engelberg, R., Dotolo, D., Silvestri, G.A., & Curtis, J.R. (2010). Nurses identification of important yet underutilized end of life care: Skills for patients with life limiting or terminal illnesses. *Journal of Palliative Medicine, 13*(6), 753–759.

Schmidt, T., Hickman, S., Tolle, S., & Brooks, H. (2004). The physician orders for life sustaining treatment program: Oregon emergency medical technicians' practical experiences and attitudes. *Journal of American Geriatric Society, 52*(9), 430–434.

Smith, T.J., Coyne, P., Cassel, B., Penberthy, L., Hopson, A., & Hager, M.A. (2003). A high volume specialist palliative care unit and team may reduce in hospital end of life care costs. *Journal of Palliative Medicine, 6*(5), 699–705.

Tilden, V., Corless, I., Dahlin, C., Ferrell, B., Gibson, R., & Lentz, J. (2010). *Advance care planning as an urgent public health concern.* Washington, DC: American Academy of Nursing.

Tilden, V., Nelson, C., Dunn, P., Donius, M., & Tolle, S. (2000). Nursing perspective on improving communication about nursing home residents preferences for medical treatments at end of life. *Nursing Outlook, 48*(3), 109–115.

Weissman, D., Meier, D., & Spragens, L. (2008). Center to advance palliative care consultation service metrics: Consensus recommendation. *Journal of Palliative Medicine, 11*(10), 1294–1298.

Wennberg, J.E., Fisher, E.S., Stukel, T.A., Skinner, J.S., Sharp, S.M., & Bronner, K.K. (2004). Use of hospitals, physician visits, and hospice care during last six months of life among cohorts loyal to highly respected hospitals in the United States. *British Medical Journal, 328*(7440), 607–610.

Wittenberg-Lyles, E., Goldsmith, J., & Ragan, S. (2011). The shift to early palliative care: A typology of illness journeys and the role of nursing. *Clinical Journal of Oncology Nursing, 15*(3), 304–310.

World Health Organization (WHO). (2011). *WHO definition of palliative care.* Retrieved from www.who.int/cancer/palliative/definition/en/

Zigmond, J. (2010). Hospice hot spot: Gentiva-Odyssey pairing bans on inevitability of aging population. *Modern Healthcare, 40*(22), 6–7.

Additional Reading

American Academy of Nursing. (2010). *Advance care planning as an urgent public health concern.* Washington, DC: Author.

Critical Thinking

1. Based on the investigation in this article, does the evidence support increased quality of life as a result of suggested solutions to end-of-life care?

2. What is the role of advance directives in end-of-life decision making and how do these directives influence treatment?

Create Central

www.mhhe.com/createcentral

Internet References

U.S. Department of Health & Human Services
www.hhs.gov/healthcare/rights

U.S. Centers for Medicare & Medicaid Services: Medicaid.gov
www.medicaid.gov/affordablecareact/affordable-care-act.html

U.S. Centers for Medicare & Medicaid Services: Medicare.gov
www.medicare.gov/about-us/affordable-care-act/affordable-care-act.html

LISA A. GIOVANNI, MSN, RN, is Director of Quality, Visiting Nurse Association, St. Luke's University & Health Network, Bethlehem, PA.

Article

Prepared by: Elaina Osterbur, *Saint Louis University*

iHubs: A Community Solution to Aging in Place

A new collaborative spurs a creative intergenerational strategy to address the unique needs of Colorado Springs' growing elder community.

BETH ROALSTAD

Learning Outcomes

After reading this article, you will be able to:

- Identify the concept of iHub.
- Discuss the benefits of iHubs.

Russ wants someone to pay attention to his complaint of an earache that has been going on for two years. Whenever he goes to the doctor, he says, they concentrate solely on his arrhythmia and cardiac health. Delores wants a cooking and nutrition class to help her cope with her newly diagnosed diabetes. Mary wants a place to go to converse with neighbors after having her Golden Circle subsidized meal.

All of these requests and others could be more easily met when the Innovations in Aging Collaborative is able to train its local community centers to create intergenerational hubs, or iHubs, that would be situated just blocks from older adults' homes, to better serve the needs of people like Russ, Delores, and Mary.

The iHub concept involves an intergenerational social gathering place focused on older adults living in a particular area of the community, but also attracting people of all ages. iHubs could be established in existing community centers or other facilities and cultural centers that also support the needs of elders.

A Young Nonprofit Tackles Aging

The Innovations in Aging Collaborative, a new nonprofit organization in Colorado Springs, Colorado, about an hour south of Denver, started out in 2008 as a volunteer effort to identify challenges and opportunities arising with Colorado Springs' rapidly growing aging population. Incorporated in December 2012, Innovations hired its first staff member and embarked upon goals set forth by community stakeholders. Our board of directors comes from multiple sectors: business leaders, the public library system, higher education, healthcare, gerontology, neighborhood leaders, and senior service organizations. Innovations' mission is to convene the community to promote creative approaches to address the challenges and opportunities of aging.

Stakeholders as well as older adults who have participated in conversations with Innovations over the past five years stressed a preference for collaboration rather than launching a new infrastructure, and they asked us to organize resources through private partnerships, public policy, and citizen efforts. They also recognized that leveraging existing resources was going to be important to the success of iHub: creating a new program requiring large investments from funders was not going to work in a community with more than 2,000 registered public charities (Summit Economics, 2013).

Aging in Colorado Springs

Colorado Springs lies at the foot of Pikes Peak, at 6,010 feet above sea level. A beautiful city that blends an urban atmosphere with quick access to mountain recreation, Colorado Springs now is facing a "silver tsunami" as is the rest of the nation, but has unique challenges. Colorado long has been a state with a young population, but between 2000 and 2010, its ages 55 to 64 group increased by an annual average of 6.1 percent, compared to a total population increase of 1.7 percent.

According to the 2010 census, Colorado Springs' El Paso County had an older-than-age-65 population of approximately 62,000. By 2020, this will double; and by 2030, the older adult population will nearly triple to 172,394, with the general population at 981,394 (Adams, 2011).

The Colorado Springs community is geographically large, making access to and delivery of services difficult. Transportation for those with mobility barriers is a huge problem—both for people who do not own (or who cannot afford) a car and for elders dependent upon public or specialized transportation. The 2013 and 2011 *Quality of Life Indicators* reports pointed out that 42 percent of our community elders experienced a transportation barrier when engaging in activities such as buying groceries and filling prescriptions, going to medical appointments, and participating in social activities (Pikes Peak United Way, 2011, 2013). Another challenge for Colorado Springs (and Colorado in general) is the low numbers of physicians, specialists, and psychiatrists for a population the size of our community (Adams, 2011).

iHubs Get Rolling

Innovations in Aging believes that a successful community integrates and involves all of its residents. To that end, we are promoting the concept of iHubs inside existing community centers and natural gathering places to support aging in place. We have hosted two significant community events, bringing together a cross section of human service professionals, nonprofit leaders, government officials, business leaders, artists, and retirees to create an open dialog to address the issues, but also to identify potential solutions to support older adults' ability to age in place. Innovations hopes to create an intimate neighborhood model to cope with challenges such as transportation, and to have easy access to wellness, fitness, arts, culture, and education programs close to home for elders aging in place.

We currently are working, with the help of our volunteer teams, through community centers to reach out to several hundred neighborhood residents to gather input and co-create programs in their community centers that meet their needs and evolve to meet the changing needs of their neighbors. For example, hosting a semi-regular veterinarian services clinic for elders' pets; launching new community-based classes from the local community college; and bringing the experience of an art gallery to the community centers through classes taught by local artists. Innovations identified certain Colorado Springs community centers as the first potential partners for collaborating to design a neighborhood-based iHub; we considered four centers, an alternative facility in a neighborhood lacking a senior center, and a virtual hub. In the end, we selected the Westside Community Center to partner with because of its internal capacity and enthusiastic leadership.

Innovations began the program at Westside with surveys, interviews, and focus groups. The goal is to gather data for two months; evaluate current programs; identify potential gaps and opportunities; invite new collaborators; implement programs; and evaluate progress at ninety days and six months. We are working with the community center to invite elders in the neighborhood to participate in surveys and focus groups. This will help the community center in its short-term and long-term planning.

The Westside Community Center is evaluating its existing programs. So far, the feedback has been very informative. We have talked about the need for transportation and medical care, but also basic concerns around home safety and maintenance. The needs are great, and our challenge will be to connect older adults to existing service providers and trustworthy enterprises to meet them all.

Russ, Delores, and Mary participated in one of our focus groups as a part of Innovations' community outreach. Many participants want to remain in their homes as long as possible and to be connected to neighbors of all ages. The group is outspoken, well-connected, and fiercely independent; 75 percent drove themselves to lunch the day of the interview, and the average age in the room was seventy eight. Innovations looks forward to engaging with more elders like these and continuing to solicit their input to shape a community action plan.

An Involved Community Can Realize the iHub Vision

We envision our city and county having several iHubs in formal community centers, but also in libraries, fitness centers, and perhaps in residential housing complexes. We need continued involvement from all levels of our community to achieve this goal—from the mayor to the children who will participate in cooking classes with people like Delores. The greater involvement and engagement of people of all ages will create a community that will be able to care for all of its citizens. This goal is lofty, but seems achievable, given the level of interest in iHubs.

References

Adams, T. H. 2011. *Aging in El Paso County*. A report compiled for Innovations in Aging Collaborative. www.innovationsinaging. org/Resources/2011+Innovations+in+Aging+Collaboration+ Report-26.html. Retrieved October 4, 2013.

Pikes Peak United Way.org. 2011. *Quality of Life Indicators Report*. www.ppunitedway.org/ourimpact/qli. Retrieved October 4, 2013.

Pikes Peak United Way.org. 2013. *Quality of Life Indicators Report*. www.ppunitedway.org/ourimpact/qli. Retrieved October 4, 2013.

Summit Economics. 2013. *Nonprofits Matter: An Economic Force for Vibrant Community*. A report compiled for the Center for Nonprofit Excellence. www.cnecoloradosprings.org. Retrieved October 4, 2013.

Critical Thinking

1. What makes iHubs different from many of the programs that senior centers and agencies offer?

2. What are the benefits of offering in iHubs in libraries, fitness centers, and communties centers?

3. Describe other ventures or iHub opportunties that could benefit your community.

Internet References

American Society on Aging
   http://www.asaging.org

Innovations in Aging Collaborative
   http://www.innovationsinaging.org/index.php/outreach

Beth Roalstad, MSW, is the executive director of the Innovations in Aging Collaborative in Colorado Springs, Colorado.

Article   Prepared by: Elaina Osterbur, *Saint Louis University*

Social Security Twist for Boomers with Public, Private Jobs

AMANDA ALIX

Learning Outcomes

After reading this article, you will be able to:

- Identify the Windfall Elimination Provision.
- Discuss how the Windfall Elimination Provision works.

Are you a Baby Boomer who has worked for both the public and private sector during your working career? If so, you are probably feeling pretty good about your retirement options, which very likely include a public pension, as well as Social Security. Unfortunately, under the Windfall Elimination Provision, you may not be eligible for all the Social Security benefits you think are coming to you.

No More "Double Dipping"

Before 1983, people who worked in both public and private jobs could collect a full pension when they retired, as well as Social Security benefits, as long as they qualified. Benefits were calculated as though the employee had been a low-wage worker throughout his or her career.

In order to make sure that lower-paid employees are given an ample monthly payment upon retiring, Social Security is calculated in favor of low wage-earners. So not only were public employees able to retire with a pension, but any additional work in which employees paid into Social Security was calculated with maximum returns in mind.

Therefore, a retired public worker with a pension could also draw a monthly Social Security benefit based upon around 55% of private-sector earnings prior to retirement—quite a bit more than the 25% that high-wage individuals typically get. The enactment of the WEP put an end to this "double dipping."

How It Works

Whether WEP applies to you depends on a few factors. The first, of course, is that you must have worked for a federal, state, or local government, employment which was covered by pension benefits, but not Social Security—in other words, you never had Social Security tax deducted from your pay. Secondly, you must have also worked in a job that was covered by Social Security, even if the employer also offered a pension plan.

If this is the case, you will have your Social Security benefits reduced according to the Social Security Administration's formula, which takes your inflation-adjusted, average monthly earnings, and divides them into three brackets: in approximate terms, the first $800, the next $3,300, and the amount above $4,100. The first amount is multiplied by 90%, the second by 32%, and anything left over, by 15%. Adding them together gives you your monthly benefit. It's that 90% bracket that the WEP uses to reduce your benefit.

A Big Exception

You are excepted from the WEP under certain circumstances— one of which is that you had 30 years or more of "substantial" earnings. In order to obtain the 90%, you will need that full 30 years; the percentage drops after that. With 20 or fewer years of substantial earnings, the multiplier is only 40%.

The SSA's Retirement Planner gives an indication of how this might work. The maximum monthly reduction for someone reaching age 62 this year, with 20 or fewer years of substantial earnings, is $408.00.

A few things affect this amount, however. One is that the WEP will never be more than one-half of your non-Social Security pension; the other has to do with cost of living adjustments.

The WEP will be calculated on your benefit amount before the yearly COLA is applied.

The age at which you take benefits also factors into the mix. The SSA chart represents a scenario for retirement at age 62, the earliest age at which you may collect. Retiring at your full retirement age—or later—will change your benefit profile accordingly.

Though you won't really know how WEP will affect you until you reach retirement age, being aware that it will be a factor will spare you any surprises later on. In addition, knowing this fact can allow you to tweak your retirement planning in order to minimize the WEP's impact.

A mix of public and private employment can influence Social Security spousal benefits, as well.

Critical Thinking

1. How does the Windfall Elimination Provision affect Social Security benefits?
2. Discuss how the Windfall Elimination Provision affects low-paid workers versus high-paid workers.

Internet References

AARP: What You Need to Know About the Windfall Elimination Provision
http://www.aarp.org/work/social-security/info-07-2013/social-security-windfall-elimination-provision.html

U.S. Social Security Administration: Windfall Elimination Provision
http://www.ssa.gov/pubs/EN-05-10045.pdf

Amanda Alix, "Social Security Twist for Boomers with Public, Private Jobs," *USA Today,* July 21, 2014.

Article Prepared by: Elaina F. Osterbur, *Saint Louis University*

Social Security Heading for Insolvency Even Faster

Trust Funds Could Run Dry in about 2 Decades

Learning Outcomes

After reading this article, you will be able to:

- Identify the reasons given for the Social Security program heading for insolvency.
- State the time when the Medicare and Social Security trust funds are expected to be insolvent.

Social Security is rushing even faster toward insolvency, driven by retiring baby boomers, a weak economy and politicians' reluctance to take painful action to fix the huge retirement and disability program.

The trust funds that support Social Security will run dry in 2033—three years earlier than previously projected—the government said Monday.

There was no change in the year that Medicare's hospital insurance fund is projected to run out of money. It's still 2024. The program's trustees, however, said the pace of Medicare spending continues to accelerate. Congress enacted a 2 percent cut for Medicare last year, and that is the main reason the trust fund exhaustion date did not advance.

The trustees who oversee both programs say high energy prices are suppressing workers' wages, a trend they see continuing. They also expect people to work fewer hours than previously projected, even after the economy recovers. Both trends would lead to lower payroll tax receipts, which support both programs.

Unless Congress acts—and forcefully—payments to millions of Americans could be cut.

If the Social Security and Medicare funds ever become exhausted, the nation's two biggest benefit programs would collect only enough money in payroll taxes to pay partial benefits. Social Security could cover about 75 percent of benefits, the trustees said in their annual report. Medicare's giant hospital fund could pay 87 percent of costs.

"Lawmakers should not delay addressing the long-run financial challenges facing Social Security and Medicare," the trustees wrote. "If they take action sooner rather than later, more

options and more time will be available to phase in changes so that the public has adequate time to prepare."

The trustees project that Social Security benefits will increase next year, though the increase could be small. They project a cost-of-living-adjustment, or COLA, of 1.8 percent for 2013; the actual amount won't be known until October. Beneficiaries got a 3.6 percent increase this year, the first after two years without one.

More than 56 million retirees, disabled workers, spouses and children receive Social Security. The average retirement benefit is $1,232 a month; the average monthly benefit for disabled workers is $1,111.

About 50 million people are covered by Medicare, the medical insurance program for older Americans.

America's aging population—increased by millions of retiring baby boomers—is straining both Social Security and Medicare. Potential options to reduce Social Security costs include raising the full retirement age, which already is being gradually increased to 67, reducing annual benefit increases and limiting benefits for wealthier Americans.

Critical Thinking

1. What do the Social Security and Medicare trustees believe is causing the problems to ultimately run out of funds?
2. What would be the effect of the Social Security and Medicare programs running out of funds?
3. What is the current average retirement benefit coming from Social Security each month?

Create Central

www.mhhe.com/createcentral

Internet References

Administration on Aging
www.aoa.dhhs.gov
American Federation for Aging Research
www.afar.org

Social Security Heading for Insolvency Even Faster: Trust Funds Could Run Dry in about 2 Decades by Terre Haute Tribune-Star

187

American Geriatrics Society
www.americangeriatrics.org

Community Transportation Association of America
www.ctaa.org

Community Reports State Inspection Surveys
www.ConsumerReports.org

Medicare Consumer Information from the Health Care Finance Association
cms.hhs.gov/default.asp?fromhcfadotgov_true

National Institutes of Health
www.nih.gov

The United States Senate: Special Committee on Aging
www.senate.gov/~aging

Article   Prepared by: Elaina F. Osterbur, *Saint Louis University*

Time for a Tune-Up

Social Security faces challenges. Retirement for future generations is at stake. Here are 10 options on the table.

JONATHAN PETERSON

Learning Outcomes

After reading this article, you will be able to:

- Discuss the 10 options that would help to shore up Social Security funds.

- Determine the probability that Congress will establish private accounts with regard to payroll taxes.

- Determine the probability that there will be a Social Security program when you reach retirement.

In just 21 years, Social Security will be able to pay only three-fourths of its promised benefits, an outlook that guarantees debate about the future of—and the meaning of—Social Security in American life. Yet the projected shortfall is not the only challenge facing the program and those who depend on it. Changes in lifestyle, demographics and the economy are bringing *insecurity* to many older Americans.

Experts have put forth a number of proposals that in some combination could sustain Social Security for the long haul, while making it more helpful and fair. Here are 10 options now on the policy table in Washington:

1. Increase the Cap

You make payroll tax contributions to Social Security on your earnings up to a limit ($110,100 in 2012). If you're like most workers, you earn less than the cap. Increasing the cap to $215,400—so that 90 percent of U.S. earnings are covered—would reduce Social Security's shortfall by about 36 percent. Eliminating it altogether would end almost all of the shortfall in one stroke. Supporters say that raising the cap would be fair and that the amount would not be onerous. The main argument against such a rise is that high earners already get less of a return on contributions than lower-income workers, because benefits are progressive by design. Also, raising the earnings base would amount to a big tax hike on high earners.

2. Raise the Payroll Tax Rate

In recent years, wage earners have paid a Social Security tax of 6.2 percent on earnings up to the income cap, as have their employers. (Congress temporarily cut the employee share to 4.2 percent in 2011 and 2012 as a way to boost the economy.)

Raising the tax rate to 6.45 percent for both employees and employers would eliminate 22 percent of the shortfall and could be phased in. Critics voice concerns about the economic impact and say employers might respond by cutting other payroll costs, such as jobs.

Other ways to raise revenues include increasing income taxes on benefits. Taxing the money that goes into "salary reduction plans," which let you divert pretax income to health care, transit and other uses, could reduce the shortfall by 10 percent. But such a move would hit consumers who may rely on such accounts.

3. Consider Women's Work Patterns

Women workers—single or married—tend to get lower benefits because they're paid less over the course of their careers and because they are more likely than men to take time off from paid employment for caregiving or child-rearing. One proposal would give workers credit for at least some of the time spent caregiving or child-rearing. At the same time, a non-married woman potentially gets a much smaller benefit (depending on her earnings history) than a nonworking wife because she can't rely on a higher-earning spouse for benefits. Measures addressing these issues would be gender-neutral, so they could also help some men. The cost of such a proposal would have to be offset, however, or it could increase the shortfall.

4. Adjust Benefits

Benefit cuts are nothing to cheer about, but they would save money. They could be structured in a way that doesn't hurt current or near-retirees and low-income individuals. Any changes could be phased in after a long lead time, giving younger workers years to adjust their financial plans.

Still, reducing benefits for modest-income people could affect their standard of living in retirement. Reducing benefits for higher earners could undermine the broad public support for Social Security as a program in which everyone pays in and everyone gets benefits.

5. Set a Minimum Benefit

People who had low incomes during their working lives—perhaps one in five earners—now may end up with benefits that are still below the poverty line. A minimum benefit might be set at 125 percent of the poverty line, indexed to wage increases to keep it adequate over time.

6. Modify the COLA Formula

Social Security benefits generally rise to keep up with the cost of living. This cost-of-living adjustment, known as the COLA, is currently based on the Consumer Price Index for Urban Wage Earners and Clerical Workers (known as CPI-W).

One proposal would switch to a different measure, the "chained CPI," which assumes consumers alter their buying patterns if a price goes up too much. Say the price of beef soars—people may switch to chicken. The chained CPI rises about 0.3 percentage point more slowly each year than the CPI-W, meaning benefits would grow more slowly, too—about 6 percent less over the course of 20 years. Adopting a chained CPI would reduce the shortfall by about 23 percent.

Another approach would substitute a formula known as CPI-E. It takes into special account the type of spending that is more common among people 62 and older, such as medical care, which continues to rise faster than other costs. This could increase benefits, expanding the shortfall by about 16 percent.

7. Raise the Full Retirement Age

The age at which you can get full Social Security benefits is gradually rising to 67 for people born in 1960 and later. Pushing it up even further would save money and provide an incentive for people to keep working.

A full retirement age of 68 could reduce the shortfall by about 18 percent. Raising it to 70 would close 44 percent. Such increases could be phased in, and proponents say this approach makes sense in an era of increased life expectancy. A healthy 65-year-old man, for example, is expected to live beyond 82. But not everyone has benefited equally from increases in longevity—lower-income, less educated workers have not gained as much as their more affluent, more educated counterparts. And a later full retirement age could be onerous for workers with health problems or physically demanding jobs. A

related proposal—longevity indexing—would link benefits to increased life expectancy.

8. Give the Oldest a Boost

Americans are living longer, and the oldest often are the poorest. They may have little savings left; usually they no longer work and any pensions they have are likely eroded by inflation. A longevity bonus, for example, a 5 percent benefit increase for people above a certain age, say 85, could help them.

9. Establish Private Accounts

Free-market advocates have long pushed to make Social Security more of a private program, in which some of your payroll taxes would go into a personal account that would rise and fall with the financial markets. Supporters believe that stock market returns could make up for benefit cuts. You would own the assets in your personal account and could pass them on to your heirs. Personal accounts could be introduced gradually and become a choice for younger workers, while retirees and near retirees could remain in the current system. Opponents worry that they would replace a guaranteed, inflation-protected benefit for workers and, potentially, family members, with more limited protections. Private accounts only pay out the amount in the account. Also, diverting money to private accounts means additional funding could be needed to pay currently promised benefits.

10. Cover More Workers

Not all workers take part in Social Security. The largest uncovered group is about 25 percent of state and local government employees who rely on state pension systems. Bringing new hires into Social Security would raise enough new revenue to trim about 8 percent of the long-term shortfall (though down the road, when these people claim benefits, costs would rise). State and local governments may oppose such a measure because it would divert dollars from public pensions that are already underfunded.

Critical Thinking

1. Why do you think that at the present time the United States Congress has not discussed adopting any of the ten options that would help to shore up the Social Security funds?

2. Do you think that it is likely that Congress will establish private accounts in which some of a person's payroll taxes paid would go into an individual's account whose earnings would rise and fall with the financial markets?

3. What do you think is the probability that there will be a Social Security program when you reach retirement age and that you will receive a monthly check from the program?

Create Central

www.mhhe.com/createcentral

Internet References

Administration on Aging
www.aoa.dhhs.gov

American Federation for Aging Research
www.afar.org

American Geriatrics Society
www.americangeriatrics.org

Community Transportation Association of America
www.ctaa.org

Community Reports State Inspection Surveys
www.ConsumerReports.org

Medicare Consumer Information from the Health Care Finance Association
cms.hhs.gov/default.asp?fromhcfadotgov_true

National Institutes of Health
www.nih.gov

The United States Senate: Special Committee on Aging
www.senate.gov/~aging

Article   Prepared by: Elaina F. Osterbur, *Saint Louis University*

Retooling Medicare?

Medicare faces challenges. Retirement for future generations is at stake. Here are 7 options on the table.

PATRICIA BARRY

Learning Outcomes

After reading this article, you will be able to:

- Describe the proposed changes in Medicare that Rep. Paul Ryan, a Wisconsin Republican, is proposing.

- Identify the specific changes in Medicare payments and benefits that Ryan's plan, known as "premium support" to its proponents, is proposing.

Politicians are eyeing Medicare as a spending program ripe for cuts to help reduce the nation's deficit. And so it follows that the future of Medicare looms as a key battleground issue in the 2012 general election. But proposals to change the popular program tend to alarm older Americans, who see Medicare as part of their retirement security. And these same older Americans vote in large numbers. So stand by to hear all candidates claim that they want to "save" Medicare for future generations—but often in very different ways.

Proposed changes to the program include raising the eligibility age to 67, raising payroll taxes and requiring better-off beneficiaries to pay more. The most politically contentious plan, devised by Rep. Paul Ryan (R-Wis.), chairman of the House Budget Committee, would limit federal spending on Medicare and alter the way the government pays for benefits. Republicans say this plan is a fiscally responsible way of extending Medicare's viability as millions of boomers enter the program. Democrats call it "the end of Medicare as we know it" and a way to shift more costs to beneficiaries.

The future of Medicare looms as a key battleground issue in the 2012 election, and older Americans vote in large numbers.

Polls show that most Americans prefer to keep Medicare as it is. "Ryan's plan is a fundamental change in the structure of the program," so it makes older voters more nervous than lesser proposals do, says Robert Blendon, professor of health policy at Harvard's School of Public Health. But whoever gains the upper political hand in November, he adds, will have to wrestle with the budget deficit—and some of those decisions will likely affect Medicare.

With that in mind, AARP asked policy experts from across the political spectrum—Henry Aaron, senior fellow of the economic studies program at the Brookings Institution; Stuart Butler, director of the Center for Policy Innovation at the Heritage Foundation; and experts at Avalere Health, a Washington health care policy and research company—to give arguments for and against some Medicare proposals. (Read these in full and contact the experts at earnedasay.org.) Here are summaries of their opposing positions on seven options that most directly affect beneficiaries:

Changing the Way Medicare Pays for Benefits

Medicare now offers two ways to receive benefits. If you're in traditional Medicare, the government pays directly for each covered medical service you use. If you're in a Medicare Advantage private plan, the government pays a set annual amount to the plan for your care. Under the Ryan plan—known as "premium support" to its proponents and as a "voucher system" to its critics—the government would allow you a certain sum of money to buy coverage from competing private plans or from a revised version of traditional Medicare.

For

This would put Medicare on a budget to hold down spending and reduce the tax burden on future generations. You'd receive a share of this budget to help you purchase your health care and have more flexibility to make choices. For example, if you wanted more generous coverage (such as seeing any doctor of your choice), you'd pay the premium difference out of your own pocket, and if the difference became too high, you could switch to a less expensive plan.

Against

The value of the voucher would be tied to some economic index—not to actual health costs, which generally rise faster than other costs. So there is a high risk that benefits would become increasingly inadequate and more out-of-pocket costs would be shifted to the consumer. Medicare already has competing private plans, through the Medicare Advantage and Part D drug programs, yet the hoped-for savings from them have not yet materialized.

Raising Medicare Eligibility Age to 67

Eligibility for Medicare has always been at age 65, except for younger people with disabilities. This proposal aims to gradually bring Medicare in line with Social Security, where full retirement age is now 66 and set to rise to 67 by 2027.

For

With more Americans living longer, and health spending on older people rising, we can't afford Medicare at age 65. Raising the eligibility age would reduce federal spending on Medicare by about 5 percent over the next 20 years.

Against

This proposal would increase other health care spending—especially costs for employer health plans and Medicaid—and uninsured people would pay full costs for a longer time. Medicare premiums would rise due to fewer people in the program to share costs.

Raising the Medicare Payroll Tax

This tax, which funds Medicare Part A hospital insurance, is currently 2.9 percent of all earnings (1.45 percent each for employers and employees; 2.9 percent for the self-employed). People who have paid this tax for a sufficient time do not pay monthly premiums for Part A.

For

Part A currently faces a small long-term deficit after 2024, when it's estimated that available funds will not fully pay for all services. Increasing the payroll tax by just 0.5 percent each for employers and employees would more than fix that problem, leaving a small surplus to act as a cushion against future shortfalls or fund extra benefits in Medicare.

Against

Raising the payroll tax would mean a higher rate of tax for each dollar earned by working Americans, slowing economic growth and increasing the tax burden on future generations.

Even workers not earning enough to pay income taxes would pay this bigger tax.

Raising Medicare Premiums for Higher-Income People

Most people pay monthly premiums for Part B, which covers doctors' services and outpatient care, and for Part D prescription drug coverage. The standard premiums pay for about 25 percent of the costs of these services, while Medicare pays the remaining 75 percent out of general tax revenues. People with incomes over a certain level—those whose tax returns show a modified adjusted gross income of $85,000 for a single person or $170,000 for a married couple—pay higher premiums.

For

The easiest way to bring in more money for Medicare would be to raise the premiums even more for higher income people—so that the wealthiest older people pay the full cost and receive no taxpayer-funded subsidy. Another option is to lower the income level at which the higher premium charge kicks in, so that more people have to pay it.

Against

Higher-income earners already have paid more into the Medicare program through higher payroll and income taxes, and now pay up to three times more for the same Part B and D coverage. If increased taxes make healthier and wealthier people drop out of the program, standard premiums would eventually become more expensive for everyone.

Changing Medigap Supplemental Insurance

About one in six people with Medicare buys private supplemental insurance, also known as medigap. It covers some of their out-of-pocket expenses under traditional Medicare, such as the 20 percent copayments typically required for Part B services. This option would limit medigap coverage, requiring people to bear more out-of-pocket costs.

For

People buy medigap to limit their out-of-pocket spending in Medicare. But because they pay less, they tend to use more Medicare services, increasing the burden for taxpayers.

Against

There is no evidence that raising medigap premiums or reducing benefits would deter people from using health services unnecessarily, and most patients can't tell whether a service is necessary or not. But there is evidence that postponing needed services leads to greater health problems that cost Medicare more to fix.

Redesigning Copays and Deductibles

Currently, Parts A and B in traditional Medicare have different copays and deductibles. Some proposals would combine the programs to have only one deductible—for example, $550 annually, and uniform copays for Part A and Part B services, plus an annual out-of-pocket expense limit, similar to employer insurance plans.

For

Simplifying Medicare benefits to make them less confusing could save Medicare up to $110 billion over 10 years. An out-of-pocket cap would provide great financial protection, especially for sicker beneficiaries, and reduce the need for medigap supplemental insurance.

Against

Some beneficiaries might pay less, but others—especially those who use few services or spend longer periods in the hospital—would pay more out of pocket than they do now, unless they have additional insurance.

Adding Copays for Some Services

Medicare does not charge copays for home health care, the first 20 days in a skilled nursing facility—rehab after surgery, for example—or for laboratory services such as blood work and diagnostic tests. Several proposals would require copays for one or all of these.

For

Added copays would discourage unnecessary use of these services. Over 10 years, copays could save Medicare up to $40 billion for home health, $21 billion for stays in skilled nursing facilities and $16 billion for lab tests.

Against

Patients without supplemental insurance could pay significantly more for these services, or might not be able to afford them. This could end up harming patients and costing Medicare even more money if postponing treatment worsened patients' health, leading to expensive emergency room visits and hospital admissions. Also, patients generally follow doctors' orders and do not know which services are medically necessary and which are not.

Critical Thinking

1. What two proposed financial changes would bring in money directly to the Medicare funds?
2. What is the benefit to people who buy Medigap supplemental insurance?
3. What could be done to assure that Medicare would have adequate funds to pay for all services in the future?

Create Central

www.mhhe.com/createcentral

Internet References

Administration on Aging
   www.aoa.dhhs.gov
American Federation for Aging Research
   www.afar.org
American Geriatrics Society
   www.americangeriatrics.org
Community Transportation Association of America
   www.ctaa.org
Community Reports State Inspection Surveys
   www.ConsumerReports.org
Medicare Consumer Information from the Health Care Finance Association
   cms.hhs.gov/default.asp?fromhcfadotgov_true
National Institutes of Health
   www.nih.gov
The United States Senate: Special Committee on Aging
   www.senate.gov/~aging